Problem Orientated
Obstetrics and Gynaecology

Problem Orientated Obstetrics and Gynaecology

Ian Symonds DM BMed Sci MRCOG
Senior Lecturer in Obstetrics and Gynaecology, School of Human Development, University of Nottingham, UK

Philip N Baker DM BMed Sci BM BS MRCOG
Professor of Maternal and Fetal Health, and Director of the Maternal and Fetal Health Research Centre, St Mary's Hospital, University of Manchester, UK

Lucy Kean DM MA MRCOG
Consultant Obstetrician (Subspecialist in Maternal and Fetal Medicine), City Hospital, Nottingham, UK

ARNOLD

A member of the Hodder Headline Group
LONDON

This edition published in 2002 by Arnold,
a member of the Hodder Headline Group,
338 Euston Road, London NW1 3BH

http://www.arnoldpublishers.com

Distributed in the USA by
Oxford University Press Inc.,
198 Madison Avenue, New York, NY10016
Oxford is a registered trademark of Oxford University Press

Whilst the advice and information in this book are believed to be true and
accurate at the date of going to press, neither the authors nor the publisher
can accept any legal responsibility or liability for any errors or omissions
that may be made. In particular (but without limiting the generality of the
preceding disclaimer) every effort has been made to check drug dosages;
however, it is still possible that errors have been missed. Furthermore,
dosage schedules are constantly being revised and new side-effects
recognized. For these reasons the reader is strongly urged to consult the
drug companies' printed instructions before administering any of the drugs
recommended in this book.

British Library Cataloguing in Publication Data
A catalogue record for this book is available from the British Library

Library of Congress Cataloging-in-Publication Data
A catalog record for this book is available from the Library of Congress

ISBN 0 340 759062

1 2 3 4 5 6 7 8 9 10

Commissioning Editor: Georgina Bentliff
Development Editor: Heather Smith
Production Editor: Anke Ueberberg
Production Controller: Martin Kerans
Cover Design: Terry Griffiths

Typeset in 9.5/12 Minion by Integra Software Services Pvt. Ltd,
Printed and bound in Malta by Gutenberg Press

What do you think about this book? Or any other Arnold title?
Please send your comments to feedback.arnold@hodder.co.uk
http://www.arnoldpublishers.com

To Avril, Nicky and David

Contents

Foreword   ix
Preface   x

Introduction   1

1 About this book   3
2 History-taking and examination in obstetrics   6
3 History-taking and examination in
  gynaecology   11

In the antenatal clinic   19

4 Abnormal antibodies: blood group   21
  incompatibility
5 Anaemia in pregnancy   25
6 Breathlessness in pregnancy   29
7 Breech presentation   33
8 Diabetes   37
9 Fetal abnormality: chromosomal   41
10 Fetal abnormality: structural   46
11 Hypertension   50
12 Infections in pregnancy   56
13 Large for gestational age   60
14 Multiple pregnancy   63
15 Previous Caesarean section   69
16 Previous fetal loss   72
17 Prolonged pregnancy   75
18 Proteinuria   77
19 Pruritus and jaundice in pregnancy   80
20 Reduced fetal movements   83
21 Small for gestational age   88
22 Substance abuse   92
23 Unstable or transverse lie   95

On the delivery suite   97

24 Abdominal pain in pregnancy   99
25 Antepartum haemorrhage   102
26 Cord prolapse   106
27 Failure to progress in the first stage   108
28 Failure to progress in the second stage   112
29 Abnormal fetal heart rate patterns
   in labour   115
30 Induction of labour   123
31 Intrauterine fetal death   126
32 Maternal collapse   130
33 Meconium   137
34 Neonatal resuscitation   139
35 Normal labour   142
36 Pain relief in labour   148
37 Postpartum haemorrhage   151
38 Preterm labour   155
39 Rupture of membranes while not in labour   159
40 Shoulder dystocia   163

On the maternity wards   167

41 Difficulty with breast-feeding   169
42 The confused or withdrawn mother   172
43 The febrile patient   175
44 Venous thrombosis   178

In the gynaecology clinic   181

45 The abnormal cervical smear test   183
46 Amenorrhoea and oligomenorrhoea   188

47 Chronic pelvic pain   194
48 Contraception   199
49 Heavy periods   205
50 Hirsutism and virilization   211
51 Infertility   214
52 Intermenstrual bleeding   219
53 Menopausal symptoms   222
54 Painful intercourse   227
55 The pelvic mass   230
56 Postmenopausal bleeding   234
57 Premenstrual syndrome   238
58 Prolapse   242
59 Recurrent miscarriage   246
60 Sterilization   248
61 Termination of pregnancy   250
62 Urinary frequency   253
63 Urinary incontinence   255
64 Vaginal discharge   259

65 The swollen or painful vulva   261
66 Vulval pruritus   265

On the gynaecology wards   269

67 Acute abdominal pain   271
68 Bleeding in early pregnancy   276
69 Postoperative complications   283
70 Vomiting in early pregnancy   287

Appendices   291

A Commonly used abbreviations   293
B Glossary of commonly used terms   296
C Self-assessment questions   305
  Index   317

Foreword

Obstetrics and Gynaecology is a fascinating specialty which for a medical student and SHO should be fun to learn. The topics are not discovered in a text book, they are found in the emergency room, on the wards, in the labour ward, and in the clinics. This book fuels the student's enthusiasm by picking up on the clinical situations encountered in clinical practice and covering in a systematic way importance, aetiology and management, with clear emphasis on the key learning points.

The General Medical Council's document 'Tomorrow's Doctors' has emphasized that as teachers we are overburdening our medical students. All curricula in the UK have recently been restructured to address 'core' knowledge. In this book the core material is centered around problems that students will encounter every day. The usefulness of this book will also extend to SHOs, as all areas of clinical practice are addressed. The difficult areas, for example breast feeding and vulval irritation, are all discussed, making this book very comprehensive.

Although they abide by the dictum of providing students with core knowledge, the authors allow the inquisitive student to go further if he or she wishes by ending each chapter with further reading and providing a glossary at the end of the book. This is heart-warming for those teachers who have a vision beyond the core curriculum and continue to inspire students on a quest to extend their knowledge. Education appears to be driven by assessment and readers will be gratified to find self-assessment questions relating to the problems that are addressed in this book.

The authors have an established reputation in undergraduate and postgraduate education and assessment, as is evident in the clear and instructive problem orientated approach of this book. I'm sure it will be a very successful learning tool for both undergraduates and postgraduate students in Obstetrics and Gynaecology. It was a pleasure to read!

Dr Janice Rymer MD MRCOG FRANZCOG ILTM
Senior Lecturer/Consultant
Guy's King's and St Thomas' School of Medicine
Guy's and St Thomas' Hospital Trust
London

Preface

In this book we have tried to select those clinical problems the student or senior house officer is most likely to encounter in obstetrics and gynaecology and provide a pragmatic outline of how to set about management. Whilst this mostly follows a pattern of diagnosis (by history, examination and investigation) and then treatment, this is sometimes modified, as would be the case in reality, by the urgency of a clinical situation.

In deciding what factual information to include we have tried to adhere to the principle of it being better to know everything that is essential rather than 50 per cent of everything. For this reason you will find that our lists of differential diagnoses and treatments are perhaps less extensive than some other textbooks. Where possible, we have tried to distinguish the common from the rarer causes of a particular sign or symptom. In addition, we have tried to identify those topics which constitute 'core' knowledge at undergraduate level. We have restricted the amount of detail on basic reproductive sciences within the main part of the text to those aspects that are essential to understanding the rationale for the management of the common clinical problems. Additional information on anatomy, commonly used terms and physiology can be found in the glossary at the end of the book.

We recognize that many women present with multiple problems and that some presenting symptoms are multifactorial in origin. We have tried to address this by clear cross-referencing within the text and by the self-assessment questions.

Ian Symonds
Philip Baker
Lucy Kean

Section 1

Introduction

1. About this book 3
2. History-taking and examination in obstetrics 6
3. History-taking and examination in gynaecology 11

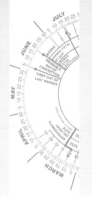

Chapter 1

About this book

How to Use This Book

Start by reading the chapters on history and examination. Subsequent chapters are organized for ease of reference in *alphabetical order*, grouped in the clinical setting in which they are most likely to be seen. Read chapters as you see cases on the wards or in the clinics while they are fresh in your mind. Those topics which contain most of the core knowledge at undergraduate level are indicated by the symbol ✐ . When you have read all the chapters, try the self-assessment questions. If you are new to obstetrics and gynaecology, additional information is provided in the glossary at the end of the book.

Organization of Chapters

Each chapter covers a single clinical problem and is divided into sections on background knowledge, diagnosis and management.

Key points from each section are summarized in boxes. The adjacent text expands on the points in the boxes and explains their significance and role in assessment and treatment.

Essential Knowledge or 'What You Need to Know'

Includes:

Definitions
Importance
Causes
Risks and complications

Definition

This describes what the chapter encompasses, the medical definition of the problem and any other terms used in that chapter.

Importance

This explains the clinical relevance of the topic. It places the problem in context, such as how common it is, the demands it makes on the health care systems and its implications for the patient.

Causes or Aetiology

Common causes
Physiological
Pathological

- Congenital
- Neoplastic
- Infective
- Iatrogenic
- Inflammatory
- Traumatic

Where necessary, this section summarizes the relevant normal anatomy or physiology. More information on normal anatomy and physiology can be found in the glossary. The common causes of a particular presenting sign or symptom are discussed. The key risk factors for the development of particular conditions and their pathophysiology are outlined.

Risks and Complications

This section describes common short-term and long-term complications of a particular problem or the common conditions causing it. These may include the effect on the fetus as well as the mother in obstetric topics and the way pregnancy itself changes the course of pre-existing medical conditions.

Diagnosis and Clinical Assessment or 'What You Need to Find Out'

Includes:

Screening
History
Examination
Investigations

Screening

Screening is the identification of (usually asymptomatic) individuals at increased risk of a particular problem from within the general population. These individuals may then have diagnostic investigations or increased monitoring, leading to earlier treatment or the use of preventative measures to reduce the morbidity or mortality associated with the condition.

History

Ask about:

- Details of the presenting complaint
- Relevant review of other systems
- Past obstetric and gynaecological history
- Medical and surgical history
- Patient needs and expectations.

This section highlights the key questions that should be included in the history for a particular presenting complaint or request. These should be asked as part of, and not instead of, a full gynaecological or obstetric history (as outlined in the chapters on history-taking and examination). An accurate history is the most important single step in the management of most of the clinical problems in this book. It gives most of the information required to make a diagnosis, with the examination and investigations serving largely to confirm this. It puts the current problem into the broader context of the patient's general physical and mental well-being as well as her current social situation, all of which are essential considerations when discussing treatment options. Finally,

the process of taking the history serves as the first step in establishing the relationship between doctor and patient.

Examination

Check:

- General condition
- Abdominal examination
- Pelvic examination.

This outlines the key features in general, abdominal and pelvic examinations that should be sought or excluded for a particular symptom. This is not a substitute for a full and systematic examination but a guide to interpreting the likely findings for a particular set of symptoms.

Investigations

Appropriate investigations may include:

- Haematology
- Biochemistry
- Immunology
- Microbiology
- Pathology
- Imaging
- Surgical.

This concerns the relevant tests required either to confirm a diagnosis or as a prerequisite for treatment. These may include blood tests, imaging, histology and surgical procedures such as laparoscopy or hysteroscopy. In some cases, investigation may be done in several stages, with the more complex, invasive or expensive tests only being used as indicated by the results of the initial basic investigations.

Management or 'What You Need to Do'

Includes:

Prevention
General measures
Medical treatment
Surgical treatment
Counselling
Follow-up

Management includes assessing the patient's condition, explaining the diagnosis and treatment and arranging suitable follow-up, not just carrying out the treatment itself.

Where the management of a particular problem is principally dependent on the diagnosis, the treatment options for the commoner causes are outlined, with reference to other chapters where the same condition or type of treatment is discussed in more detail. In other cases it will be determined by a more general approach, applicable to several diagnoses, or by the patient's need for fertility, contraception etc.

Priorities

This highlights when the situation demands an alternative approach to the 'usual' sequence of history, examination, investigation, diagnosis and then treatment.

Prevention

This includes measures taken for the general population, as well as those people identified by screening as being at high risk, to prevent, or ameliorate the effects of, a particular condition.

General Measures

Not all symptoms require treatment. A woman presenting with postmenopausal bleeding needs investigation to exclude malignancy, but in the majority of cases this will not be the final diagnosis and all that will be required is explanation and reassurance. Even where treatment is desired or required, this need not involve medication or surgery. Advice about changes in lifestyle or weight, or help to enhance coping mechanisms will form an essential part of the management of many problems and in some cases is the mainstay of 'treatment'.

Medical Treatment

This may be divided into first-line and second-line treatment. The principal contraindications and side-effects of each are noted, where these have a significant effect on deciding which drug to use and what information needs to be given to patients. As well as oral and parenteral medication, this may include medical devices such as the levonorgestrel intrauterine system.

Surgical Treatment

This section concentrates on those procedures that are in common use at present and includes both open and endoscopic operations. It includes details of any contraindications and important complications of treatment.

Counselling

Effective communication with the patient and her relatives is an essential part of the management of all the problems in this book. This section highlights those cases where there are key points of information about a specific treatment or condition that need to be given to the patient, often to allow her to make an informed choice between different courses of action.

Follow-up

This outlines, where appropriate, the length and frequency of follow-up required for a particular condition or after a particular treatment. The risk of recurrence and, for malignancy, the 5-year survival are given.

Learning Points

- **Summarizes the points that need to be committed to memory. This is usually because they are of critical importance in the understanding or management of the problem, but it may also include facts that need to be learnt because they are counterintuitive.**

Further Reading

In this section, key review papers and chapters in books are listed, as well as guidelines published by the Royal College of Obstetricians and Gynaecologists. The other chapters of the book that relate to the current topic or which contain sections giving more details about particular conditions and treatments of relevance to the problems discussed in the chapter in question are listed under 'See Also'.

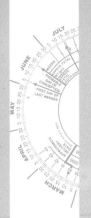

History-taking and examination in obstetrics

Introduction

The following describes the way in which you might take a history from a woman admitted to the antenatal ward or delivery suite with a problem during pregnancy or when seen for the first time in the booking clinic. It is usually not necessary to recap the full history during a routine visit to the antenatal clinic or when the woman is admitted in labour, as most of the necessary information will already be on record in her notes from the booking visit. The way in which the history is taken will also be modified by the clinical situation. In an emergency, it may be necessary to omit most of the questions below until the patient's clinical condition is stabilized.

History

Start by introducing yourself and explaining who you are. Confirm the name and age of the patient and how many weeks pregnant she is (gestation) by counting back from the estimated date of delivery to the present date.

Estimated date of delivery

The average duration of pregnancy is 266 days from conception. The expected date of delivery (EDD) can be calculated by adding a year and 7 days to the date of the last menstrual period (LMP) and subtracting 3 months. Remember this only works for a 28-day cycle (as you are assuming ovulation occurred 14 days after that date) and needs to be adjusted by adding an additional week for a 35-day cycle. If the date of the last period is uncertain or if the gestational age on an early ultrasound scan differs by more than a week from that predicted by the LMP, the EDD will usually be calculated from the early scan.

Presenting Complaint

Unless this is a routine booking or follow-up clinic visit, ask about any new symptoms, including details of their onset and duration, and any other associated symptoms. In addition, always ask about pain, bleeding and fetal movements.

Present Pregnancy

Next, ask about other details of the current pregnancy, including at what gestation the patient booked for antenatal care. This will tell you how reliable ultrasound dating of the pregnancy is likely to be, and the amount of antenatal care the patient will have had. Ask about any screening tests for fetal chromosomal or structural abnormalities carried out in the second trimester (see Chapters 9 and 10) and the results of these, if known. Check to see if there have been any other problems earlier in the present pregnancy and if these required admission to hospital. In particular, ask about any history of high blood pressure or bleeding.

Previous Obstetric History

Ask about:

Dates of previous pregnancies and outcomes
Mode of deliveries and birthweights, if known
Current health of previous children

Any antenatal problems
Puerperal problems
Change of partner

One of the key predictors of risk in any pregnancy is the outcome of previous pregnancies. Ask about the number of previous pregnancies and outcomes, including method of delivery, birthweight, if known, and any antenatal problems. Conditions such as pre-eclampsia, gestational diabetes and abruption are more likely to occur in women who had these in a previous pregnancy. First pregnancies are more likely to be complicated by hypertension and low birth-weight, whereas postpartum haemorrhage occurs more often in women who have had more than four previous pregnancies. Conditions in which a paternal genetic contribution affects outcome, such as iso-immunization and pre-eclampsia, will be affected by a change of partner. Finally, ask about postnatal problems, especially depression and venous thrombo-embolism, as there is a significant risk of recurrence of these conditions in the puerperal period.

Commonly used terms

Parity – number of children delivered after 24 weeks
Gravidity – number of times pregnant
Primigravida – a woman in her first pregnancy
Nullipara – a woman having had no deliveries after 24 weeks' gestation
Multigravida – a woman in her second or subsequent pregnancy
Grand multipara – a woman having had five or more pregnancies of more than 24 weeks

Previous Medical History

Relevant details from the past medical history include:

- cardiac disease
- thromboembolic disease
- endocrine disease (diabetes)
- anaesthetic problems
- current medication and allergies.

Most women of child-bearing age will have few, if any, significant medical problems, but where these do exist they are often significantly affected by the physiological changes of pregnancy. This especially applies to cardiac disease (mostly congenital in Western-born women, but there is still a significant incidence of rheumatic heart disease in those from the developing world) and diabetes. Pregnancy is associated with an increased risk of venous thrombosis, so a past history of deep vein thrombosis or pulmonary embolus is important, especially if this was associated with a previous pregnancy or taking the combined contraceptive pill. Check if she has ever had an anaesthetic and, if so, if there were any problems with this – she may need an anaesthetic at short notice during pregnancy. Ask about current medication and any allergies.

Social and Family History

Ask about:

Occupation
Home circumstances
Support
Smoking
Family history

Ask about occupation or partner's occupation. Perinatal mortality rates are higher in social classes IV and V. Ask about support at home – whether a woman will agree to be admitted to hospital may have more to do with making arrangements to look after any other children than the current obstetric problem. Smoking is associated with an increased risk of growth restriction and an increased perinatal mortality. Ask about other recreational drug intake, including alcohol consumption, as this may affect fetal development or be associated with neonatal withdrawal symptoms after delivery (see Chapter 22). Ask if there is any family history of hereditary disease, thrombosis, hypertension or diabetes.

Examination

General Examination

Check:

General condition, weight, height
Pulse, blood pressure
Anaemia
Goitre
Heart sounds
Oedema (feet, sacrum, fingers)

Even while you are introducing yourself and asking about the presenting symptoms, you should be assessing the patient's general condition. Does she appear in pain and, if so, is it intermittent as with contractions or constant? Does she appear pale and sweaty? Check pulse and blood pressure, and look for signs of anaemia and oedema. Remember that oedema of the feet and ankles is normal in later pregnancy. Look for pitting oedema over the back whilst you are listening to the chest. A soft systolic murmur over the left sternal edge, or flow murmur, is a normal finding in pregnancy. Blood pressure should be taken with the patient semi-recumbent or slightly tilted onto her left side, taking the diastolic as where the sounds disappear (V sound). Always ask for urinalysis, to look for the presence of protein and glucose. Breast examination is no longer routinely carried out unless indicated by symptoms.

Abdominal Examination

Key steps in antenatal abdominal examination are:

Inspection for distension, scars, striae, linea nigra, fetal movements

Palpation for symphysis–fundal height
- Fetal – lie, presentation, station, position, uterine tenderness, liquor volume
- Organomegaly, tenderness, peritonism

Auscultation for fetal heart sounds

Make sure the patient is comfortable and is not lying flat on her back. This can precipitate syncope by causing aortocaval compression by the uterus. Ask about any areas of discomfort. Look for scars, striae gravidarum and any signs of fetal movement. Next find the top of the symphysis pubis and measure to the top of the uterus with the tape facing downwards. Turn the measure over and read off the symphysis–fundal height in centimetres. After 20 weeks there is an approximate correlation with the gestation in weeks in a singleton pregnancy (Figure 2.1). However, use of a symphysis–fundal height chart, such as included in the National Maternity Record, is preferable. Gently palpate along either side of the uterus, noting any areas of tenderness and whether the uterus reacts to touch by contracting. If the uterus is soft, you should be able feel the smooth, firm edge of the fetal back and determine its relation to the long axis of the uterus (the lie). This will be longitudinal, transverse or oblique (Figure 2.2). Next try to locate the fetal head. If the lie is longitudi-

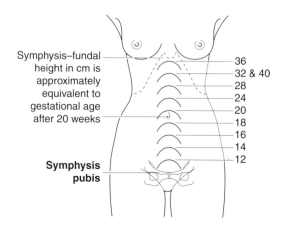

Figure 2.1 Uterine size related to gestational age (weeks after last menstrual period)

nal, this will be either in the midline just above the symphysis pubis (cephalic) or at the fundus of the uterus (breech). This is the presentation. If the presentation is cephalic, see how many fifths of the head you can feel above the bony pelvis (if you can feel less than three-fifths of the head, it is said to be engaged). Don't worry too much about the position (the relationship between the fetal occiput and the maternal pelvis). If you can't make out fetal parts at all, this may indicate absent or very increased liquor volume.

Finish the abdominal examination by palpating the rest of the abdomen for any areas of tenderness (especially over the liver and epigastrium) and feel for any enlargement of the liver.

Listen for fetal heart sounds and make a note of the rate. This can be done with a Pinnard's fetal stethoscope after about 20 weeks, and after 14 weeks using a portable Doppler ultrasound. The heart sounds are best heard midway between the umbilicus and the anterior superior iliac spine, on the side where the baby's back is in a cephalic presentation and at the level of the umbilicus for a breech. If the heart sounds you hear are higher than you expect, recheck that you have the presenting part correct.

Pelvic Examination

Indications for vaginal examination during pregnancy

Suspected labour

Suspected rupture of membranes

Assessment of pelvis and cervix when planning delivery

Never carry out vaginal examination in the presence of vaginal bleeding until placenta praevia has been excluded.

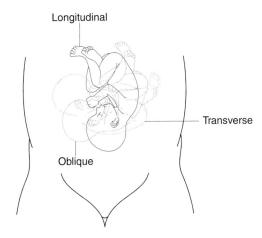

Longitudinal

Transverse

Oblique

Figure 2.2 Fetal lie is the relationship between the long axis of the fetus and the uterus

Pelvic examination is no longer a routine part of antenatal examination. It forms an essential part of the management of labour in assessing the progress and onset of labour as well the position and presenting part of the fetus (see Chapter 35).

Prior to labour, the principles of vaginal examination are the same as outlined for gynaecological examination (see Chapter 3).

Presenting Your Findings

Start by introducing the patient by name, age and current gestation in weeks from the LMP. Give the number of the present pregnancy and the main reason for admission. Give details of the presenting complaint, then details of the rest of the current pregnancy, including the expected date of delivery and results of any early prenatal diagnostic tests. Give details of any other problems during the current pregnancy not already covered in the presenting complaint. Summarize the number of previous pregnancies and their outcomes and then give details of any problems. Present the remainder of the history in a logical, structured way, not skipping back and forward between items. At the end of your history, give a summary in one sentence.

Example of a typical history

This is Miss Smith, a 23-year-old lady who is 32 weeks into her second pregnancy and who was admitted last night as an emergency with vaginal bleeding. Miss Smith has had three episodes of painless vaginal bleeding over the last 6 months of between a tablespoon and a cupful in amount. The first of these was after intercourse, but the last two have been unprovoked. She has no other symptoms and reports no changes in fetal movements. Her last menstrual period was on September 16, giving her an estimated date of delivery of June 23, confirmed by ultrasound scan at 12 weeks. She declined serum screening but did have a normal fetal anomaly scan at 19 weeks. The pregnancy had been uneventful until the current problem. Three years ago, she had a normal vaginal delivery at 38 weeks of a 3.5-kg healthy male infant with no antenatal problems. She normally has a regular 28-day menstrual cycle and was using the combined pill for contraception until 12 months ago. She has no previous gynaecological history of note and her last cervical smear, 2 years ago, was negative. She is not on any medication and has no known allergies. She lives with her partner and has family who can help look after her first child if she needs to stay in hospital. She does not smoke or drink.

In summary, Miss Smith is a 23-year-old lady presenting with a painless antepartum haemorrhage at 32 weeks into her second pregnancy.

When you are asked to examine a pregnant patient, start by asking her permission and checking that she is comfortable and not lying too flat. Unless your are asked only to discuss one particular part of the examination, always start by commenting on the patient's general condition and checking her pulse and blood pressure. For abdominal examination, list the findings on inspection then measure the symphysis–fundal height. Palpate the uterus for the lie, presentation and position of the fetus and then feel for any tenderness in the epigastrium and right upper quadrant. Keep your eyes on the patient's face throughout the examination for any sign that you are hurting her. Listen for the fetal heart tones and count the rate over 15 seconds. Ask if a urinalysis has been performed.

Example of presentation of clinical findings

On general examination Miss Smith looked well. She was not clinically anaemic. Her blood pressure was 110/70 and her pulse 88 and regular. Examination of the cardiovascular and respiratory systems was unremarkable except for a soft systolic murmur at the left sternal edge consistent with a flow murmur. The abdomen was symmetrically distended, consistent with pregnancy with striae gravidarum and a linea

(cont.)

(cont.)

nigra. There were no scars or visible fetal movements. The symphysis–fundal height was 31 cm, consistent with the stated gestational age. There was a single fetus with a longitudinal lie; cephalic presentation and the presenting part was five-fifths palpable. The uterus was soft and non-tender. The fetal heart rate was 150 and regular. There were no signs of active bleeding. A vaginal examination was not performed. Urinalysis showed a plus of blood but no protein.

Learning Points

If This is a Booking Visit

- **Take a full previous obstetric, medical, surgical, social and family history**
- **Arrange ultrasound confirmation of gestation and calculate the EDD**
- **Perform a general medical and abdominal examination**
- **Check urinalysis, weight, height**
- **Send midstream urine sample for culture**
- **Take blood for full blood count (FBC), blood group serology, rubella, syphilis, hepatitis (human immunodeficiency virus, HIV)**
- **Counsel about screening for neural tube defects and trisomy**
- **Assign risk and plan management**

For Follow-up Visits Remember to

- **Confirm current gestation**
- **Ask about problems, fetal movements, pain and bleeding**
- **Perform an abdominal examination**
- **Check blood pressure and urinalysis**
- **Send blood for FBC, serum antibodies 28 and 36 weeks if Rh-negative**
- **Arrange ultrasound scan if indicated**

See Also

History-taking and examination in gynaecology (Chapter 3).

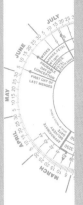

History-taking and examination in gynaecology

Introduction

An accurate history is the essential starting point for both the diagnosis and management of most gynaecological disorders.

All doctors will develop their own system for history-taking and this will be modified by the specialty in which they practise and the nature of the presenting complaint. The most important elements are to be comprehensive and systematic. In an emergency situation it may be necessary to defer taking a full history and concentrate on that information required for an immediate diagnosis and treatment.

History

Always start by introducing yourself and explaining who you are. Check the patient's name and whether she prefers to be addressed as 'Mrs' or 'Miss' if you are unsure about her marital status. Ask about age and occupation. The age of the patient will influence the likely diagnosis for a number of presenting problems. For example, irregular vaginal bleeding is more likely to be due to infection in the young and malignancy in the older woman. Occupation may be relevant to both the level of understanding that can be assumed and the impact of different gynaecological problems on the patient's life. What is the principal reason for the patient being here? Was she referred by her GP for a routine outpatient appointment or has she just arrived as an emergency? The immediate priorities for assessment and management may

be very different for a woman referred with a long history of heavy periods and one admitted with a life-threatening bleed in early pregnancy, even though the presenting 'symptom' is the same in both cases.

Presenting Complaint

Ask about:

Onset and duration of main complaint
Associated symptoms and relationship to menstrual cycle
Previous treatment and response

Start by allowing the patient to describe in her own words the history of her present symptoms. After they have given their history several times, patients may start to anticipate questions and give the information they think the doctor wants to hear. Specific questions relating to the commonest presenting complaints are dealt with in more detail in later chapters.

Key questions common to most situations will include the onset and duration of symptoms, whether they are associated with any other symptoms and, in women of reproductive age, whether they vary with the menstrual cycle. Ask the patient whether she has had similar problems in the past and, if so, whether any treatment or investigation was undertaken and the response to previous treatment. Remember that patients are less likely to volunteer negative responses. There may be several symptoms or problems. Try to separate these out and work through the details of each separately.

Previous Gynaecological History

Relevant items in the gynaecological history

Previous investigations or treatment
Contraceptive history
Sexual history
Cervical smear
Menstrual history

Ask about any previous gynaecological problems and treatments. For all women of reproductive age, ask about contraception if they are sexually active. This is important not only to determine the possibility of pregnancy but because the method of contraception used may itself be relevant to the presenting complaint (e.g. irregular bleeding may occur when taking the contraceptive pill or when an intrauterine device is present). For women over the age of 20, check the date and result, if known, of the last cervical smear. Details of taking a sexual history are covered in more detail in Chapter 54.

Menstrual history

Date of the last menstrual period (LMP) – was it on time and normal?
Length of bleeding
Interval between start of periods
Heaviness of bleeding – clots, flooding (night), anaemia
Pain and its relationship to the bleeding
Intermenstrual bleeding
Age of menarche

Unless it has already been covered in the presenting complaint, ask about the date of the LMP and whether it was normal and occurred at the expected time. Ask about the normal length of menstrual cycle. Remember that this is the number of days from the first day of bleeding to the first day of the following period, not the interval between the end of one period and the start of the next. If the menstrual cycle varies, note the minimum and maximum lengths. The menstrual cycle is commonly abbreviated as:

$$K = X/Y$$

where Y is the number of days of the cycle and X is the duration of bleeding in days.

The heaviness of bleeding is very subjective. Ask about the presence of clots, the amount of sanitary protection used and flooding (i.e. staining of clothes or sheets despite using sanitary protection) and treatment for anaemia. Ask about pain during or preceding menstruation and the presence of bleeding between periods (intermenstrual bleeding). Finally, ask about the age of menarche.

Previous Pregnancies

Check for:

How many (gravidity)?
Outcome (parity)
Surgical deliveries (birthweight)

The amount of detail needed on previous pregnancies will depend on the presenting problem. In most cases, the number of previous pregnancies and their outcome (miscarriage, ectopic, abortion or delivery after 24 weeks) are all that is required; for more details see the chapters on infertility (Chapter 51) and recurrent miscarriage (Chapter 59). Gravidity (G) is the number of times the woman has been pregnant and parity (P) the number of infants delivered of more than 24 weeks' gestational age or 500 g birthweight. This may be abbreviated as:

$$GxPy^{+z}$$

- where x is the number of pregnancies, y the parity and z the number of pregnancies ending before 24 weeks.

Previous Medical History

Ask about:

Previous abdominal surgery
Major cardiovascular/respiratory disease
Endocrine disease
Thromboembolic disease
Breast disease

Ask about previous medical problems, especially any other endocrine disease and major cardiovascular/respiratory disease and venous thromboembolism. Ask about previous operations, especially abdominal surgery and any anaesthetic problems. Women with a history of breast cancer are more at risk of ovarian and uterine carcinoma.

Drugs and Allergies

Ask about current medication, especially sex steroids and their antagonists and anticoagulants. Check for any allergies.

Social and Family History

Ask about:

Home circumstances
Support
Smoking
Family history

A strong family history of ovarian and/or breast cancer is associated with an increased risk of developing ovarian cancer. Ask about what support the patient has at home and at work. This will have a bearing on the arrangements she will need to make to come into hospital and the support she will require after discharge. Ask about smoking and consumption of alcohol.

Examination

The intimate nature of gynaecological examination means that it is especially important to ensure privacy. The examination should ideally take place in a separate area to that in which the consultation is held. The patient should be allowed to undress in privacy and, if necessary, empty her bladder first. Before starting the examination explain what will be involved in vaginal examination and also explain that the patient can ask for the examination to be stopped at any stage. A chaperone should generally be present, although the patient has a right to refuse this.

General Examination

Key features

General condition, weight, height
Pulse, blood pressure
Anaemia
Goitre
Breast examination (if indicated)
Secondary sex characteristics, body hair

Assess the patient's general condition, including signs of poor peripheral perfusion (pallor, cold extremities, sweating) and pain. Check weight, height, pulse and blood pressure. Look for features of anaemia and thyroid disease. Breast examination should be performed if there are symptoms (Figure 3.1). As you carry out your examination, make a note of the secondary sex characteristics and distribution of body hair.

Abdominal Examination

Key steps

Inspection – distension, scars
Palpation – masses, organomegaly, tenderness, peritonism, nodes, hernial orifices
Percussion – ascites

Expose the area between the xiphisternum and pubic symphysis, keeping the rest of the patient covered. Begin by inspection, looking for any swelling or scars. Remember to look in particular in the umbilicus for scars from previous laparoscopies, and in the suprapubic region where transverse incisions from Caesarean sections and most gynaecological operations are found. Ask the patient to indicate any areas of discomfort and then, starting away from these

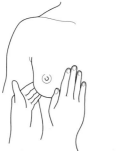 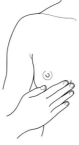 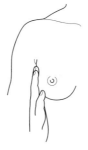 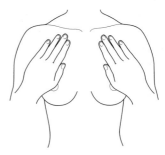

Figure 3.1   Breast examination should include systematic examination of the four quadrants of the breast and axillary tail

areas, gently palpate the abdomen, looking for any masses and tenderness. If there is a mass, try to determine if it is fixed or mobile, smooth or regular, hard or fluctuant. Try to determine if it arises from the pelvis (you shouldn't be able to palpate the lower edge above the pubic bone). Check the hernial orifices and feel for any enlarged lymph nodes in the groin. Finally, see if you can palpate the edge of the liver or spleen and either kidney. If there are areas of tenderness, note whether these are associated with any guarding or rebound. If there is generalized abdominal distension, look for evidence of ascites by percussion (the flanks should be dull to percussion and this area of dullness will move as the patient rolls onto her side). A full bladder will also be dull to percussion. Auscultation of bowel sounds is indicated in patients with postoperative abdominal distension or acute abdominal pain.

Pelvic Examination

Key steps

Explanation, comfort, privacy, chaperone
Inspection of external genitalia
Speculum examination, smear, swabs
Bimanual examination
Rectal examination, if indicated

Before starting a pelvic examination, make sure that the patient understands what is involved and why it needs to be done. A chaperone should generally be present although the patient has a right to decline this. The patient should understand that she has the right to stop the examination at any point.

Start the examination with a careful inspection of the vulva, parting the lips of the labia minora with the left hand to look at the external urethral meatus. Look for any discharge, redness, ulceration and old scars. Speculum examination is normally carried out with the patient in the supine position using a bivalve or Cusco's speculum (Figure 3.2). It is a good idea to have this warmed to room temperature and lubricated with a small amount of KY jelly. Holding the lips of the labia minora open with the left hand, insert the speculum into the introitus with the widest part of the instrument in the transverse (not anteroposterior) position, as the vagina is widest in this direction. When the speculum reaches the top of the vagina, gently open the blades and visualize the cervix. Look for any

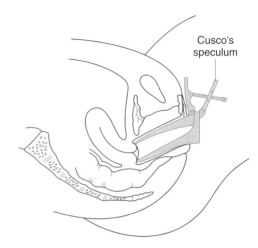

Figure 3.2 Insertion of a Cusco's speculum

discharge or bleeding from the cervix, any areas of ulceration and any polyps. Remember that the appearance of the cervix is changed after childbirth, with the external os more irregular and slit-like. The commonest finding is of a so-called erosion or ectropion. This is an area of cervical epithelium around the cervical os that appears a darker red colour than the smooth pink of the rest of the cervix. It is not an erosion at all but normal columnar epithelium extending from the endocervical canal onto the ectocervix. This is a normal finding in women of reproductive age, especially during pregnancy and whilst taking the contraceptive pill. If the clinical history suggests possible infection (see Chapter 64), take swabs from the vaginal fornices and cervical os and place in transport medium to look for *Candida*, *Trichomonas* and *Neisseria*, and take a separate swab from the endocervix for *Chlamydia*.

Taking a cervical smear

This should be done mid-cycle at least 3 months after pregnancy and not during menstruation. Explain the purpose of the test and warn the patient that she may notice some spotting afterwards. After inserting a speculum as above, wipe away any discharge or blood. Note the appearance of the cervix. A 360° sweep should be taken with a suitable spatula pressed firmly against the cervix at the junction of the columnar epithelium of the endocervical canal and the squamous epithelium of the ectocervix. The sample should be spread evenly across a glass slide labelled with the patient's name and identification number and sprayed with a suitable fixative solution.

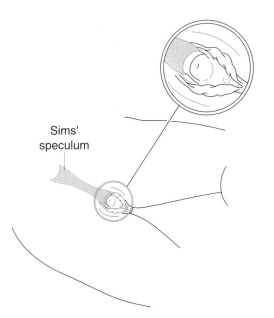

Sims'
speculum

Figure 3.3 Examination using a Sims' speculum

If the presenting complaint is of urinary incontinence or prolapse, examine the anterior vaginal wall using a Sims' speculum (Figure 3.3). To do this, ask the patient to lie on her left side facing away from you with her legs drawn up towards her chest. Ask her to lift her right leg (or get an assistant to hold the leg) and part the buttocks with your left hand. Insert the speculum with the right hand, angling it slightly back toward you. Ask the patient to bear down or cough and look for any leakage of urine or movement of the anterior vaginal wall. Using a pair of sponge-holding forceps, it should be possible to displace the anterior vaginal wall up a little so you can see the cervix.

Bimanual examination involves palpation of the pelvic organs between one hand placed on the lower abdomen and two fingers of the other hand in the vagina (Figure 3.4). It is usually carried out with the patient in the supine position or whilst in lithotomy. Part the lips of the labia with the left hand and insert the index and middle fingers of the right hand into the vagina until you can feel the cervix. This is usually 2–3 cm across and has a consistency like the tip of your nose. Now gently displace the uterus upwards and anteriorly and see if you can feel the fundus with your other hand. Assess the size of the uterus, whether it is mobile, and its position in relation to the vagina (Figure 3.4). A retroverted uterus is a normal finding in 10–15 per cent of women, although if the uterus is fixed in this position it may indicate pelvic pathology. The uterus tends to be more difficult to assess or may be palpable through the posterior fornix and the cervix may be more anterior. Examine each vaginal fornix again, feeling for any swelling (Figure 3.5). In a thin woman, it may be possible to palpate the ovaries, which are about 4–5 cm in size. Note whether there is any tenderness and whether this is worse when you try to move the cervix (cervical excitation). The uterus is normally described in terms of the equivalent sized pregnant uterus (Figure 3.6). It is not normally palpable by abdominal examination until 12 weeks. If enlarged, it may also be described as uniform or irregular in shape.

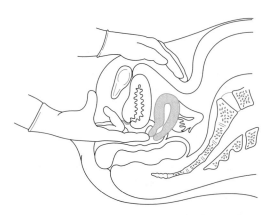

Figure 3.4 Bimanual examination of the uterus

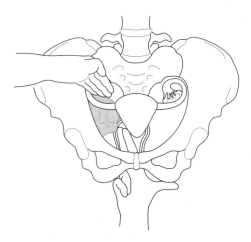

Figure 3.5 Bimanual palpation of an adnexal mass

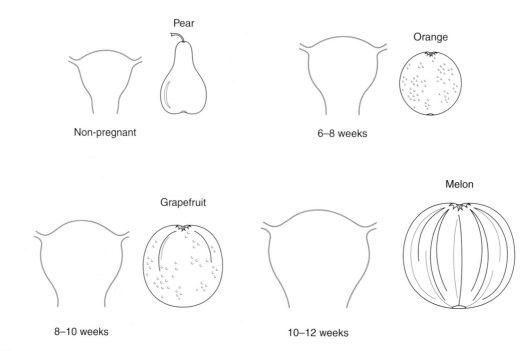

Figure 3.6 Assessment of uterine size up to 12 weeks

Presenting Your Findings

For a student, presenting your findings is a way of demonstrating both your ability at history-taking and your understanding of a particular problem. This is your chance to impress, so don't muck it up! Before you even start it is worth taking a few minutes to look through your notes and plan your presentation. Clearly, you must not omit important items of information (which may include negative responses to specific closed questions), but equally you should be prepared to leave out information that is not relevant to the current gynaecological problem or its treatment. There is usually no need to mention that a 57-year-old lady with vaginal prolapse had her ingrowing toenail removed 20 years ago unless she had an adverse reaction to the anaesthetic. Start by introducing the patient by name and age and give the main reason for admission. If there are several problems, say so, and deal with each in turn. If the history consists of a long narrative of events, try to summarize these rather than recapping each event. Present the remainder of the history in a logical, structured way, not skipping back and forward between items. This should always include the date of the last menstrual period and cervical smear. At the end of your history, give a summary in no more than one or two sentences.

Example of a typical history

This is Mrs Brown, a 53-year-old housewife who has been referred by her general practitioner to the clinic because of postmenopausal bleeding. Mrs Brown has had three episodes of painless vaginal bleeding over the last 6 months. Her last menstrual period was 3 years ago and prior to this she had a regular 28-day menstrual cycle. She has no previous gynaecological history of note and her last cervical smear was 2 years ago and was negative. She has had three pregnancies with uncomplicated normal vaginal deliveries at term. She underwent a left mastectomy 7 years ago for breast cancer and was last seen at the follow-up clinic

6 months ago when there was no evidence of recurrent disease. She has no history of diabetes or hypertension and had no problems with the general anaesthetic at the time of the mastectomy. She is currently taking tamoxifen and has no known allergies. She lives with her husband, who is well. She does not smoke or drink.

In summary, Mrs Brown is a 53-year-old lady with a 6-month history of postmenopausal bleeding on tamoxifen.

Examination technique has been covered above, but if you are presenting findings from an examination you have previously performed, the same principles apply. Unless you are asked only to discuss one particular part of the examination, always start by commenting on the patient's general condition, including pulse and blood pressure. For abdominal examination, list the findings on inspection and palpation and percussion (if there is abdominal distension or a mass). Try to distinguish whether a mass is arising from the pelvis and, if so, describe it in terms of a pregnant uterus (e.g. a mass reaching the umbilicus would be a 20-week size pelvic mass). If there are areas of tenderness, specify whether they are associated with signs of peritonism (guarding and rebound). On pelvic examination, describe the findings on inspection of the vulva and then of the cervix (if a speculum examination was carried out). Describe the size, position and mobility of the uterus and any tenderness. Finally, say whether there were any palpable masses or tenderness in the adnexae.

Example of presentation of clinical findings

On general examination Mrs Brown looked well. She was not clinically anaemic and her body mass index was 31. Her blood pressure was 130/90 and her pulse 88 and regular. She has a scar on the chest consistent with a previous mastectomy and the remaining breast appears normal. There were no palpable masses in the breast or lymphadenopathy. Examination of the chest and heart was unremarkable. On abdominal examination there were no visible scars or distension. On palpation, the abdomen was soft and non-tender with no palpable masses and no organomegaly. On pelvic examination, the external genitalia were normal, apart from an old scar on the perineum consistent with a previous tear or episiotomy. On speculum examination, the cervix and upper vaginal mucosa appeared healthy. She had a normal-sized, mobile, anteverted uterus and there were no palpable adnexal masses.

Learning Points

- **Introduce the patient by name**
- **Start the history with a clear indication of the presenting complaint or the reason why the patient is in the ward or clinic**
- **Include details of the social history**
- **Summarize your findings**
- **Don't appear disorganized or waffle**
- **Don't simply read back your notes**
- **Don't reprise past history or systems review if not relevant**
- **Don't use abbreviations or medical terms you can't define**

See Also

History-taking and examination in obstetrics (Chapter 2)

Further Reading

Royal College of Obstetricians and Gynaecologists. Intimate Examinations: Report of a Working Party. RCOG Press, London, 1997.

Section 2

In the antenatal clinic

4. Abnormal antibodies: blood group incompatibility 21

5. Anaemia in pregnancy 25

6. Breathlessness in pregnancy 29

7. Breech presentation 33

8. Diabetes 37

9. Fetal abnormality: chromosomal 41

10. Fetal abnormality: structural 46

11. Hypertension 50

12. Infections in pregnancy 56

13. Large for gestational age 60

14. Multiple pregnancy 63

15. Previous Caesarean section 69

16. Previous fetal loss 72

17. Prolonged pregnancy 75

18. Proteinuria 77

19. Pruritus and jaundice in pregnancy 80

20. Reduced fetal movements 83

21. Small for gestational age 88

22. Substance abuse 92

23. Unstable or transverse lie 95

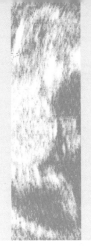

Chapter 4

Abnormal antibodies: blood group incompatibility

Importance

If enough fetal blood cells leak into the maternal circulation, the antigens on the fetal cells may provoke a maternal antibody response. Some of these antibodies are capable of crossing the placenta and react with the fetal erythrocytes, causing haemolysis and anaemia. Haemolytic disease of the newborn may occur, and severe disease may cause fetal death. Several blood groups are capable of producing fetal risk, but the Rhesus (Rh) group has caused the most problems. With an adequate prophylactic anti-D gamma globulin programme, fewer than 1 in 500 pregnancies will be affected by Rh incompatibility.

Causes

The Rh blood group is the most complex human blood group. The Rh antigens are grouped in three pairs: Dd, Cc, Ee. The major red cell antigen in this group (D) is of prime concern. The fetus receives half of its genetic component from the mother and half from the father; the fetus may therefore have a different blood group from its mother. A woman who is lacking the Rh factor may carry an Rh-positive fetus. If sufficient fetal red cells pass into the maternal circulation, maternal antibodies to the Rh antigen may develop, cross the placenta, and cause haemolysis.

ABO incompatibility is three to four times more common than Rh incompatibility. However, ABO incompatibility is rarely responsible for severe anaemia; the usual clinical problem is early jaundice, which usually requires phototherapy rather than exchange transfusion. The condition is characterized by involvement in first pregnancies, and is unpredictable in subsequent pregnancies.

Other red cell antigens (Kell, Duffy, M) are rarely responsible for incompatibility reactions, but do have the potential to cause significant neonatal morbidity.

Screening

On the first antenatal clinic visit, all pregnant women should be screened for the ABO and Rh groups. They should also undergo antibody screening using the indirect Coombs' test or enzyme (e.g. papain) techniques. (Occasionally rarer Rh subtypes (C, c, E, e) or red cell antigens other than Rh (D), A and B, may be involved; these include the Kell, Duffy, and Kidd antigens.) The incidence of Rh-negative women is relatively high in Caucasian populations (up to 15 per cent).

If no red cell antibodies are found on initial testing, Rh-negative women should be re-tested during the pregnancy. Some centres recommend re-testing at 30, 36 and 40 weeks' gestation, others at 28 and 34 or 36 weeks' gestation. Umbilical cord samples are also sent to determine the Rh status of the baby, to determine whether antibodies are present and to ensure optimal prophylaxis (as below).

Screening of Rh-positive women varies. In some centres, Rh-positive women are only tested at the booking visit unless other red cell antibodies are detected or if they have had previous blood transfusions. In other centres, all Rh-positive women are screened at the booking visit and at 28 and 36 weeks' gestation.

Diagnosis and Clinical Assessment

History

A history taken from a Rh-negative woman may indicate whether her baby is likely to suffer from haemolytic disease of the newborn.

Ask about:

Previous blood transfusion

Previous affected pregnancies (number, severity, treatment required)

Whether the father of this pregnancy is the same as previous pregnancies

The first pregnancy represents a 'sensitizing' experience and the baby is not usually affected. Women who have had a blood transfusion may be an exception to this.

Examination

Examination of the mother rarely contributes to a diagnosis or risk assessment of haemolytic disease of the newborn.

Investigation

The following investigations may be indicated:

Paternal blood ABO group and Rh genotype

Antibody level

Ultrasonography

Cordocentesis

Amniocentesis

ABO incompatibility conveys a protective effect; fetal cells of a different ABO group from that of the mother are destroyed before sensitization can occur. The father may be heterozygous for the Rh factor (in which case his children may be either Rh-positive or Rh-negative). If the father is Rh-positive homozygous and ABO-compatible, the risks are four- to five-fold greater than if he is Rh-positive heterozygous and ABO-incompatible.

Positive antibody testing provides an indication that the baby may be affected. In general, titres below 4 IU/mL indicate that serious fetal disease is unlikely. Increasing titres provide a reasonable guide to severity, particularly in 'first affected' pregnancies.

Ultrasound appearances which would suggest *haemolytic disease* include:

- placental thickness
- increased abdominal/head circumference ratio
- altered relative diameters of intrahepatic and extrahepatic veins.

Signs of *cardiac failure or 'hydrops'* (suggestive of severe disease) include:

- generalized skin oedema (>5 mm)
- pleural effusion
- pericardial effusion
- ascites.

If Rh antibodies are absent, the *differential diagnosis of fetal 'hydrops'* includes:

- chromosomal abnormality, e.g. trisomies
- cardiovascular malformation
- cardiac arrhythmias
- α-thalassaemia
- twin–twin transfusion
- infections, e.g. parvovirus.

The antibody titre and the severity of haemolytic disease in previous pregnancies determine the need for invasive tests.

In cordocentesis, a fetal blood sample is taken from the umbilical vein, at the insertion into the placenta. The fetal haemoglobin, haematocrit, blood group, direct Coombs' test and bilirubin level provide an accurate indication of the fetal condition. The procedure is associated with considerable fetal mortality (2 per cent), but can be combined with intrauterine transfusion (discussed below).

Amniocentesis is described in Chapter 9. The test is a safer option than cordocentesis once fetal viability has been established. The level of bilirubin (which reflects the degree of fetal red blood cell destruction) is determined by spectrophotometry. The fetal risk is calculated by comparing the optical density values obtained with standard reference charts (such as the Liley chart).

Management

Priorities

Determine whether a pregnancy is at risk of sensitization by screening

Prevent the development of abnormal antibodies in unsensitized pregnancies by anti-D prophylaxis

Identify sensitized pregnancies and assess the risk

Management of sensitized pregnancies

Prevention

Indications for prophylactic therapy include:

Miscarriage

Ectopic pregnancy

Chorionic villous biopsy/amniocentesis

Trauma

Placental abruption

External cephalic version

Childbirth

Transfer of fetal cells to the maternal circulation can occur in situations in which placental integrity is disturbed; of these, the most important is childbirth. Prophylaxis is not required for miscarriage occurring before 12 weeks unless the uterus is instrumented.

Factors increasing fetal red cell transfer to the mother at the time of birth include:

- Caesarean section
- multiple pregnancy
- manual removal of placenta
- stillbirth
- placenta praevia.

The introduction of anti-D immunoprophylaxis has reduced the perinatal mortality due to haemolytic disease of the newborn by a factor of 1000; 125 IU of anti-D will absorb 1 mL of fetal blood in the maternal circulation. The amount of fetomaternal haemorrhage, and thus the amount of anti-D required, can be assessed by the Kleihauer test. This test is based on the principle that fetal cells remain stable in an acid pH, whereas adult haemoglobin is eluted from the maternal cells. Less than 1 per cent of deliveries are associated with a fetomaternal haemorrhage of more than 4 mL, and thus 500 IU is sufficient in over 99 per cent of cases.

The guidelines for postnatal prophylaxis in the UK are:

Collect maternal blood for Kleihauer testing

Administer 500 IU anti-D intramuscularly to all Rh-negative mothers giving birth to Rh-positive babies (or to babies of unknown status)

Administer the dose as soon as possible after birth and always before 72 hours

Administer more anti-D if the Kleihauer test indicated a fetomaternal haemorrhage of more than 4 mL

A dosage of 250 IU anti-D in early pregnancy and 500 IU in late pregnancy should be administered for the indications detailed above. In some centres, prophylactic injections are given to all Rh-negative women at 28–30 weeks' gestation; this further reduces the risk of sensitization in late pregnancy.

Close collaboration among the obstetrician, biochemist, haematologist and paediatrician is necessary.

Management of the Sensitized Pregnancy

The couple should be informed about the nature of the problem, the tests that are available, and the management options. The management options depend on the severity of the fetal condition.

Management options include:

Intrauterine transfusion

Intensive fetal surveillance

Elective delivery

Exchange transfusion after delivery

Intrauterine transfusion is considered when the haemolytic disease is so severe that the fetus is unlikely to survive long enough to allow delivery at 30–32 weeks. The procedure involves fresh, packed, group O Rh-negative blood being transfused into the umbilical or hepatic vein of the fetus, or into the peritoneal cavity.

Serial ultrasound scans will facilitate detection of signs of fetal hydrops. In addition, the ultrasound scans will form part of the careful assessment of fetal well-being (Chapter 20).

The decision regarding the optimal timing and mode of delivery will depend on the degree of haemolytic disease and the assessment of fetal well-being. If the baby is only considered to be mildly affected, delivery will be effected at 37–40 weeks; if there is severe disease, delivery at 32 weeks may be planned. Communication between obstetric and neonatal staff is essential.

Exchange transfusion is indicated on the basis of anaemia or hyperbilirubinaemia. The blood of the baby is exchanged with donor blood in repeated aliquots of 10–20 mL.

Neonatal complications are those of preterm delivery and hyperbilirubinaemia, which include neural deafness and intellectual impairment, and those associated with exchange blood transfusions, which include viral and bacterial infections, disturbances in electrolytes, cardiac arrhythmias and neonatal death.

Follow-up

After a pregnancy has been complicated by Rh incompatibility, there are serious implications for future pregnancies. All babies will be affected by the condition, at increasingly earlier gestations.

Learning Points

- **Blood group incompatibility arises when the fetus inherits blood group factors from the father which are absent in the mother**

- **The number of affected fetuses has fallen dramatically since the introduction of anti-D prophylaxis**
- **A number of complex management decisions are necessary if moderate or severe fetal haemolysis occurs**

See Also

Fetal abnormality: chromosomal (Chapter 9)
Reduced fetal movements (Chapter 20)
Preterm labour (Chapter 38)

Further Reading

National Blood Transfusion Service Immunoglobulin Working Party. Recommendations for the use of anti-D immunoglobulin. *Prescribers' Journal* 1991; 30: 137–45.

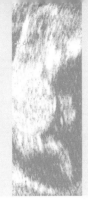

Chapter 5

Anaemia in pregnancy

Definition

Anaemia in pregnancy is variously defined as a haemoglobin concentration < 11.0 g/dL, or as < 11.5 g/dL in the first half of pregnancy and/or < 10.5 g/dL in the second half of pregnancy.

Importance

Anaemia is a common condition (present in 2–20 per cent of pregnant women). It is associated with increased mortality and morbidity of both mother and baby, with increased incidences of maternal infections, cardiac failure, premature labour and intrauterine growth restriction. It is important to diagnose the type of anaemia and treat it accordingly.

Causes

Common diagnoses

Iron deficiency anaemia
Folic acid deficiency anaemia
Haemoglobinopathies

In pregnancy, the blood volume increases by 35 per cent as the uteroplacental bed and venous dilatation cause an expansion of the vascular space. Whilst the red cell volume rises by 25 per cent, the plasma volume increases by 45 per cent. This results in a haemodilatation and the 'physiological anaemia of pregnancy'.

Iron deficiency is the commonest cause of anaemia in pregnancy. The serum iron falls in pregnancy, but the iron-binding capacity of serum proteins increases, allowing greater storage of iron. An additional 800 mg of iron is required in pregnancy, due to the expanded red cell volume (400 mg), the fetus (300 mg) and the placenta (100 mg). Normally only 10 per cent of dietary iron is absorbed, but this increases to 20 per cent in pregnancy. Total iron stores are 1200 mg (excluding red cells) but may be decreased.

Causes of decreased iron stores

Excessive loss – previous pregnancies, menorrhagia, antepartum haemorrhage, hookworm infestation, multiple pregnancies
Poor dietary intake
Malabsorption syndromes

Folic acid is necessary for amino acid metabolism and is required by dividing cells; large amounts (up to 400 μg each day) are needed in pregnancy. A deficiency of folic acid has also been implicated in the pathogenesis of neural tube defects and may predispose to placental abruptions. The causes of folic acid deficiency are similar to those of iron deficiency; folic acid is present in green vegetables. The demand for folic acid is increased in any woman taking anticonvulsant therapy. Vitamin B_{12} deficiency is extremely rare in pregnancy.

The haemoglobinopathies are classified as either quantitative defects (thalassaemias) or qualitative defects in which an abnormal form of haemoglobin is produced (such as in sickle cell disease). Thalassaemias can involve the alpha or beta haemoglobin chain.

Beta-thalassaemias predominantly affect women of Mediterranean origin and can be heterozygous (minor) or homozygous (major). In beta-thalassaemia minor, a haemolytic anaemia results in a shortened red blood cell life span and the haemoglobin concentration typically falls to below 10 g/dL in the third trimester. Inheritance is autosomal recessive, and there is a 1 in 4 chance of the child suffering from beta-thalassaemia major if the partner also has beta-thalassaemia minor. In the UK, the carrier rate is only 1 in 10 000, but in Cyprus the carrier rate is 1 in 7. In beta-thalassaemia major, severe anaemia necessitates blood transfusions. The management problem is one of iron overload from the transfused cells; this results in hepatic, endocrine and myocardial damage, and often causes death in the teens.

Alpha-thalassaemia predominantly affects women from Southeast Asia. Four gene loci code for the alpha chain. In alpha-thalassaemia trait, one alpha gene (alpha$^+$) or two alpha genes (alpha^0) are deleted. Women with alpha-thalassaemia trait (particularly alpha^0) can become markedly anaemic in pregnancy. When three genes are deleted, a tetramer of beta chains (haemoglobin H) can be detected and anaemia may be severe. When all four genes are deleted, a tetramer of fetal gamma chains forms (haemoglobin Barts); this condition results in severe fetal anaemia and a hydropic stillbirth.

Over 250 structural variants of haemoglobin have been described, but the most important is sickle cell haemoglobin (haemoglobin S), most commonly found in African-American women. The heterozygous state (sickle cell trait) is not associated with major morbidity. In homozygous sickle cell disease, sickling crises may occur in which there is haemolysis and tissue ischaemia. Haemoglobin SC disease (there are two abnormal haemoglobin forms, S and C) is similar to sickle cell anaemia in terms of complications.

Diagnosis and Clinical Assessment

Screening

The haemoglobin value and red cell indices should be checked at the booking clinic visit; this initial test will detect pre-existing anaemia (usually iron deficiency or an inherited disorder). Haemoglobin electrophoresis should be performed, if indicated by the ethnic origin of the pregnant woman. If a haemoglobin variant of thalassaemia is identified, blood from the partner should also be examined. The risk to the baby of a serious haemoglobin defect can then be assessed early in pregnancy. If there is a significant fetal risk, the option of antenatal diagnosis (chorionic villous biopsy or fetal blood sampling) should be considered.

The haemoglobin estimation should be rechecked at about 28 weeks' gestation. The later tests are important in detecting iron deficiency and folic acid deficiency anaemias. If the haemoglobin concentration indicates anaemia, a clinical assessment should be performed, with history, examination and further investigations as indicated.

History

Ask about:

Diet and medication
Any gastrointestinal disorders
Previous menstrual and reproductive history
Any history of blood loss
Ethnic origin

Examination

Key features

Skin bruising
Koilonychia
Hepatosplenomegaly
Lymph node enlargement
Mouth and gum changes
Peripheral neuropathy

Investigations

Appropriate investigations may include:

Blood film
Iron studies
Haemoglobin electrophoresis
Reticulocyte count
Serum folate and B$_{12}$
Bone marrow aspirate
Renal function tests

A hypochromic microcytic picture on the blood film suggests iron deficiency or thalassaemia. Iron deficiency anaemia will be confirmed by a low serum iron, raised serum transferrin and low serum ferritin. The reticulocyte count will be raised in blood loss or haemolysis. Iron deficiency may mask the macrocytosis of folic acid deficiency, although examination of the blood film may reveal oval macrocytes among iron-deficient microcytic cells. Serum folate estimations are unreliable and the definitive diagnosis of folic acid deficiency in pregnancy may involve a bone marrow aspirate.

Electrophoresis will distinguish beta-thalassaemia from iron deficiency anaemia. In beta-thalassaemia minor, there is an elevation of haemoglobin A_2 (excess alpha chains combine with delta chains as there is a lack of beta chains). Alpha-thalassaemia trait can be identified by DNA analysis of nucleated cells. If the woman is of African-American descent, electrophoresis to screen for a qualitative change in haemoglobin production (such as the sickle cell variant) should be performed.

Renal function tests should be performed, as chronic renal disease is present in a significant minority of pregnant women with a haemoglobin concentration below 9 g/dL.

Management

Prevention

The place of routine iron and folate supplementation in pregnancy is controversial. Although the physiological requirements in pregnancy exceed the usual intake of most healthy women, even in the developed world, there is little evidence from controlled trials to support routine supplementation. In areas where iron and folate deficiencies are prevalent, prophylactic supplementation may be indicated. A range of preparations is available, but a dose of 270 mg ferrous sulphate and 300 μg folic acid would be typical.

Iron Deficiency

The haemoglobin level should rise by 1 g every 7–10 days with ferrous sulphate 600 mg daily. Side-effects of iron administration are dose related. Although some women have gastric symptoms, the main complaint is constipation (usually resolved by increased dietary fibre). Slow-release forms are more expensive and only have fewer side-effects because much of the iron is not released and is excreted unchanged. The most common reason for a failure of therapy is poor compliance. Management of iron deficiency anaemia in late pregnancy is a particular challenge, as a satisfactory response must be obtained within a reasonable time. The increase in haemoglobin concentration is no greater with parenteral as compared with iron therapy. Intramuscular injections of iron sorbitol citrate should be reserved for women with a genuine intolerance to oral iron. Intravenous administration of iron dextran is rarely prescribed in pregnancy; the initial intravenous infusion should be slow, as anaphylactic reactions can occur. If is there is not enough time to achieve a reasonable haemoglobin at delivery, a blood transfusion should be arranged. If there is no response to iron therapy, other causes of anaemia should be considered.

Folic Acid Deficiency

Severe megaloblastic anaemia is uncommon. Initial treatment should be with 5 mg folic acid tablets taken daily. In malabsorption states, intramuscular injection is occasionally required.

Haemoglobinopathies

There is no specific treatment to correct the abnormal haemoglobins of sickle cell and sickle cell C disease. Repeat transfusions reduce the likelihood of crises by maintaining a high proportion of haemoglobin as haemoglobin A (composed of alpha and beta chains) and by reducing the stimulus to erythropoiesis (and production of more sickle cells). The target to aim for is a haemoglobin concentration of 10.5–12.5 g/dL with 60 per cent as haemoglobin A. Folic acid supplementation should be instigated, but iron administration may cause haemosiderosis and should only be given if there is a certainty that the woman is iron deficient. In sickle cell disease, crises should be prevented (by avoiding hypoxia, dehydration and infection).

Iron therapy should also be avoided in thalassaemias. Folic acid should be routinely prescribed, and blood transfusions may be necessary.

Learning Points

- The common causes of anaemia in pregnancy are iron deficiency, folic acid deficiency and the haemoglobinopathies
- The place of routine iron and folate supplementation in pregnancy is controversial
- Treatment of anaemia in pregnancy should be after a diagnosis has been made

Further Reading

Letsky EA. Anaemia in pregnancy. In: Studd J, ed. *Progress in Obstetrics and Gynaecology*, vol. 6. Churchill Livingstone, Edinburgh, 1987, pp. 23–58.

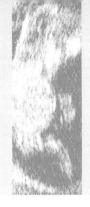

Breathlessness in pregnancy

Importance

The conditions responsible for causing breathlessness in pregnancy include major causes of maternal mortality, particularly pulmonary embolism and cardiac disease. Any complaint of breathlessness should be investigated thoroughly.

Causes

Causes include:

Physiological
Anaemia
Pulmonary embolism
Asthma
Chest infection
Congenital heart disease
Rheumatic heart disease
Paroxysmal supraventricular tachycardia

Rarer causes include ischaemic heart disease, myocarditis, cardiomyopathy, pulmonary hypertension, pneumothorax and sarcoidosis.

The physiological increase in the ventilatory requirements of a pregnant woman is largely met by an increase in tidal volume rather than respiratory rate. However, this extra respiratory work may be perceived as 'shortness of breath', especially in the second half of pregnancy.

Asthma is the commonest disease affecting the lungs in pregnancy, and affects 1 per cent of women. The effect of pregnancy on asthma is very variable, although there is a tendency for the condition to improve. Progesterone induces a relaxation of smooth muscle and the higher levels of endogenous

corticosteroids may be therapeutic. Nevertheless, asthma may present for the first time in pregnancy. Occasionally, prolonged periods of maternal hypoxia can lead to intrauterine growth restriction.

Chest infections are usually secondary to upper respiratory viral infections. Responsible organisms include bacteria (such as haemolytic streptococci or *Haemophilus*), *Mycoplasma* and the varicella virus. Varicella infection may result in a severe pneumonia with chest infection.

Congenital heart defects are the most prevalent form of cardiac disease in pregnancy. These defects include patent ductus arteriosus, septal defects and great vessel anomalies; defects can occur in combination. Rheumatic heart disease remains a problem in poor socioeconomic conditions where streptococcal infections are common. Paroxysmal supraventricular tachycardia is relatively common in women of reproductive age and attacks occur more frequently in pregnancy.

Pulmonary embolism is discussed in Chapter 44 and anaemia is discussed in Chapter 5.

Diagnosis and Clinical Assessment

History

Ask about:

Past medical history
Exacerbating or predisposing factors
Associated symptoms

It is essential to elicit a precise history of any past medical condition which may be responsible for the breathlessness.

The pattern of attacks or an exposure to irritants or allergens may suggest an asthmatic aetiology. A reduced exercise tolerance is typical of cardiac insufficiency. This reduced exercise tolerance forms the basis of the New York Heart Association classification (Table 6.1).

Coffee, anxiety or tobacco may precipitate a supraventricular tachycardia. The history may elicit features which predispose to a thromboembolic event, such as an operative delivery or prolonged bed rest.

Associated wheezing is typical of asthma, but can also be found following a pulmonary embolism. The presence of associated symptoms such as fever, chills, pleuritic chest pain or a cough will suggest a chest infection. Nocturnal dyspnoea is a feature of cardiac disease. A woman with a supraventricular tachycardia is usually aware that her heart is beating quickly and may feel faint. Chest tightness or pain may indicate a pulmonary embolism.

Examination

On general examination, clubbing and cyanosis with a raised jugular venous pulse are features of cardiac insufficiency. Cardiomegaly, hepatomegaly and peripheral oedema should be sought (although oedema is found in the majority of uncomplicated pregnancies). A rapid (> 150 beats/min) and regular pulse indicates a supraventricular tachycardia.

On chest auscultation, the presence of a murmur or murmurs suggests a valvular lesion, although a pulmonary ejection systolic murmur is commonly present in normal pregnancies. Fine basal crepitations indicate left-sided cardiac failure, whereas coarse crepitations suggest a diagnosis of a chest infection. Cases of asthma are associated with an expiratory wheeze.

Investigation

Depending on the history and examination findings, relevant investigations may include:

Electrocardiogram (ECG)
Echocardiogram
Cardiac catheter studies
Peak expiratory flow rate
Sputum and blood culture, serological tests
Chest X-ray
Isotope lung studies

Any patient with cardiac disease should be formally assessed with respect to the nature and severity of the lesion. Investigations may include an ECG, X-ray, echocardiogram and even cardiac catheter studies. As much information as possible regarding cardiac function and the pressure across valves should be obtained. A tachycardia with a complex of normal configuration is typical of supraventricular paroxysmal tachycardia.

Peak expiratory flow will be reduced in cases of asthma.

If a chest infection is suspected, sputum should be sent for culture and sensitivity, and blood cultures should be performed in severe cases. Serological tests may indicate a recent viral infection (see Chapter 12).

In acute attacks of asthma, the lungs appear hyperinflated on X-ray. In cases of pneumonia, the X-ray appearances are of mottled opacities in affected lung fields. The classical chest X-ray features following pulmonary embolism are of single or multiple pulmonary opacities. However, the definitive diagnosis is usually made after isotope lung scanning (see Chapter 44).

Table 6.1 New York Heart Association classification of exercise tolerance

Grade	Definition
Grade 1	Normal exercise tolerance
Grade 2	Breathless on moderate exertion (heavy housework)
Grade 3	Breathless on less than moderate exertion (light housework)
Grade 4	Breathless without significant activity

Management

The management plan is wholly dependent upon the diagnosis made.

Asthma

The management of asthma is similar to that of a non-pregnant woman. The drugs used in asthma (beta-sympathomimetics, theophyllines, chromoglycate and steroids) are relatively safe; adverse effects will be reduced by inhaled rather than oral medication. Attacks may be severe; hospitalization and intense monitoring may be necessary.

Chest Infection

The treatment for a chest infection is also similar to that of a non-pregnant woman. Failure to respond to penicillins or cephalosporins should raise the possibility of organisms such as *Mycoplasma* (which usually responds to erythromycin) or viral pneumonia.

Cardiac Disease

> **Key features**
>
> Pre-pregnancy assessment: treatment should be optimized
> Joint management with a cardiologist
> Termination of pregnancy if prognosis very poor
> Detailed ultrasound scan at 20 weeks' gestation
> Anticoagulation prophylaxis
> Iron and folate supplementation
> Serial ultrasound scans
> Plan management of labour: antibiotics, analgesia, short
>   second stage, oxytocin

Women with cardiac disease should be assessed by a cardiologist before pregnancy. Medical treatment should be optimized and any necessary surgery should be performed before pregnancy. Women with grade 1 and 2 disease (New York Heart Association classification) can be reassured that with the appropriate care, they should tolerate pregnancy well. Grades 3 and 4 account for only 10 per cent of cases, but 85 per cent of maternal mortality. Pregnancy should be advised against (and adequate contraceptive measures ensured) if conditions with a particularly poor prognosis in pregnancy are identified. Such conditions include pulmonary hypertension, Marfan's syndrome with aortic involvement, or grade 4 disease.

If pregnancy occurs in the presence of these conditions, termination should be considered. Regular antenatal clinic visits should be arranged, and these should be planned in conjunction with a cardiologist. A detailed ultrasound scan should be arranged at 20 weeks' gestation in order to check for fetal anomalies, with particular focus on cardiac lesions. Anticoagulation prophylaxis against thromboembolic disease should be considered for women predisposed to this complication (e.g. women with pulmonary hypertension or prosthetic heart valves). Iron and folate supplementation should be prescribed in order to prevent the potential aggravation of cardiac compromise by anaemia. Serial ultrasound scan assessment of fetal growth and wellbeing should be performed.

A plan for the management of labour should be established after consultation with cardiologist and anaesthetist colleagues. Induction of labour should only be performed for obstetric indications, as spontaneous labour should be more efficient and thus place less demand on cardiac reserve. A vaginal delivery will usually be the preferred mode of delivery, although there are exceptions to this (pulmonary hypertension, coarctation of the aorta). Other components of the intrapartum management plan may include amoxycillin prophylaxis against bacterial endocarditis, and avoidance of excess intravenous fluids. Epidural anaesthesia is contraindicated in certain conditions (aortic stenosis, hypertrophic obstructive cardiomyopathy). The lithotomy position should be avoided because of the risk of increased venous return precipitating pulmonary oedema. Ergometrine is contraindicated and a slow injection of Syntocinon should be given to avoid postpartum haemorrhage.

Massage of the carotid sinus for a few seconds may terminate an attack of paroxysmal supraventricular tachycardia. If it does not do so, a sedative and retiring to bed may be all that are required; many women then awake to find that the attack is over.

The management of pulmonary embolism is discussed in Chapters 32 and 44.

Learning Points

- **Causes of breathlessness in pregnancy are many and varied. They include physiological changes, pulmonary embolism, asthma, chest infection, cardiac disease and supraventricular tachycardia.**

Rare causes include ischaemic heart disease, myocarditis, cardiomyopathy, pulmonary hypertension, pneumothorax and sarcoidosis
- Key features of the management of cardiac disease include pre-pregnancy assessment, joint management with a cardiologist, prophylaxis against thromboembolism and anaemia, serial assessment of fetal well-being and a detailed interpartum management plan established in conjunction with an anaesthetist

See Also

Maternal collapse (Chapter 32)
Venous thrombosis (Chapter 44)

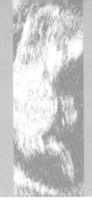

Chapter 7

Breech presentation

Importance

A breech presentation is where the caudal pole of the baby (the breech) presents in the inlet of the pelvis. The incidence of breech presentation at term is approximately 3 per cent, and at 29–32 weeks is approximately 14 per cent. The management of breech presentation at term is one of the most controversial aspects of obstetric practice; in particular, the role of the vaginal breech delivery has been questioned.

Aetiology

Predisposing factors include:

Multiparity
Multiple pregnancy
Placenta praevia or pelvic tumours
Fetal anomaly (e.g. hydrocephalus) or uterine anomaly
Fetal macrosomia or contracted maternal pelvis
Neurological disorders

Diagnosis and Clinical Assessment

The incidence of breech presentation decreases with increasing gestational age; the majority of cases of breech presentation at 30 weeks' gestation will be cephalic presentations at delivery. The time when diagnosis is most important is after 34 weeks' gestation.

History

The history is of limited value in the diagnosis of a breech presentation. However, there are certain features of the history that should increase the index of suspicion regarding a breech presentation.

Ask about:

Breech presentation at earlier gestation
Breech presentation at previous delivery
Uterine fibroids
Uterine malformation

If a breech presentation has been identified at an earlier gestation, the woman should be reviewed to ensure that spontaneous version has occurred. The incidence of breech presentation is increased if previous pregnancies have been complicated by a breech presentation; in some cases this is due to the presence of uterine fibroids or a congenital uterine anomaly.

Examination

Key findings

A soft, yielding, irregular mass is over the pelvis
A ballottable fetal head is palpable in the fundus
The fetal heart is detected above the umbilicus

The fetal head in the fundus is often associated with tenderness on palpation and shows characteristic ballottability. A failure to elicit the ballottability may be due to extended fetal legs, oligohydramnios, bicornuate uterus, obesity, an anterior placenta or a fetal head which has moved under the costal margin. If there is doubt regarding the fetal presentation after 34 weeks' gestation, the diagnosis should be confirmed by a pelvic examination or an ultrasound scan.

Investigation

An ultrasound scan should be arranged in order to:

Confirm the presentation
Determine the type of breech

(cont.)

(cont.)
Exclude a fetal anomaly
Exclude hyperextension of the neck
Estimate liquor volume and placental site
Estimate fetal weight

The majority of breech presentations (60 per cent) are extended ('frank', with the fetal legs extended at the knee), flexed breech ('complete', with the fetal legs flexed at the knee) is the next in frequency, and a small minority of cases (< 5 per cent) are footling breech presentations ('incomplete', with one fetal leg extended and the other flexed) (Figure 7.1).

Fetal malformations such as anencephaly and hydrocephalus are rare, but breech presentations occur in about 15 and 25 per cent, respectively. Other anomalies such as skeletal or muscle deformities, or chromosomal abnormalities are occasionally present. Hyperextension of the neck (the 'star-gazing' fetus) can cause spinal cord and brain injuries at vaginal delivery.

Most authorities have recommended the abandonment of X-ray pelvimetry measurement of pelvic diameters – it does not appear to be a helpful determinant of the success of attempted vaginal delivery. Clinical pelvimetry is probably only useful if the maternal pelvis is grossly contracted (e.g. road traffic accident, rickets).

Management

If a breech presentation is found on examination after 34 weeks' gestation, an explanation of the finding, and of the need for careful assessment, should be given to the pregnant woman and her partner. The first option to consider is to attempt to turn the baby to a cephalic presentation by external cephalic version (ECV). If ECV is not performed, or is unsuccessful, the next step is to determine the planned mode of delivery.

External Cephalic Version

Current evidence indicates that ECV performed at term and particularly with tocolysis is a safe procedure for carefully selected women. In such patients, it seems likely that benefits outweigh the risks (of premature labour, fetomaternal haemorrhage, cord accidents).

Contraindications to ECV

Absolute
- Multiple pregnancy
- Antepartum haemorrhage
- Placenta praevia (or any other need for Caesarean section)
- Ruptured membranes
- Significant fetal abnormality

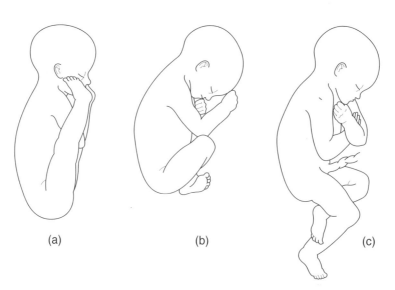

(a)　　　　(b)　　　　(c)

Figure 7.1　Types of breech presentation: (a) extended, (b) flexed, (c) footling

Relative

- Previous Caesarean section
- Intrauterine growth restriction (IUGR)
- Rhesus isoimmunization

ECV is more difficult in nulliparous or obese women, when the fetal legs are extended, the uterus is irritable, or when the amniotic fluid volume is reduced.

The tocolytic employed is usually a small intravenous dose of ritodrine (0.2 mg/min) or terbutaline (0.5 μg/min). A preliminary ultrasound scan will localize the placenta and show the disposition of the fetus. A variety of techniques are described – these involve disengagement of the breech by abdominal pressure, encouraging the baby to somersault into a cephalic presentation, and maintaining the position of the baby for a few minutes. After ECV, the fetal heart-rate pattern should be continuously monitored and an injection of anti-D gamma globulin should be given to Rhesus-negative women.

For patients who present with a previously undiagnosed breech in labour, consideration can be given to performing ECV if they are in the early stages and the membranes are still intact.

Decision Regarding Mode of Delivery

The issue of the safest method for delivery of a breech presentation has vexed obstetricians for many years.

Perinatal and neonatal morbidity and mortality rates are higher after vaginal breech deliveries than after vaginal cephalic deliveries. However, breech presentations are associated with increased incidences of congenital anomalies, IUGR and either polyhydramnios or oligohydramnios. The results of the recently completed term breech trial showed that vaginal delivery carried an increase in the risk of fetal morbidity or mortality regardless of parity or experience of the person delivering the baby. The overall risk of fetal damage in the vaginally delivered group was approximately 1 per cent. There are some criticisms of the trial which slightly weaken the findings, but overall it is now possible to counsel mothers that the risks of vaginal delivery are higher than for elective Caesarean section. However, for some women a 1 per cent risk of fetal morbidity may not appear large and they will wish to attempt a vaginal delivery.

Factors that are associated with a more favourable outcome for vaginal delivery are listed in Table 7.1.

In the term breech trial, the maternal morbidity for mothers randomized to elective Caesarean section was not higher than for the group randomized to vaginal delivery, perhaps in part because only 54 per cent of women randomized to vaginal delivery actually delivered by this method.

Therefore the potential problems must be discussed with the mother, but in general, her wishes should be followed. Women should be advised that the chance of vaginal delivery in subsequent pregnancy if the fetus is cephalic is approximately 70–80 per cent, and thus a

Table 7.1 Criteria for deciding mode of delivery

Favourable for vaginal delivery	Unfavourable for vaginal delivery
Previous delivery of normal-sized infant	Nulliparity
	Other indication for Caesarean section
Estimated fetal weight 2–3.8 kg	Estimated fetal weight > 3.8 kg
Extended breech presentation	Footling breech presentation Hyperextended neck
Normal liquor volume	Oligohydramnios/polyhydramnios
Maternal desire for vaginal delivery	Maternal desire for Caesarean section
Gestation > 33 weeks	Previous Caesarean section
Grossly contracted pelvis (clinical examination)	

Caesarean section this time does not preclude a vaginal delivery in more favourable circumstances.

Vaginal Breech Delivery

There is no evidence to suggest that induction of labour or augmentation is contraindicated, although many units do not practise these. Epidural analgesia is encouraged in many units as it prevents bearing down efforts before the cervix is fully dilated. This has to be balanced against the problems produced by epidural analgesia, such as less efficient uterine activity as the second stage approaches and poorer maternal effort. This has a greater impact on primigravidae, and in many units the vaginal delivery rate for trial of breech labour is less than 50 per cent.

The conduct of a breech delivery has a number of differences from a cephalic delivery. An episiotomy is cut and the breech is allowed to deliver spontaneously. The legs can be flexed to aid delivery. Once the trunk is delivered, the arms are swept across the fetal chest and delivered. It is vital to keep the breech in a back upper-most position, to prevent the chin from being caught under the symphysis. Allowing the breech to hang encourages flexion of the fetal head. Once the nuchal line is seen, the head can be delivered, either by the use of forceps or by flexing the head over the perineum with one hand on the mandible and one on the malar eminence. This is called Mariceau–Smellie–Veit manoeuvre. It is reserved for cases where there is a lax perineum. Using forceps allows a controlled delivery of the head, without sudden compression and expansion.

Postnatal Care

Postnatally all babies who have been persistently breech, even if ECV was successful, should have their hips carefully examined. The risk of congenital dislocation of the hips is much higher in these babies, especially for extended breeches and girls.

Learning Points

- The incidence of breech presentation decreases with increasing gestational age; most cases of breech presentation at 30 weeks' gestation will be cephalic presentations at delivery
- If a breech presentation is found on examination after 34 weeks' gestation, an ultrasound scan should be arranged in order to confirm the presentation, determine the type of breech, exclude a fetal anomaly and hyperextension of the neck, and estimate liquor volume, placental site and fetal weight
- The management options are external cephalic version, elective Caesarean section, or trial of vaginal delivery

See Also

Unstable or transverse lie (Chapter 23)

Further Reading

Hannah ME, Hannah WJ, Hewson SA, Hodnett ED, Saigal S, Willan AR. Planned caesarean section versus planned vaginal birth for breech presentation at term: a randomised multicentre trial. Term Breech Trial Collaborative Group. *Lancet* 2000; 356: 1375–83.

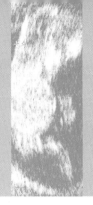

Chapter 8

Diabetes

Importance

About 0.5 per cent of pregnant women will have been diagnosed as having diabetes before they become pregnant. Gestational diabetes occurs in about 3 per cent of pregnancies in the UK but can complicate up to 20 per cent of pregnancies in the Middle East. Long-term follow-up studies indicate that a significant minority (30–50 per cent) of these women develop diabetes in later life. Diabetes may result in serious pregnancy complications.

Aetiology

The effect of pregnancy hormones on carbohydrate metabolism places a stress on pancreatic beta-cell function. This leads to an increase in insulin requirements in women with pre-existing diabetes, or may lead to diabetes developing in pregnancy (gestational diabetes).

Complications

The complication of diabetes in pregnancy may affect either the pregnancy or the diabetes.

Complications affecting the pregnancy

Congenital anomalies
Miscarriage
Macrosomia
Pre-eclampsia
Polyhydramnios
Iatrogenic preterm delivery
Infection
Neonatal problems

Complications affecting the diabetes

Hypoglycaemia and ketoacidosis
Increased insulin requirements
Nephropathy
Retinopathy

There is a twofold increase in congenital anomalies. The most common abnormalities are neural tube defects, but cardiovascular, renal tract and gastro-intestinal anomalies can also occur. Sacral agenesis is very rare, but it is almost a pathognomonic finding in infants of diabetic mothers. Women with diabetes are also more prone to spontaneous miscarriage, especially women with diabetes of long duration and established small vessel disease, and women in whom control of the disease is poor. Congenital malformations and miscarriage appear to be related to diabetic control around the time of organogenesis; these complications are therefore not increased in women with gestational diabetes.

Macrosomia is more common in the infants of mothers with diabetes than in uncomplicated pregnancies, even with the best diabetic control currently available. This complication leads to an increased incidence of shoulder dystocia (Chapter 40). Diabetes is not associated with intrauterine growth restriction unless the diabetes is complicated with microvascular disease.

Pregnant women with insulin-dependent diabetes are at greater risk of developing pre-eclampsia (Chapter 11) and polyhydramnios (Chapter 13) and of iatrogenic preterm delivery (Chapter 38) compared with the general population.

Infections including candidiasis and urinary tract infections are increased. Pregnant women with diabetes are also at a greater risk of post-Caesarean section febrile morbidity and uterine infection.

Neonatal problems include respiratory distress syndrome and hypoglycaemia, in addition to the increased risk of congenital malformations, birth injury (from macrosomia) and prematurity. These complications are more likely, and more severe, when there is poor control of the diabetes.

With changing insulin requirements, hypoglycaemia and ketoacidosis are more common than in non-pregnant women with diabetes. This is particularly so if early pregnancy is characterized by nausea and vomiting, or if there is any superimposed illness.

Nephropathy (manifest by proteinuria, Chapter 18) without significant hypertension and a normal serum creatinine is not associated with a poor fetal outcome. The prognosis worsens in the presence of hypertension or impaired renal function. Although the majority of women with renal disease do not experience a deterioration of renal function during pregnancy, some women do suffer a deterioration that does not improve after pregnancy. There is also concern about the effects of pregnancy on women with proliferative retinopathy; pregnancy appears to be associated with a deterioration in the condition.

Diagnosis and Clinical Assessment

Screening for Gestational Diabetes

Gestational diabetes is defined as glucose intolerance appearing during pregnancy, and is a biochemical manifestation rather than a disease.

Recommended protocol

Urine should be tested for glycosuria by dipstick testing at every antenatal visit

Timed random laboratory blood glucose measurements should be made whenever glycosuria (1 + or more) is detected, at the antenatal booking visit and at 28 weeks' gestation

A 75 g oral glucose tolerance test (GTT) with laboratory blood glucose measurements should be performed if the timed random blood glucose concentrations are > 6 mmol/L in the fasting state or 2 hours after food, or > 7 mmol/L within 2 hours of food

---

Additional indications for a glucose tolerance test include:

- family history of diabetes in a first-degree relative
- obesity (e.g. >90 kg)
- history of pregnancy complicated by stillbirth, polyhydramnios or fetal macrosomia.

History

Symptoms such as polyuria and polydipsia are indicative of diabetes in pregnancy.

Examination

Findings on examination are rarely helpful in establishing a diagnosis of diabetes in pregnancy (although ketoacidosis may occasionally be found). However, once a diagnosis has been made, regular, careful examinations to exclude any complications of the disease are essential.

Investigation

The diagnosis of diabetes in pregnancy is made on the basis of the GTT (Table 8.1).

Glucose Tolerance Test

The pregnant woman should have fasted overnight. After a fasting blood sample has been taken, a glucose load of 75 g is given orally and the blood sample is repeated 2 hours after the glucose load.

Management

Principles include:

Preconceptual care
Education
Dedicated antenatal care

Management of the diabetes

Assessment of glucose levels
Dietary control
Glucagon
Insulin
Monitoring of any diabetic complications

Management of the pregnancy

Screening for fetal anomaly
Assessment of fetal growth and well-being
Timing and mode of delivery
Plan for labour and delivery

Table 8.1 WHO criteria for the 75 g oral glucose tolerance test (GTT) during pregnancy

	Plasma glucose (mmol/L)	
	Fasting	2 hour
Normal	< 6	< 7.8
Gestational impaired glucose tolerance	6–7	7.8–11.1
Diabetes	> 7	> 11.1

Perinatal and maternal mortalities have declined appreciably since pregnant women with diabetes have been managed by dedicated teams for antenatal care with a consultant diabetologist, a nurse specializing in diabetes, a dietician and a consultant obstetrician. Frequent antenatal visits are necessary, depending on the degree of control and the development of any complications; pregnant women with diabetes should be seen weekly in the third trimester.

Preconceptual Care

Increasingly, women with diabetes wish to discuss the implications of pregnancy before they conceive. All who care for diabetic women should be aware of, and be prepared to discuss, the significance of the pregnancy to the woman with diabetes, the risks to the fetus and neonate, and the importance of good control of the diabetes (optimizing preconceptual glucose levels can significantly reduce the risk of structural fetal abnormalities). Since diabetes is a chronic and progressive disease, the advice may need to include a discussion of the fact that postponement of pregnancy until a later age may worsen the prognosis. Women can be reassured that there is no evidence of any long-term adverse effects on the development or intelligence of their offspring, and that the risk of their children developing juvenile diabetes is less than 2 per cent. Folate 5 mg daily should be prescribed for 2 months prior to conception, in order to reduce the incidence of neural tube defects.

The most important person in the care of a pregnant woman with diabetes is the pregnant woman herself. The greater the degree of understanding and input from the woman, the greater the likelihood of good diabetic control. Ideally, education regarding the reasons for meticulous care in pregnancy should commence preconceptually; it should certainly be a major facet of antenatal care.

Management of the Diabetes

Glucose levels can be monitored at home using a reflectance meter. Blood glucose measurements should be performed before each meal, and 90 minutes after meals. The aim should be fasting glucose levels between 4 and 6 mmol/L and postprandial (90 min) levels below 7.0 mmol/L. Fructosamine or glycosylated haemoglobin levels give a guide to control over the preceding weeks. Problems with plasma glucose control may require admission and monitoring.

Dietary control is also important. A programme of three meals and several snacks should be suggested in order to limit periods of hyperglycaemia and hypoglycaemia. Complex carbohydrates or starches (grains and legumes) are preferable to concentrated sucrose-type sweets. Dietary control may be sufficient to control glucose levels in pregnancies complicated by gestational diabetes.

The insulin requirement of most insulin-dependent women increases in the second half of pregnancy, and many non-insulin-dependent women will require insulin for the first time during their pregnancy. To attain good glycaemic control, most patients will require multiple injections. The 'basal-bolus' regime is used in many centres. This entails a small dose of medium-acting or long-acting insulin in the evening to ensure constant basal insulin levels and bolus doses of short-acting insulin before each meal in an effort to mimic a physiological pattern of insulin secretion. Pumps for continuous subcutaneous infusion of insulin are available, but are expensive and complex to use.

Because of the risk of hypoglycaemia, especially in the first trimester, all insulin-dependent diabetic women should be provided with a glucagon 'kit' early in pregnancy. Monitoring of diabetic complications includes regular ophthalmological examination to assess retinal vascular changes. If there is evidence of deteriorating retinopathy, intensive laser treatment can maintain visual acuity. Serial tests of renal function should also be performed, particularly if there is any evidence of hypertension or proteinuria. Urine cultures should be repeated regularly.

Management of the Pregnancy

An early ultrasound scan to confirm the gestational age should be performed. A detailed ultrasound scan should be arranged at 18–20 weeks' gestation (Chapter 10). Pregnant women with insulin-dependent diabetes do not have an increased risk of Down's syndrome. Maternal serum screening for Down's syndrome is invalid due to lower levels of α-fetoprotein observed in diabetic pregnancies.

Fetal growth should be assessed by serial ultrasound scans from 28 weeks' gestation. The frequency of tests of fetal well-being (Chapter 20) depends on the gestational age, severity of the disease, and the presence of other factors which may influence fetal well-being, such as pre-eclampsia.

Delivery

The timing of delivery will be expedited if complications such as pre-eclampsia or fetal compromise ensue. However, there is no valid reason to terminate an otherwise uncomplicated pregnancy in a woman with diabetes before term. The pregnancy should not proceed beyond 39 weeks' gestation. Although the mode of delivery should be determined by obstetric indications, Caesarean section rates are three to five times higher than in the general pregnant population. The only increased hazard of vaginal delivery in women with diabetes is that of birth trauma to the infant. An elective Caesarean section should be performed if the estimated fetal weight on ultrasound scan is > 4.5 kg. If an elective Caesarean section is performed, it should be at 09.00 h. The morning dose of insulin should be omitted, and a dextrose and insulin infusion should be administered until the woman is able to tolerate oral nutrition.

If a vaginal delivery is anticipated, a plan for the management of labour should be discussed antenatally. Infusions of dextrose, insulin and potassium should be administered in labour. The blood glucose measurements should be performed hourly and the insulin infusion rate increased or decreased as appropriate. If a woman is in preterm labour, it should be remembered that both tocolytic (such as ritodrine) and steroid therapies are insulin antagonists and will cause marked hyperglycaemia. Epidural analgesia is recommended and continuous fetal heart rate monitoring should be performed. A paediatrician should be present at delivery. The insulin infusion should cease with the delivery of the placenta, and plasma glucose levels will determine subsequent requirements. Breast-feeding is to be encouraged.

Learning Points

- **Definitions of diabetes in pregnancy and screening strategies for gestational diabetes vary**
- **Complications of diabetes in pregnancy can affect either the diabetes or the pregnancy**
- **Management of diabetes in pregnancy should be multidisciplinary and should start with pre-conceptual care**

See Also

Fetal abnormality: structural (Chapter 10)
Large for gestational age (Chapter 13)
Shoulder dystocia (Chapter 40)

Further Reading

Enkin M, Keirse MJNC. Gestational diabetes and diabetes in pregnancy. In: Chalmers I, ed. *A Guide to Effective Care in Pregnancy and Childbirth*. Oxford University Press, Oxford, 1990, pp. 41–43, 105–110.

Pregnancy and Neonatal Care Group. Report. *Diabetic Medicine* 1996; 13: S43–53.

Fetal abnormality: chromosomal

Importance

Chromosomal disorders arise in the stages of gamete formation or early in embryonic cleavage; they are associated with 40–50 per cent of miscarriages and a lesser number of perinatal deaths, malformed or small-for-dates infants. Disorders of the autosomes and sex chromosomes occur with equal frequency, but the former are more damaging. Down's syndrome is the most common congenital cause of intellectual impairment and may also present with structural abnormalities.

Causes

Trisomy 21 (Down's Syndrome)

Down's syndrome (trisomy 21 or a translocation affecting chromosome 21) is the commonest chromosomal anomaly (1.3 per 1000 births).

Clinical features

Face – upward slanting eyes, prominent epicanthic folds, flat nasal bridge, protruding tongue
Brushfield's spots – speckling of the iris on ophthalmoscopic examination
Limbs – single palmar creases, short, broad hands, wide spaces between first and second toes
Heart defects – atrial/ventricular septal defects (40 per cent)
Duodenal atresia
Umbilical hernias
Mental retardation

Other Chromosomal Anomalies

Trisomy 18 (Edwards' syndrome) is the next most common autosomal chromosomal anomaly (1 in 7000 births). Characteristic features include a small jaw (micrognathia), a prominent occiput, deformed ears, flexed, deformed hands and 'rocker-bottom' feet. Trisomy 13 (Patau's syndrome) is characterized by microcephaly, microphthalmia, cleft lip/palate, heart defects, and polydactyly with overlapping fingers.

Many sex chromosome abnormalities are not associated with an abnormal phenotype at birth and are not diagnosed until later life. Turner's syndrome (45X) occurs in 1 in 5000 births and may be recognized by antenatal ultrasound (cystic hygroma or fetal hydrops) or after delivery by a webbed neck, coarctation of the aorta, and hands and feet that are swollen by lymphoedema.

Diagnosis and Clinical Assessment

Screening

The majority of Down's syndrome babies are born to women below the age of 35, and alternative risk predictor methods of supplementing the information from maternal age alone have been proposed.

Increased risk of chromosomal abnormality may be identified by:

Advanced maternal age
Previous history of chromosomal abnormality
Risk predictor tests – biochemical and ultrasound
Structural abnormalities identified on ultrasound scan
Intrauterine growth restriction (IUGR)

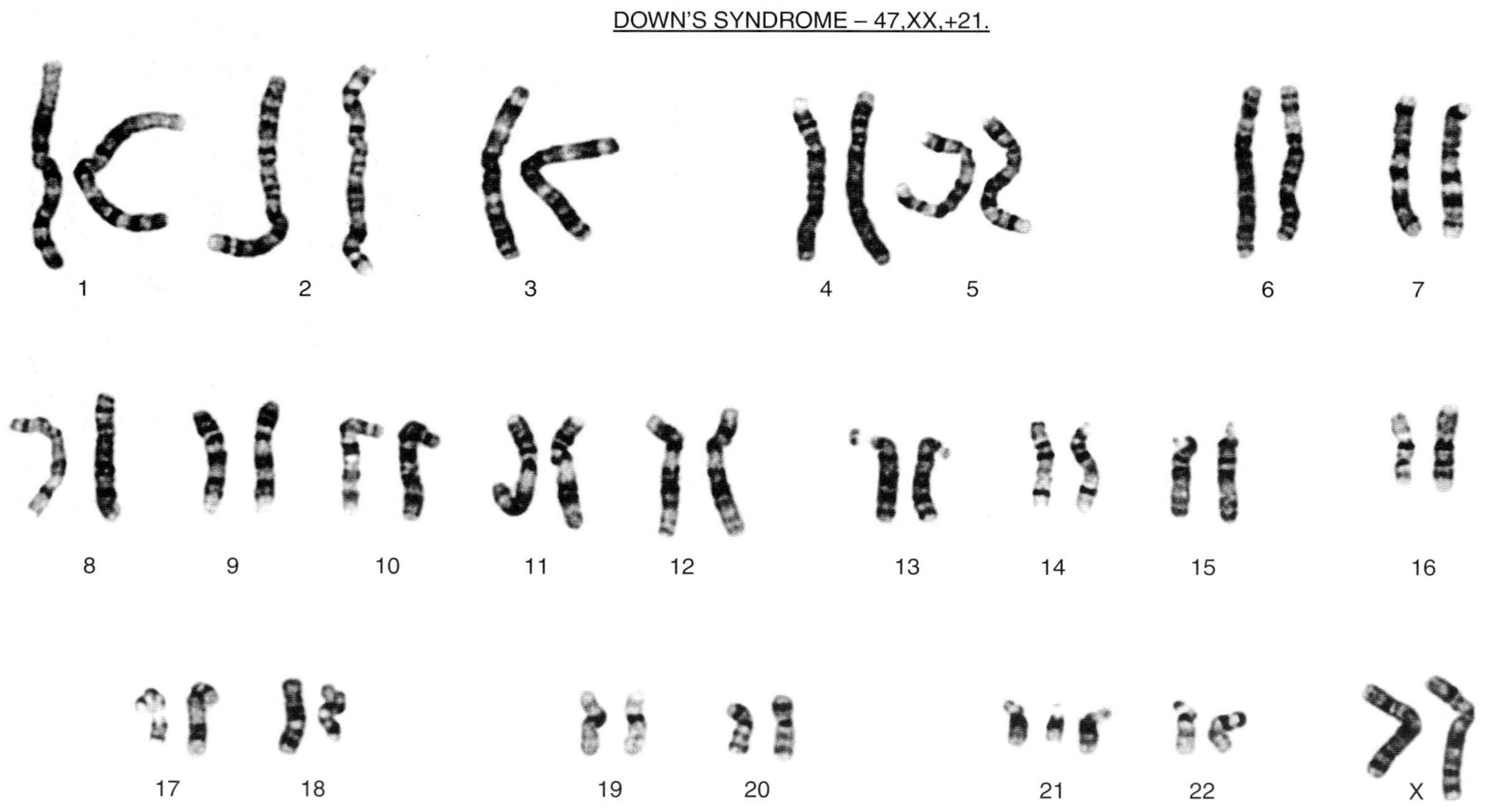

DOWN'S SYNDROME – 47,XX,+21.

Figure 9.1 Karyogram of Down's syndrome (trisomy 21). (We are grateful to the Cytogenetic Services, Nottingham City Hospital, for supplying this figure.)

Maternal Age

The risks of trisomy 21 are closely related to maternal age and, at mid-trimester, range from about 1 in 3000 at 18 years to about 1 in 200 at 37 years, 1 in 70 at 40 years and 1 in 20 at 45 years. (The corresponding figures at birth will be lower due to an increased pregnancy loss rate.) The options of screening tests and prenatal diagnostic tests (see below) should be discussed with all women over 35 years of age.

Previously Affected Pregnancy

The evaluation of a couple who have a previous history of a child born with Down's syndrome is performed in conjunction with a clinical geneticist. A careful history should be taken. Pertinent features include a history of all pregnancies, including stillbirths and miscarriages, whether consanguinity exists, and a detailed family history. It may be necessary to obtain medical records of other relatives. It is important to establish whether the chromosomal complement of the child was determined:

- If the child had trisomy 21 (Figure 9.1), the couple should be quoted a risk of 1 in 100, or twice the maternal age-related risk, whichever is the higher. Five per cent of cases of Down's syndrome result from a translocation, i.e. the number of chromosomes is normal, but additional chromosome 21 material is present. If the child had a translocation, the parental chromosomes should be checked. If one parent has a translocation involving chromosome 21 (commonly affecting chromosome 14), the parent will be normal as the translocation is balanced. However, during gametogenesis, the sperm or ovum may receive both the normal chromosome 21 and the translocated material. If the father is a carrier, the risk in a subsequent pregnancy is 2 per cent, whereas if the mother is a carrier, the risk is 10 per cent (these risks are not influenced by maternal age).
- If the chromosomal analysis of the child is unavailable, the couple should undergo karyotypic studies to determine if either has a balanced translocation.

Biochemical Screening Tests

The main biochemical screening test is 'the triple test' and is performed at 15–17 weeks' gestation. The triple test relies on evidence that there are lower levels of serum α-fetoprotein and unconjugated oestriol and raised human chorionic gonadotrophin (HCG) in Down's syndrome pregnancies as compared with normal pregnancies. However, there is much overlap between the measurements in normal and Down's syndrome pregnancies; the triple test is not diagnostic, merely providing a risk which can be compared with that based on maternal age alone. Careful counselling before any risk predictor tests are performed should be mandatory.

Ultrasound

Various ultrasound screening tests have been advocated. These include the use of a thickened nuchal skinfold as indicative of an increased risk of Down's syndrome (Figure 9.2). The 18–20-week detailed ultrasound scan (Chapter 10) may identify fetal structural defects associated with Down's syndrome; these include cardiac defects, the 'double bubble' indicative of duodenal atresia, and the abdominal wall defect of exomphalos. 'Soft markers' of a chromosomal anomaly may also be seen. The presence of two or more markers conveys a risk of 1 in 100.

Soft markers of chromosomal anomalies

Choroid plexus cysts
Nuchal skin fold > 6 mm
Echogenic (bright) foci in the heart or bowel
Renal pelviceal dilatation > 4 mm

The incidence of Down's syndrome is also increased in pregnancies complicated by IUGR (Chapter 21), particularly when the growth restriction is symmetrical (i.e. brain sparing is absent), and in pregnancies associated with polyhydramnios (Chapter 13).

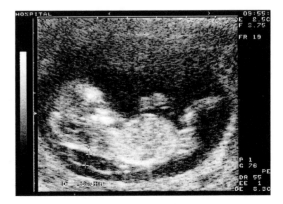

Figure 9.2 Increased nuchal translucency, identified by ultrasound screening

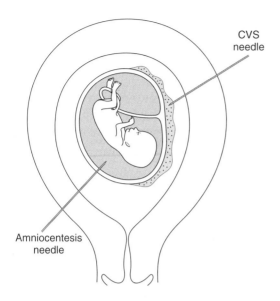

Figure 9.3   Amniocentesis and chorionic villous sampling (CVS)

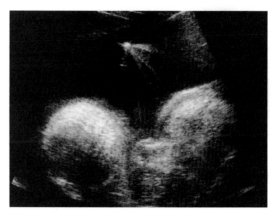

Figure 9.4   Amniocentesis being performed under ultrasound guidance. The bright echo at the top of the image indicates the tip of the needle

Prenatal Diagnostic Testing

If an increased risk is identified, couples require careful counselling which should be non-directive and include accurate information as to the options available.

Options include:

No action – couples may not wish to contemplate termination of pregnancy, even if an abnormality was found

Additional risk assessment using non-invasive biochemical or ultrasound methods

Invasive methods of providing a diagnosis

Chorionic Villous Sampling (CVS)

This involves the use of a cannula (or biopsy forceps) under ultrasound guidance, to take a small biopsy (5–10 mg) from the chorion frondosum (Figure 9.3). Samples can be taken transabdominally or transcervically. CVS can be performed in the first trimester. It enables rapid, direct karyotypic analysis because of the higher mitotic activity of trophoblasts compared with amniocytes, and results are obtained within 24 hours. There is a 1–2 per cent incidence of placental mosaicism, where a discrepancy between chorionic and fetal karyotypes exists; this necessitates further investigation by amniocentesis. Randomized, controlled studies suggest that the miscarriage rate is slightly higher after CVS than after amniocentesis, and is between 1 and 4 per cent (see Table 9.1). An additional concern regarding the safety of CVS was raised by reports of fetal limb abnormalities following the procedure. Subsequent reports indicate that this complication does not occur when CVS is performed after 9 weeks.

Amniocentesis

This is a procedure in which a sample of about 15 mL of amniotic fluid is obtained by fine-needle aspiration through the maternal abdominal wall, under ultrasound control (Figure 9.4). The major problem with the technique is the additional risk of miscarriage associated with the procedure, which is

Table 9.1   Comparison of the techniques of amniocentesis and chorionic villous sampling

Amniocentesis	Chorionic villous sampling
Lower miscarriage rate (0.5–1 per cent)	Higher miscarriage rate (1–4 per cent)
Usually performed later (15–17 weeks)	Performed earlier (after 10 weeks)
Longer time to obtain result (2–3 weeks)	Shorter time to obtain results (24 h)
	Risk of placental mosaicism

between 0.5 and 1 per cent. Other drawbacks include the anxious 2–3-week time interval between taking the sample and obtaining the result. As amniocentesis is not usually performed until 15 weeks' gestation, an abnormal result is not obtained until a relatively late stage in the pregnancy. Culture failure occurs in about 2 per cent of cases, and leads to further delay.

Management

The finding of a normal karyotype should provide reassurance for the couple, but does not exclude any genetic or structural fetal abnormality. An abnormal result necessitates further careful, non-directive counselling.

Continued Pregnancy

The couple may not wish to proceed with a termination of pregnancy. If a pregnancy is not terminated, or if a diagnosis of Down's syndrome was not suspected antenatally, the clinical diagnosis after delivery is usually straightforward (see above). The diagnosis should be confirmed by checking the baby's karyotype from blood lymphocytes.

Termination of Pregnancy

If the parents do choose to proceed with a termination, the method used depends on the gestational age.

Late First Trimester

These women are usually managed by dilatation of the cervix and evacuation of the uterus using suction curettage.

Mid-trimester

A combination of medical and surgical procedures is usually undertaken. A combination of prostaglandins and anti-progesterone agents (mefipristone) can be used to induce labour. After expulsion of the conceptus, curettage is usually performed to prevent delayed haemorrhage or infection from retained products of conception. Alternatively, the termination may be performed surgically, by dilatation and evacuation; although this method is quicker, it requires an experienced operator when performed in the second trimester.

Learning Points

- The risks of trisomy 21 (Down's syndrome) are closely related to maternal age
- Biochemical and ultrasound risk predictor tests for Down's syndrome are not diagnostic; they merely provide additional risk assessment to maternal age alone
- Counselling regarding prenatal diagnostic tests should be non-directive

See Also

Fetal abnormality: structural (Chapter 10)
Large for gestational age (Chapter 13)
Small for gestational age (Chapter 21)

Further Reading

Beischer NA, Mackay EV, Colditz PB. The abnormal fetus. In: *Obstetrics and the Newborn.* WB Saunders, London, 1997, pp. 161–74.

Fetal abnormality: structural

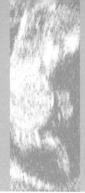

Importance

Two to three per cent of babies will have a significant congenital malformation, many of which will have a structural component. Whilst some of these defects will be relatively easy to diagnose antenatally by ultrasound scan (such as anencephaly), many will be much more difficult to identify (such as subtle cardiac lesions). Much depends on the expertise of the ultrasonographer and the threshold of suspicion, i.e. whether the scan is a routine screening test or is being performed because of high-risk features. In the UK, the incidence of neural tube defects is about 4/1000 births. Forty per cent of fetuses with neural tube defects are miscarried, and 20 per cent are still-born; with surgery, 50 per cent of the remainder survive 5 years, but only 1–2 per cent have no residual handicap.

Causes

Structural abnormalities affecting the fetus range from relatively minor problems (such as an additional digit) to conditions that are incompatible with life (such as anencephaly). The aetiologies are usually multifactorial; there may be a genetic predisposition that is revealed by an additional adverse factor (a dietary deficiency or an environmental agent). The classical example of this is neural tube defect, which is the example used in this chapter. Neural tube defects commonly allow herniation of the meninges and spinal cord, often resulting in partial or complete paralysis – called spina bifida.

Diagnosis and Clinical Assessment

Screening

Over 90 per cent of infants with a neural tube defect are born to parents with no family history of the condition. Because there is often no family history, major interest has been focused on screening methods.

Biochemical Screening Test: Maternal Serum α-Fetoprotein

α-Fetoprotein (αFP) is the major protein in early life and is raised in both the amniotic fluid and maternal serum when the fetus has an open neural tube defect. The screening programme was developed when it was apparent that almost all open neural tube defects result in abnormally high levels of maternal serum αFP. Maternal serum αFP levels rise until 30 weeks' gestation and then decline. Between 15 and 20 weeks' gestation, levels rise by about 15 per cent each week. (αFP is usually expressed as multiples of the median: values over 2.5 multiples of the median are taken as abnormal.) An elevated maternal serum αFP is not diagnostic of a neural tube defect (as detailed below). If the maternal serum αFP level is raised, a careful explanation regarding the variety of potential causes of this elevation should be given, emphasizing the fact that the test is not just for spina bifida.

> **Causes of a raised maternal serum αFP**
>
> Wrong gestational age (i.e. more advanced than anticipated)
> Multiple pregnancy
> Fetomaternal haemorrhage
> Fetal death
> Neural tube defects

Other fetal abnormalities, including abdominal wall defects, congenital nephrosis, bowel obstruction, renal tract abnormalities, sacrococcygeal teratoma

Placental/umbilical cord tumours

Maternal liver disease

Ultrasound Screening Tests

Protocols differ as to whether all patients should have a detailed ultrasound scan, or whether it should be just those deemed to be at particular risk (on the basis of other screening tests, maternal age, family history, etc.), and in the parameters that are included in a detailed ultrasound scan. With the improved resolution of fetal ultrasound scanning techniques, increasing numbers of fetal abnormalities are detected. Fetal anomaly scans are usually performed at 18–20 weeks' gestation.

Basic measurements to establish gestational age and exclude gross abnormalities should include:

Biparietal diameter

Head circumference

Anterior and posterior ventricular horns

Cerebral hemispheres

Femur length

Nuchal fold thickness

There are also 'soft markers' for chromosomal abnormalities (Chapter 9).

History

A careful history should be taken. In particular, the gestational age should be checked (the dates from the last menstrual period should be confirmed by ultrasound dating). Any bleeding in early pregnancy should be noted. The incidence of neural tube defects varies markedly according to ethnic group and geographic, temporal and socioeconomic factors; a deficiency of folic acid has been found to increase the incidence. However, a previous history conveys an increased risk: if one previous child has a neural tube defect, the incidence rises to 4–5 per cent; if two or more are affected, the risk is 10 per cent. Other influences discerned from the history include insulin-dependent diabetes and anti-epileptic therapy.

If any structural abnormalities are identified on ultrasound, ask about:

Exposure to infection (e.g. rubella)

Medication (e.g. thalidomide)

Drug abuse (e.g. cocaine)

Previous history

Family history

Examination

Examination of the pregnant woman plays little part in the identification of increased risk, although if an abnormality such as a congenital cardiac defect or a neural tube defect is identified, the fetus is at increased risk.

Investigation

Ultrasound

A detailed fetal anomaly scan should be performed, with particular reference to the fetal spine (Figure 10.1). The ultrasound scan will exclude many of the causes of a raised maternal serum αFP.

For a detailed anomaly scan, the following structures should be identified:

- cerebellum
- longitudinal and transverse sections of the spine
- four-chamber view of the heart
- chest, diaphragm and stomach (to exclude diaphragmatic hernia)
- abdominal wall and cord insertion
- kidneys and bladder
- four limbs and the digits.

Amniocentesis (see Chapter 9)

With advances in the resolution of ultrasound scans, this invasive procedure is rarely indicated. If, however, there are problems in visualizing fetal anatomy (for whatever reason), amniocentesis and measurement of amniotic fluid αFP should be performed. If amniocentesis is indicated, acetylcholinesterase (AChE) should be measured. AChE is present in high concentrations in the fetal cerebrospinal fluid and should not normally be found in the amniotic fluid. As discussed in Chapter 9, the identification of a structural anomaly or two or more 'soft markers' by ultrasonography should lead to a consideration of the fetal karyotype.

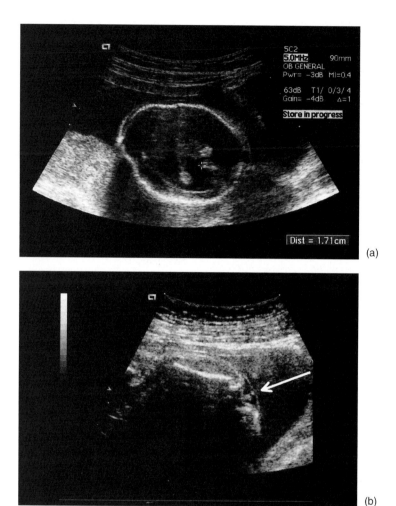

(a)

(b)

Figure 10.1 (a) Hydrocephalic fetal head with increased ventricle size and 'lemon'-shaped head. (b) Lumbosacral neural tube defect (indicated by arrow)

Karyotype analysis should also be considered because of the known association between open neural tube and ventral wall defects and certain trisomies (13 and 18).

Management

Prevention

The need for preconceptual folic acid supplementation should be stressed. The recurrence rate is significantly reduced by folic acid supplementation (5 mg/day) which should be commenced prior to the pregnancy.

Counselling

If a neural tube abnormality is found on ultrasound scan, each abnormality should be considered on an individual basis:

- Careful, non-directive counselling should be provided. Parents must be allowed to make their own decisions on the basis of accurate information.
- All members of the health care team should be informed, including the general practitioner and the community midwife.
- Referral to a tertiary centre should be considered if there is doubt regarding the nature or extent of the lesion. Ultrasonography has the advantage of

enabling assessment of motor function (by observing fetal leg movements) and thus prognosis.

- If serious fetal structural abnormalities are detected, the couple need to be carefully counselled regarding the option of termination of pregnancy (Chapter 61).

Management of the Ongoing Pregnancy

If the pregnancy is continued, the aim should be to protect exposed neural tissue at and following delivery. Caesarean section, delicate handling and expert neonatal care may facilitate this. Treatment consists of closing the spinal defect within the first few days after delivery and dealing with any subsequent problems as necessary.

If maternal serum αFP levels are elevated, and yet no abnormalities are detected, the fetus remains at risk of intrauterine growth restriction. Serial third trimester estimations of fetal growth and biophysical profile should be planned.

Learning Points

- The aetiologies of structural abnormalities such as neural tube defects are usually multifactorial
- Values of maternal serum αFP over 2.5 × multiples of the median are taken as abnormal
- The causes of a raised maternal serum αFP
- The components of basic and detailed ultrasound anomaly scans

See Also

Fetal abnormality: chromosomal (Chapter 9)

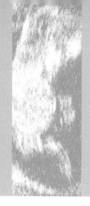

Hypertension

Importance

The hypertensive disorders of pregnancy are a major cause of maternal mortality and morbidity and perinatal mortality and morbidity (the disorders are responsible for the occupancy of approximately one-sixth of special care baby unit cots).

Classification

The three major disorders

Chronic or pre-existing hypertension

Non-proteinuric pregnancy-induced hypertension

Proteinuric pregnancy-induced hypertension or pre-eclampsia

Classification suffers from a lack of uniformity in definition. A simple approach is as follows:

- *Chronic hypertension* is defined as a persistently elevated blood pressure of 140/90 mmHg or greater, before 20 weeks' gestation. Diagnosis may be difficult in patients who present for the first time after the first trimester, due to the physiological decrease in blood pressure which occurs in mid-pregnancy.
- *Pregnancy-induced hypertension (PIH)* is defined as two successive blood pressure recordings greater than 140/90 mmHg, at least 6 hours apart, in a previously normotensive woman, after the 20th week of pregnancy (alternative definitions incorporate rises in blood pressure, typically of 30/15 mmHg).
- *Pre-eclampsia* is defined as PIH with the addition of significant proteinuria (greater than 300 mg or

500 mg/L in a 24-hour urine collection, in the absence of a urinary tract infection).

Chronic Hypertension

Importance

Chronic hypertension occurs in about 1–2 per cent of pregnant women, depending on the population studied. The two most important pregnancy complications are superimposed pre-eclampsia (five- to ten-fold increased incidence) and placental abruption (fivefold increased incidence). Other risks include an exacerbation of hypertension, renal failure and cerebrovascular accidents. Perinatal mortality is related to the severity of the hypertension.

Aetiology

Common causes

Essential hypertension

Renal disease

Endocrine disorders

Collagen vascular diseases

Essential hypertension accounts for 90 per cent of cases; secondary causes include renal disease (glomerulonephritis, nephropathy), diabetes with vascular involvement, thyrotoxicosis, phaeochromocytoma and collagen vascular disease (systemic lupus erythematosus, scleroderma).

Diagnosis and Clinical Assessment

At the antenatal booking visit, patients with chronic hypertension should be divided into two groups: low-risk and high-risk cases (Table 11.1). A careful past

Table 11.1 Risk features for chronic hypertension

Low risk	High risk (any of the following)
Blood pressure < 160/105 mmHg	Blood pressure > 160/105 mmHg
Essential hypertension	Secondary hypertension
Maternal age < 40	Maternal age > 40

medical history (specifically enquiring about cardiac, thyroid and renal disease, diabetes, and the outcome of any previous pregnancies) should be taken from all women with chronic hypertension.

Baseline investigations – serum urea, urate and electrolytes, urine analysis and culture, and 24-hour urine collection for protein and creatinine clearance – should be performed in all patients.

Management

Management plan

Low-risk patients
- Discontinuation of any antihypertensive medication
- Assessment of fetal size

High-risk patients
- Additional booking clinic investigations
- Close monitoring and surveillance
- Ultrasound assessment of fetal growth and biophysical profile
- Consideration of the timing and mode of delivery

Low-risk Patients

Frequent review will be needed in the weeks following discontinuation of any antihypertensive medication; however, antihypertensive therapy only needs to be restarted in a minority of women. If it is necessary to restart medication, suitable and safe choices include: methyldopa, labetalol, and nifedipine (angiotensin-converting enzyme inhibitors or diuretics should be avoided; these drugs can have serious effects on the fetus).

If there is any concern about the clinical assessment of fetal size, serial ultrasound measurement of fetal growth should be performed on a monthly basis. If there are no complications, and medication has not been necessary, induction of labour before 41+ weeks' gestation is not indicated.

High-risk Patients

Additional investigations at the antenatal booking visit should include a chest X-ray, an electrocardiogram (especially if there is a long history of hypertension) and antinuclear antibodies.

These patients should be very closely monitored; surveillance should include frequent antenatal clinic visits and joint management by obstetricians and physicians. Periods of hospitalization may be necessary. Serial ultrasound scan assessment of fetal growth and biophysical profile should be performed. The timing and mode of delivery should be carefully considered and will depend on maternal and fetal well-being and the presence of any complications. The use of antihypertensive medication is an indication for delivery at, or before, 38 weeks' gestation.

Non-proteinuric Pregnancy-induced Hypertension

Importance

The condition is common, affecting up to 10 per cent of first pregnancies. PIH in the absence of proteinuria is not associated with increased maternal or perinatal mortality. Oedema in pregnancy is a physiological finding, and the presence of oedema in a patient with non-proteinuric PIH is not associated with a worse outcome.

Management

- Exclude chronic hypertension
- Reassurance
- Surveillance

Women with non-proteinuric PIH are usually asymptomatic. Chronic hypertension should be excluded by ensuring that there was no hypertension prior to pregnancy or in early pregnancy.

Reassurance regarding the lack of any maternal or perinatal complications should be given. Non-proteinuric PIH does not merit in-patient admission or induction of labour. Unless blood pressure measurements rise to levels at which there is a danger of a cerebrovascular accident (in which case, emergency treatment on the labour ward should be followed by urgent delivery), antihypertensive therapy is not indicated. With the exception of the emergency situation, antihypertensive therapy does not benefit either mother or baby. Ultrasound assessment of fetal growth should not be performed unless clinical findings suggest that this investigation is indicated.

Whilst the PIH remains non-proteinuric, the risks are minimal. Nevertheless, close surveillance is necessary to ensure that proteinuria does not develop. Increased surveillance could include frequent antenatal clinic visits, the community midwife visiting on a daily basis, and attendance at an antenatal day-case assessment unit.

Criteria for referral to the hospital antenatal clinic

Proteinuria develops on dipstick testing
Blood pressure measurements are persistently
   > 150/100 mmHg
Symptoms suggestive of pre-eclampsia (see below) develop

Pre-eclampsia

Importance

Pre-eclampsia is a multisystem disorder which is responsible for a high proportion of antenatal admissions, inductions of labour and Caesarean sections. The incidence of pre-eclampsia is between 2 and 4 per cent of first pregnancies. Maternal complications range from renal failure to eclampsia, and fetal complications include growth restriction and prematurity. Pre-eclampsia is thus both common and dangerous, and is unpredictable in its onset, progress and complications.

Complications

Maternal
- Cerebrovascular accident
- Eclampsia
- Pulmonary oedema
- Renal failure
- Disseminated intravascular coagulation (DIC)
- Liver failure

Fetal
- Intrauterine growth restriction (IUGR)
- Intrauterine fetal death

Table 11.2   Predisposing factors to pre-eclampsia

General	History of pre-eclampsia in a previous pregnancy
Genetic	Family history ($\times$ four-fold incidence if first-degree relative)
Hyperplacentosis	Multiple pregnancy
	Hydatidiform mole
	Hydrops fetalis
Immunological	Primigravida
	Change of partner
Vascular disease	Chronic hypertension
	Renal disease
	Diabetes mellitus
	Collagen vascular diseases

Aetiology

A simplified pathogenesis of the disease is outlined in Figure 11.1 There is a genetic predisposition to the disease (which is reflected in the increased incidence if a relative suffered from pre-eclampsia) (see Table 11.2). The genetic predisposition leads to an abnormal interaction between invading trophoblast cells (of fetal origin) and the decidua (which is rich in immunologically active cells). Faulty interplay between the unique antigens on the trophoblast cells and the decidua leads to defective invasion of the muscular layer of the spiral arteries in the decidua and myometrium.

A failure to convert the spiral arteries to low-resistance vessels leads to a diminished uteroplacental blood supply. (Pre-eclampsia and intrauterine growth restriction share a common pathogenesis.) Uteroplacental hypoperfusion results in the release of a potent circulating factor (as yet unidentified) and then widespread activation of endothelial cells (hence the multisystemic nature of the disease). The widespread endothelial activation results in:

- decreased endothelial production of the vasodilators such as prostacyclin;
- platelet activation (and increased production of the vasoconstrictor thromboxane A_2)
- increased sensitivity to vasoconstrictor agents such as angiotensin II.

A vicious circle is set up, with vasospasm leading to further ischaemia and further vasospasm.

Diagnosis and Clinical Assessment

The diagnosis of pre-eclampsia must be established. Any pregnant woman who presents with hypertension and proteinuria must be assessed, either as an in-patient or on an outpatient surveillance unit.

History

Patients with pre-eclampsia are usually asymptomatic; if symptoms develop, they may indicate worsening of the condition. The most sinister symptom is epigastric pain which may reflect subcapsular liver haemorrhages and must never be ignored. Other symptoms, such as headaches, breathlessness, drowsiness and visual disturbances, are less specific but may be helpful.

Examination

Serial blood pressure measurements will determine the presence or absence of PIH (defined above), and automated blood pressure measuring devices may facilitate this determination. Other clinical signs such as epigastric tenderness and hyperreflexia (up to three beats of clonus may be normal in pregnancy) may reflect a deterioration in the condition.

Investigation

A midstream urine specimen should be sent for microscopy and culture (to exclude a urinary tract infection) and the protein content of a 24-hour urinary collection should be measured. If the level of proteinuria is insignificant (< 300 mg/24 hours), management should be on an outpatient basis.

Pre-eclampsia rarely occurs in a multiparous woman whose first pregnancy was uncomplicated; unless there has been a change of partner, any such diagnosis should be treated with great suspicion. The differential diagnosis should include chronic hypertension and underlying renal disease.

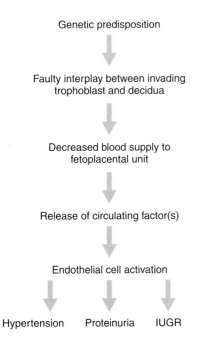

Figure 11.1   A simplified pathogenesis of pre-eclampsia

Management

Prevention

Low-dose aspirin prophylaxis has not been found to be effective in preventing recurrent pre-eclampsia, although it may be of some benefit if the previous pregnancy was complicated by severe, early-onset disease. In this case, a thrombophilia screen should also be performed, as the incidence of underlying thrombotic tendencies is increased in such patients and may warrant anticoagulant therapy.

> **Priorities**
>
> Establish a diagnosis
> Assess and monitor the maternal and fetal condition
> Consider therapy
> Consider delivery

Assessment and Monitoring

Once a diagnosis of pre-eclampsia has been made, the condition of the mother must be assessed and monitored.

History and Examination

The development of any symptoms (above) may indicate a deterioration in the maternal condition. The most important clinical signs are serial blood pressure recordings and daily dipstick assessment of proteinuria. The community midwife and general practitioner should be alerted to the possibility of recurrent disease. The patient should be referred back to the hospital if hypertension or persistent proteinuria occurs.

Fetal surveillance should include clinical parameters such as maternal perception of fetal movement and clinical assessment of symphysis–fundal height.

Investigations of Maternal Well-being

Laboratory tests will identify complications of this multi-organ disease and should include:

- Full blood count – the platelet count and haematocrit are particularly pertinent. If the platelet count is abnormal ($< 100 \times 10^9$), a clotting screen should be performed.
- Blood tests of renal function – serum uric acid measurement (normally < 350 mmol/L) is often the most sensitive index, and detects tubular damage before abnormalities in urea, electrolytes and creatinine are apparent.
- 24-hour urine collection for measurement of protein and creatinine clearance.

- Liver function tests – the first parameter to become abnormal is usually the transaminase.

A marked deterioration in any of these parameters may indicate a need for emergency treatment and delivery of the baby.

Investigations of Fetal Well-being

Tests of fetal well-being should be performed on in-patients with pre-eclampsia. These should include fetal heart rate monitoring, ultrasound measurement of fetal growth, ultrasound assessment of biophysical profile (particularly amniotic fluid estimation) and Doppler measurement of umbilical artery blood flow velocity. Tests of fetal well-being are discussed in Chapter 20. A deterioration of any of these parameters may indicate a need to deliver the baby.

Therapy

Patients with pre-eclampsia should be advised regarding the nature and complications of pre-eclampsia. It can be extremely frustrating for an asymptomatic patient to remain in hospital, often with no clear idea of how long her in-patient stay will be. Similarly, a husband of a pre-eclamptic patient on the intensive care unit, or a couple with a baby on the special care baby unit, will often appreciate an explanation of the aetiology and pathogenesis of the disease.

> **Therapeutic options**
>
> Bed rest
> Antihypertensive medication
> Steroids

All therapeutic modalities are palliative and the disease continues to progress until the baby has been delivered. There is little evidence that many of the suggested therapies improve either maternal or perinatal outcome. In particular:

- Bed rest is of little or no benefit; patients with pre-eclampsia should be admitted in order to monitor the disease progression and ensure that there is no rapid deterioration in maternal or fetal condition, not to impose bed rest.
- Once a diagnosis of pre-eclampsia has been made, low-dose aspirin is not helpful.
- Antihypertensive therapy can reduce blood pressure and thus some of the maternal risk. However, it will not alter the multisystemic disease process and may mask the clinical sign of

hypertension; the identification of disease progression is then more difficult. Antihypertensive therapy is rarely indicated unless the blood pressure rises to levels at which there is concern that the pregnant woman will suffer a cerebrovascular haemorrhage (i.e. over 160/110 mmHg), in which case emergency management is necessary. Outside the emergency situation, if antihypertensive therapy is deemed appropriate, suitable agents are labetalol, nifedipine, methyldopa and hydralazine. Diuretics are of little value and are potentially harmful.

Delivery

The timing of delivery in pregnancies complicated by pre-eclampsia can be very difficult. Once a diagnosis of pre-eclampsia has been made, delaying delivery can only be harmful to the mother (although the later the gestation, the greater the chance of a successful induction of labour). Where there is obvious placental involvement with intrauterine growth restriction, delivery before the fetal biophysical parameters become abnormal may lead to the baby suffering problems due to prematurity. On the other hand, if delivery is delayed, the mother's condition may deteriorate and the chance of fetal hypoxic injury increases.

In general:

- *At term* (>37 weeks' gestation), delivery should be arranged. Unless there are other complications or contraindications, a vaginal delivery should be planned.
- *Between 33 and 37 weeks' gestation*, the bias should be towards delivering the baby (by Caesarean section).
- *At gestations below 33 weeks*, expectant management with close surveillance is often indicated.

As the gestation advances, the threshold for delivery falls. It is in this group of patients that antihypertensive agents may be of value in advancing the gestation at which the baby is delivered. Patients should be managed on a day-to-day basis, and unfortunately it is rarely possible to provide women with pre-eclampsia with a long-term or even a medium-term plan. If premature delivery is contemplated, steroids should be prescribed to enhance fetal surfactant production (there is some evidence that steroid administration also provides a short-term improvement in the maternal condition).

Recurrent Disease

There is a 25 per cent recurrence rate, although in successive pregnancies pre-eclampsia tends to be less severe and present at progressively later gestations.

Management in subsequent pregnancies

Consider low-dose aspirin therapy

Thrombophilia screen

Increased surveillance

See Also

Maternal collapse (Chapter 32)
Proteinuria (Chapter 18)
Small for gestational age (Chapter 21)

Further Reading

Lindheimer M, Roberts JM, Cunningham G (eds). *Chesley's Hypertension in Pregnancy.* Appleton Publishing, New York, 1999.

Chapter 12

Infections in pregnancy

Importance

Maternal and perinatal deaths from infection are now rare in the developed world, although viruses and drug-resistant bacteria present a major challenge. The pregnant woman is predisposed to infection in three classical sites: the uterus, the urinary tract and the breast. These are discussed in separate chapters on urinary tract problems, ruptured membranes, difficulty with breast-feeding and the febrile patient. This chapter will focus on generalized maternal infections, particularly those which lead to complications affecting the fetus.

Causes

Toxoplasma, rubella, cytomegalovirus (CMV) and herpes simplex comprise the 'TORCH' infections that can cause a classical syndrome affecting the fetus (Table 12.1).

Clinical features of the TORCH syndrome

Intrauterine growth restriction
Hepatosplenomegaly
Jaundice
Petechiae
Anaemia
Pneumonia
Mental retardation

Rubella infection is important because of its high prevalence and its very damaging effects on the fetus. If the infection occurs in the first trimester, fetal abnormalities (deafness, cardiac defects and cataracts) are common; the classical TORCH syndrome may also be seen.

CMV affects 1:500 pregnancies and is the leading cause of congenital infection in many countries. CMV may present with the classical TORCH syndrome and is one of the commonest causes of psychomotor retardation in children.

As the varicella zoster virus is highly contagious, most women have been in contact with it and problems in pregnancy are rare. However, varicella infections in the first half of pregnancy can cause fetal growth restriction, brain atrophy and limb or eye anomalies. Infections in the second half of pregnancy can cause herpes zoster of the infant and maternal pneumonia may be a serious complication.

Parvovirus B19 infection can lead to intrauterine growth restriction, stillbirths and preterm labour. The greatest risk is in the second trimester when targeting of the erythroid precursor cells in the fetal bone marrow can lead to severe anaemia and fetal hydrops.

Table 12.1 Common causes of infection in pregnancy

Category	Cause of infection
Viruses	Rubella
	Cytomegalovirus
	Varicella
	Parvovirus
	Measles
	Hepatitis
	Herpes simplex
	Human immunodeficiency virus (HIV)
Bacteria	Syphilis
Protozoa	Toxoplasmosis

Measles infection is caused by a paramyxovirus. Infection results in a small increased risk of miscarriage and congenital anomaly, and a significant risk of neonatal mortality if the infection is within a week of delivery. Herpes simplex infection of the newborn results from transmission at birth. The condition varies from involvement of only the skin, to involvement of the eye and nervous system, to widespread dissemination.

The human immunodeficiency virus (HIV) resides in the T4 immune cell and reduces effective immune function. Pregnancy has little effect on the progression or development of acquired immune deficiency syndrome (AIDS). However, transmission to the baby can be transplacentally and at or after delivery, and occurs in approximately 30 per cent of cases.

Hepatitis infections are discussed in Chapter 19. A number of other viral infections can be passed from mother to fetus (influenza, mumps, Coxsackie B virus, vaccinia virus), but are either less common or have few effects on the fetus

Syphilis is caused by the spirochete *Treponema pallidum*. Fetal infection may result in preterm birth, growth restriction, stillbirth or a neonatal syndrome (features include hepatosplenomegaly, pneumonia, anaemia, jaundice, skin lesions and osteochondritis).

Toxoplasmosis can result in the classical TORCH syndrome; central nervous system damage is particularly prominent, with calcification a late result.

Diagnosis and Clinical Assessment

Screening

At the antenatal booking clinic, the following screening tests for infection, or lack of immunity to infection, should be performed (depending on the population):

- antibody to rubella
- antibody to other TORCH and parvovirus infections
- test for syphilis – rapid plasma reagin (RPR) or *Treponema pallidum* haemagglutination (TPHA)
- hepatitis B status (Chapter 19)
- HIV status.

Approximately 90 per cent of pregnant women are rubella immune on testing.

The advantage of checking antibodies to the TORCH infections is that, if a woman has been found to be negative for antibody, any subsequent non-specific febrile illness should be treated with suspicion.

If women screen positive for syphilis, a more detailed study is made to confirm the presence of the disease by specific antitreponemal testing.

Routine blood testing for HIV is indicated in some areas. Counselling regarding the testing and the implications of any positive result should be available.

History

Ask about:

History of previous infection

Timing of exposure to infection

Extent of exposure to infection

Extent and timing of any symptoms

An accurate history is essential in making a diagnosis and assessing the risks to the pregnancy. Whilst a previous rubella or measles infection conveys immunity to further infections, individuals infected with CMV harbour the virus for life and reactivation can occur (with or without clinical manifestations). Unlike rubella, CMV can affect successive pregnancies. The risk of transmission from mother to baby at the time of birth is high in primary herpes infections, but very low in a woman with recurrent genital herpes, even when the virus is being shed at the time of delivery.

Determination of the timing of exposure to infection will enable the relationship between exposure to infection and any subsequent signs or symptoms to be assessed. Incubation periods for the viral infections are typically in the order of 2 weeks. In addition, it should facilitate a more accurate consideration of the risk to the fetus. For example, the risk of fetal damage from a rubella infection is 80 per cent in the first month of the pregnancy, 30 per cent in the second, 5–10 per cent in the third and fourth, and most unlikely after this time.

The likelihood and extent of any exposure to infection must be determined. Rubella infection is spread by droplet and infected subjects are contagious for 1 week before and 2 weeks after the appearance of the fine rash. CMV is transmitted by close physical contact with an infected individual or via infected blood, urine, saliva or breast milk. The depth of risk assessment for HIV will vary with the social setting, but risks are related to unsafe sex or drug practices. Toxoplasmosis is spread by handling infected cat faeces or by eating vegetables contaminated following contact with contaminated faeces; poorly cooked meat provides another source of infection.

A history of any suspicious symptoms should always be elicited. Many viral infections are subclinical, but there may be symptoms of malaise or fever. Similarly, toxoplasmosis may present with minimal symptoms.

Examination

Few of the signs of viral infection are specific and many infections are subclinical. However, if a viral infection is suspected, a careful examination for any pyrexia, lymphadenopathy, joint swelling or skin rash should be made. The fine rash of rubella can be distinguished from the coarser rash of measles. The vesicular lesions occurring in an acute attack of herpes genitalis are so typical that diagnostic confusion is rare.

Investigations

The choice of investigation depends upon the suspected infection:

If rubella is suspected, blood samples should be taken 2–3 weeks apart for determination of antibody levels – a fourfold rise indicates a recent infection. The majority of women will already be rubella-immune. If the woman presents more than 2 weeks after possible exposure and the antibody levels are high, the IgM titre should be checked (IgM antibody is only present for 6 weeks and indicates a primary infection). The diagnosis can also be made by isolating the virus in urine, blood or pharyngeal swabs. Serological tests are also available for other TORCH infections. The diagnosis of CMV is made from viral culture of secretions or the demonstration of 'owl's eyes' inclusions in urine. Parvovirus IgM is detected within 3 days of any rash and persists for up to 3 months.

Specific diagnosis of herpes genitalis requires viral identification in cultures from active lesions.

Management

Prevention

If found not to be immune to rubella, women should avoid contact with infected sufferers, be given immunoglobulin if any contact occurs and be immunized in the puerperium. In the United States, universal vaccination of young children has led to a marked decline in the reported incidence of congenital rubella.

In women not immune to one or more of the 'TORCH' infections, general hygiene measures should be emphasized at the booking clinic; close contact with chronic excreters (chronically infected children or immunosuppressed individuals) should be avoided if possible. Pregnant women should also be warned of the possible dangers of contracting toxoplasmosis if cats or their litter are handled, food hygiene is not scrupulous, or undercooked meat is eaten.

Treatment

Management is determined by:

Diagnosis
Gestational age
Assessment of fetal risk
Wishes of the pregnant woman and her partner

A clear explanation of the diagnosis, the risks to the fetus and the available management options is essential. In many cases, reassurance that any fetal damage is unlikely may be all that is required. However, in other cases, the assessment of risk may be difficult and it is often helpful to involve a microbiologist or virologist in management discussions. If a TORCH or parvovirus infection is suspected, a detailed ultrasound scan may provide evidence of a fetal anomaly.

Rubella

As discussed above, the risk of fetal damage from a rubella infection is 80 per cent in the first month of the pregnancy. If maternal infection in early pregnancy is confirmed, termination should be discussed (confirmation of fetal infection by invasive tests is an option). Routine use of immune serum globulin for post-exposure prophylaxis is not recommended, but may have a role where maternal rubella occurs and termination of pregnancy is not an option.

Other TORCH Infections

As with rubella, if maternal infection in early pregnancy is confirmed, termination should be discussed. Approximately 50 per cent of fetuses will be infected following maternal CMV; 5–10 per cent of cases are symptomatic and, of these, the majority result in major sequelae. The virus can be isolated from the urine of infected newborn infants.

Parvovirus

If a maternal infection is diagnosed, symptomatic treatment of arthralgia and fatigue should be prescribed. The fetus should be screened using ultrasound scans for hydrops. If hydrops develops, an *in utero* blood transfusion should be considered (see Chapter 4).

Herpes Simplex

Any patient who gives a history of previous herpes simplex infections should be reassured. Recurrent episodes of infection are very unlikely to cause effects in the fetus and serial viral cultures of asymptomatic women who have had previous infections are no longer recommended. Since the fetus is infected during passage down the birth canal at vaginal delivery, the presence of active lesions at the time of delivery is an indication for Caesarean section. If the membranes are ruptured longer than 4 hours, the advantage of a Caesarean section is lost.

Human Immunodeficiency Virus

HIV-positive women should be screened for other sexually transmitted diseases, CMV and toxoplasmosis. Helper T-lymphocyte (CD4 +) counts should be serially monitored. Counts < 500/mm^3 should suggest that patients are seen by an HIV specialist. Counts < 200/mm^3 require antibiotic prophylaxis against *Pneumocystis carinii* pneumonia. Any overt opportunistic infection should be treated. Vertical transmission to the fetus is reduced by Caesarean section, avoidance of breast-feeding and treatment with zidovudine (AZT).

Syphilis

If syphilis is diagnosed, treatment with an adequate course of penicillin should be prescribed. Infected women should be screened for other sexually transmitted infections and contact tracing should be instigated.

Learning Points

- Toxoplasma, rubella, cytomegalovirus, and herpes simplex comprise the 'TORCH' infections that can cause a classical syndrome affecting the fetus
- Antenatal screening tests for infection, or lack of immunity to infection, include antibodies to TORCH and parvovirus infections, tests for syphilis, and hepatitis B and HIV status
- If a TORCH infection is suspected, blood samples should be taken 2–3 weeks apart for determination of antibody levels – a fourfold rise indicates a recent infection. If it is more than 2 weeks after possible exposure and antibody levels are high, IgM titres should be checked
- Management of any infection is determined by the diagnosis, the gestational age, assessment of fetal risk and the wishes of the pregnant woman and her partner

See Also

Substance abuse (Chapter 22)
Difficulty with breast-feeding (Chapter 41)
The febrile patient (Chapter 43)
Ruptured membranes while not in labour (Chapter 39)

Further Reading

Enkin M, Kierse MJNC, Chalmers I. *A Guide to Effective Care in Pregnancy and Childbirth.* Oxford University Press, Oxford, 1989, pp. 89–100.

Beischer NA, Mackay EV, Colditz PB. Infections in pregnancy. In: *Obstetrics and the Newborn.* WB Saunders, London, 1997, pp. 294–310.

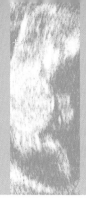

Large for gestational age

Importance

In the second half of pregnancy, the symphysis–fundal height measurement (in cm) should approximate to the gestational age (in weeks). Recently, maternity records have incorporated more accurate symphysis–fundal height charts. A measurement greater than 3 cm more than that anticipated from the gestation is 'large for gestational age' and merits investigation. In a significant minority of cases, pregnancy complications (with varying implications) will be identified.

Causes

Causes of large-for-dates pregnancy

Incorrect dates
Obesity
Multiple pregnancy
Large for gestational age or macrosomic fetus
Polyhydramnios
Uterine/extrauterine causes – fibroids, ovarian cyst, ascites

Multiple pregnancy is discussed in Chapter 14.

Although the terms are not strictly synonymous, large-for-gestational-age and macrosomic fetuses are variously defined as those with birthweights in excess of 4500 g, or birthweights above the 90th or 95th centiles for gestational age. The correlations with morbidity and mortality are improved when definitions are used which correct the birthweights for variables such as parity, maternal height and weight, ethnic origin and infant sex.

Factors that predispose to large-for-gestational-age fetuses include:

- maternal diabetes
- maternal obesity

- previous large-for-gestational-age fetus
- fetal hydrops
- genetic and congenital conditions such as Beckwith–Wiedemann syndrome.

Maternal diabetes is discussed in Chapter 8. Maternal obesity is associated with a fivefold increase in the incidence of large-for-gestational-age fetuses. Immune and non-immune causes of fetal hydrops are discussed in Chapter 4. Beckwith–Wiedemann syndrome results from pancreatic islet cell hyperplasia.

Polyhydramnios is defined as an amniotic fluid volume above the normal range for gestational age, or as a fluid volume greater than 2 L in the third trimester. Using the latter definition, the incidence of polyhydramnios in singleton pregnancies is approximately 1 per cent. Polyhydramnios may arise acutely, but the development is usually chronic. It represents an imbalance between the input (or production) and the output of amniotic fluid, can be associated with a variety of fetal (20 per cent) or maternal (20 per cent) disorders, or may be idiopathic (60 per cent). The majority of severe cases are caused by a fetal abnormality.

Disorders associated with polyhydramnios

Maternal diabetes
Multiple pregnancy (especially monovular twins)
Fetal anomaly, e.g. neural tube defect, oesophageal atresia
Fetal hydrops

Complications

The complications of multiple pregnancy are discussed in Chapter 14.

Increased Caesarean section rate

Increased operative delivery rate

Shoulder dystocia

Perineal trauma

Postpartum haemorrhage

Birth injury

The most common reason for Caesarean section is poor or unsuccessful progress in labour. Perineal trauma is more likely and is related to the increased incidences of operative delivery and shoulder dystocia. A combination of inadequate labour progress, a distended uterus and perineal trauma leads to the increased incidence of postpartum haemorrhage.

Consequences of polyhydramnios

Maternal discomfort

Unstable fetal lie

Increased incidence of preterm labour

Rupture of membranes may result in cord prolapse, fetal malpresentation, placental abruption

Postpartum haemorrhage

Preterm labour results from the increased uterine distension and an increased incidence of premature rupture of membranes.

Diagnosis and Clinical Assessment

History

In large-for-gestation pregnancies, it is rare that the history is particularly informative. Any history of maternal diabetes should be sought. The birthweights of any existing children should be noted. A history of rapid abdominal enlargement may suggest acute polyhydramnios.

Examination

The palpation of more than two fetal poles will suggest a multiple pregnancy. Maternal body weight and height above the normal range will predispose to a large-for-gestational-age fetus. In the presence of polyhydramnios, clinical findings are variable and depend on the pressure within the uterus. In some cases, the uterus may be very tense, with fetal parts difficult to palpate and the fetal heart difficult to hear. Alternatively, if the pressure within the uterus is low, ballottement and palpation of the fetus may be easier than normal.

Investigation

The use of ultrasonography is crucial to the identification of a cause for the large-for-gestational-age symphysis–fundal height measurement. Multiple pregnancies may be identified.

Measurements of femur length and of head and abdominal circumferences should be made. These measurements can be compared with reference charts that correlate ultrasound assessment of fetal growth with gestational age. The measurements can also be used to calculate the estimated fetal weight (accurate to ± 10 per cent).

The diagnosis of polyhydramnios is made by ultrasound scan. In addition to subjective assessment, a 'deepest pocket' measurement of over 8 cm or an amniotic fluid index over 20 cm is diagnostic. (The amniotic fluid index is the sum of the largest vertical pockets in the four uterine quadrants.)

Management

The management of multiple pregnancy is discussed in Chapter 14.

Large-for-gestational-age Fetus

Underlying conditions such as maternal diabetes (Chapter 8) or fetal hydrops (Chapter 4) should be managed appropriately. Serial ultrasound scans will enable assessment of fetal growth. Decisions regarding the timing and mode of delivery will depend on the past obstetric history (parity, previous birthweights), the degree of macrosomia, the gestational age, whether the cervix is favourable for induction, and the wishes of the woman. If the estimated fetal weight is in excess of 5 kg, the risks of shoulder dystocia are such that elective Caesarean section should be considered. The management of shoulder dystocia is discussed in Chapter 40.

Polyhydramnios

Management

Identify and treat (if possible) any underlying disorder

Consider amniocentesis and/or indomethacin

(cont.)

(cont.)
Perform a vaginal examination after rupture of membranes
Examine the baby carefully

Maternal glucose tolerance should be checked (Chapter 8). If maternal diabetes is diagnosed, there is some evidence that increased control of carbohydrate metabolism reduces amniotic fluid volume. The ultrasound investigation which diagnosed poly-hydramnios may indicate a fetal abnormality; a neural tube defect may be identified, absence of fluid in the stomach is suggestive of oesophageal atresia, and a double bubble indicates duodenal atresia. If fetal size measurements indicate growth restriction, there is an increased likelihood of a chromosomal abnormality and invasive investigation of the fetal karyotype should be considered (see Chapter 9).

In acute cases associated with marked maternal discomfort, therapeutic amniocentesis may be help-ful. The resulting respite is often brief and the proced-ure may precipitate preterm labour. Amniocentesis may be combined with tocolytic therapy, especially at early gestations. The prostaglandin synthase inhibitor indomethacin is another option. Indomethacin reduces fetal kidney production, but after 34 weeks the drug may cause premature constriction of the ductus arteriosus and attenuation of fetal cerebral blood flow.

After the membranes have ruptured, a vaginal examination should be performed in order to confirm the presenting part and to exclude cord prolapse.

After delivery, a neonatal examination should be carefully performed in order to identify any associated abnormality; a catheter should be passed into the stomach to exclude oesophageal atresia.

Learning Points

- Causes of a symphysis–fundal height that is large for gestational age include incorrect dates, obesity, multiple pregnancy, large-for-gestational-age fetus, polyhydramnios, fibroids, ovarian cyst, and ascites
- An ultrasound examination is crucial to the iden-tification of any cause for the large-for-dates pregnancy
- Complications and management depend on the underlying cause

See Also

History-taking and examination in obstetrics (Chapter 2)
Abnormal antibodies: blood group incompatibility (Chapter 4)
Diabetes (Chapter 8)
Small for gestational age (Chapter 21)
Multiple pregnancy (Chapter 14)
Shoulder dystocia (Chapter 40)

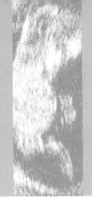

Multiple pregnancy

Importance

Although the incidence of twin pregnancies in Caucasian races is only 1 in 80 (1 in 50 in African-Americans, 1 in 150 in Asians), twin pregnancies account for over 10 per cent of perinatal deaths, and maternal morbidity and mortality rates are also increased.

Types of Twin Pregnancy

Zygosity

Twins are often described as dizygotic (biovular) when two ova are fertilized. The babies are not identical and although the placentae may be fused, they will have different circulations. Alternatively, twins may be monozygous (monovular) when a single ovum is fertilized. The babies will be identical.

Chorionicity

Twins are dichorionic if there are two placental circulations, and monochorionic when a single placenta is shared. All dizygotic twins will be dichorionic (Figure 14.1). The chorionicity of monozygotic twins depends on the stage at which cleavage into two embryos occurs (Table 14.1).

Complications (Table 14.2)

The degree to which the risk is increased depends on the type of twin pregnancy. Many of the complications of twin pregnancy are only increased if there is

monochorionicity. All the complications of twin pregnancies are increased in higher-order multiple births; the preterm delivery rate rises exponentially with the number of fetuses, as does the perinatal morbidity and mortality.

Diagnosis and Clinical Assessment

The diagnosis of a twin pregnancy is usually made in the antenatal booking clinic, following a routine ultrasound scan. In centres where routine ultrasound scans are not available, the average gestational age at diagnosis is 33 weeks.

History

Ask about:

Previous or family history
Preconceptual use of ovulation-inducing drugs (clomiphene, gonadotrophins) or the use of assisted reproduction techniques such as *in vitro* fertilization (IVF)
Excessive vomiting
High maternal age
High parity

The above features should lead to an increased suspicion of a multiple pregnancy. The increasing use of ovulation-inducing drugs and a rise in the number of women over 35 years old becoming pregnant have led to an increase in the incidence of multiple pregnancies.

Examination

The following features should lead to an increased suspicion of a multiple pregnancy:

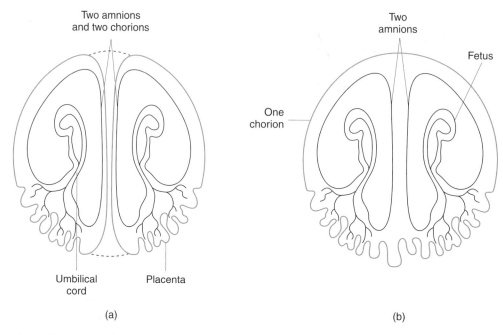

Figure 14.1 (a) Dichorionic twins. Each fetus has its own placenta, chorion and amnion – four layers separate the twins. (b) Monochorionic twins. The twins share one placenta and chorion, but usually have individual amniotic sacs – two layers separate the twins

Table 14.1 Chorionicity of monozygous twins

Stage at which cleavage occurs	Chorionicity
< 4 days (1/3 cases)	Separate amnions and chorions, i.e. dichorionic, diamniotic
5–10 days (2/3 cases)	Separate amnions, single chorion, i.e. monochorionic, diamniotic
11–13 days (1/100 cases)	Single amnion and chorion, i.e. monochorionic, monoamniotic
> 13 days (1/60 000 cases)	Conjoint or Siamese twins

Table 14.2 Complications of twin pregnancy

Maternal	Fetal
Hyperemesis	Miscarriage
Anaemia	Abnormalities
Pressure symptoms: varices, striae, oedema and dyspepsia	Prematurity
Pregnancy-induced hypertension and pre-eclampsia	Intrauterine growth restriction
Preterm labour or preterm prelabour rupture of membranes	Twin–twin transfusion
Antepartum haemorrhage	Malpresentation
Polyhydramnios	

- a symphysis–fundal height > 3 cm larger than expected for the gestational age after 22 weeks (the differential diagnosis of 'large for dates' is discussed in Chapter 13);
- the presence of more than two fetal poles.

Investigations

A raised maternal serum α-fetoprotein level may be due to a multiple pregnancy. If there is reasonable doubt that a multiple pregnancy is present, an ultrasound scan should be performed in order to establish the diagnosis. If no ultrasound scan has been performed in pregnancy, it should be standard practice to palpate the abdomen before giving an oxytocic drug in the third stage of labour.

Chorionicity is best determined by an ultrasound scan:

- if two placental sites are seen, the pregnancy is dichorionic;
- if the fetal genders differ, the pregnancy is dichorionic;
- if one placental site is seen, and the fetal genders are the same, the distinction depends on the separation and thickness of the membranes: in a dichorionic pregnancy, the membranes will be thicker (two layers of amnion and two layers of chorion) and separate over the placenta (Figure 14.2).

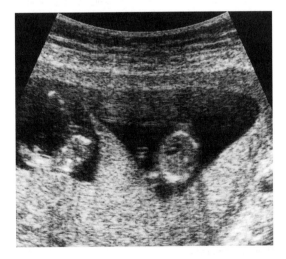

Figure 14.2 Ultrasound example of dichorionic pregnancy. These images were taken at 8 weeks' gestation and illustrate two fetuses divided by a thick membrane (demonstrating separation over the placenta: lambda sign)

Management

Priorities

Confirm the diagnosis
Establish the risk by determining chorionicity
Identify and manage complications
Plan mode of delivery ± labour

At the Antenatal Booking Clinic

- Prescribe prophylactic iron and folate supplementation
- Arrange a detailed second trimester ultrasound scan for fetal anomalies
- Consider prenatal diagnostic tests
- Plan subsequent antenatal care.

Maternal anaemia is partially due to haemodilution, but the additional demands of a twin pregnancy result in a 40 per cent reduction in iron stores. As maternal α-fetoprotein levels are elevated in twin pregnancies, the normal reference range is unhelpful (although a level > 5 multiples of the median may be used).

The increased risk of structural abnormalities (cardiac, spinal cord) particularly relates to monochorionic twins. The increased incidence of chromosomal abnormalities (such as Down's syndrome) merely relates to the increased age of women carrying twin pregnancies.

In cases at increased risk of chromosomal abnormality, invasive prenatal diagnostic testing is possible. The use of coloured dyes can ensure that both amniotic sacs are sampled at amniocentesis. However, the implications of identifying an abnormal karyotype are complex; termination of an abnormal twin will place the other twin at risk. Invasive testing should only be performed after very careful counselling.

Although antenatal care may be shared between hospital and community practitioners, the frequency of antenatal clinic visits should increase, in order to identify complications at an early stage. In uncomplicated cases, women should be reviewed every 2 weeks until 30 weeks' gestation, and then weekly until delivery. Women should be referred back to the hospital at an early stage if any symptoms of preterm labour develop.

In general, the higher the number of fetuses, the greater the perinatal mortality and morbidity. (In recent years, selective fetal reduction in cases of higher orders of multiple pregnancy has been introduced. The technique involves an injection of potassium chloride into the fetal heart under ultrasound control.)

At Subsequent Antenatal Visits

- Measure blood pressure and test urine for protein
- Assess fetal growth
- Check maternal haemoglobin level
- Check for signs and symptoms of preterm labour.

Twin pregnancies are associated with three-fold to five-fold increases in both non-proteinuric pregnancy-induced hypertension and pre-eclampsia. Fetal growth restriction occurs in 25–30 per cent of twin pregnancies. Clinical assessment cannot distinguish between the growth of different twins; serial ultrasound scans of fetal growth should be arranged. If growth restriction is identified, fetal well-being should be carefully assessed (see Chapter 20). A discrepancy in the growth of the twins may indicate twin–twin transfusion.

Twin–twin transfusion (this complication is restricted to monochorionic twins)

Vascular connections exist between the placental circulations of monochorionic twins. In 20–30 per cent of cases, blood is lost from one twin to the other

The *donor* twin is growth restricted and suffers from anaemia and hypoxia. There is also oliguria and resulting oligohydramnios

The plethoric *recipient* twin may develop cardiac failure and thrombotic problems due to hyperviscosity. Polyuria can cause acute polyhydramnios

Antenatal treatment options include:

Serial amniocentesis of the polyhydramniotic sac ± indomethacin to decrease fetal urine output

Laser photocoagulation of the abnormal vessels endoscopically

The diagnosis is confirmed by a difference in the fetal haematocrits and haemoglobin concentrations.

Prematurity is the greatest cause of perinatal mortality, and over 10 per cent of twin pregnancies end before 32 weeks' gestation. These infants have a higher incidence of respiratory distress syndrome and a higher mortality rate than singleton infants, even after correcting for differences in gestational age. Infants from multiple pregnancies, when born alive, have gestational age-specific mortality rates that are comparable to singleton infants who are at least 1–2 weeks less mature.

If any uterine activity is noted, prompt attendance at the hospital labour ward should be advised. Interventions aimed at reducing the incidence of preterm labour have not been found to be successful. These have included cervical cerclage, bed rest in hospital and beta-mimetic tocolytic agents. The intrapartum management of preterm labour is discussed in Chapter 38.

Plan the Mode of Delivery

For triplet and higher orders of multiple pregnancy, the planned mode of delivery will usually be by Caesarean section. The mode of delivery for twins will depend on the presentation of the first twin. In over 70 per cent of cases, the presenting part of the first twin is cephalic. In the absence of other complications, a vaginal delivery is usually planned in such cases. If the first twin is not cephalic, Caesarean section is usually performed.

Factors affecting risk of vaginal delivery

Type of twin pregnancy

Presentation

Gestation

Intrauterine growth restriction (IUGR)

Hypertension

Fetal abnormality

Previous Caesarean section

Monoamniotic pregnancies represent an extremely high-risk group. Cord entanglement can occur as the fetuses share the same sac. These pregnancies are usually delivered by Caesarean section. Monochorionic twin pregnancies are also a higher risk group, but if the pregnancy has progressed normally with no signs of twin-to-twin transfusion syndrome, a vaginal delivery may be possible. Dichorionic twins are the lowest risk group. Many of these can be safely delivered vaginally.

Preterm labour is much more of a problem for twin pregnancies. There are no hard and fast rules about the best mode of delivery for the preterm fetuses in this case. If the pregnancy is 34 weeks or more, this should be managed as a term pregnancy. At very early gestations, below 26 weeks, Caesarean section confers no benefit and vaginal delivery would usually be anticipated. Between these gestations lies a grey area. Caesarean section is advocated by many, but a vaginal delivery if both fetuses are cephalic is equally acceptable.

The place of elective induction at 38 weeks' gestation is controversial, with the benefit unproven.

In the third trimester, a discussion of the need for continuous fetal heart rate monitoring and the advantages of epidural anaesthesia will assist those responsible for intrapartum care.

Management in Labour

Management in labour should be directed at those factors that can particularly complicate a twin pregnancy.

> **Principles of management**
>
> Define presentations
> Continuous monitoring of both fetuses
> Monitor progress
> Suitable analgesia
> Intravenous access

The presentation of the first twin is usually easily defined on vaginal examination. If the presentation of the second twin is in doubt, ultrasound scanning will help.

In order to monitor both fetuses simultaneously, the first twin is usually monitored via a scalp electrode and the second twin via a transabdominal ultrasound transducer. Both traces can be recorded on the same monitor, thus ensuring that two different heart rate patterns are seen. Continuous fetal monitoring in established labour is performed. If there is doubt about the well-being of the second twin, delivery should be by Caesarean section, as there is no other method to ascertain fetal condition. If the first twin shows suspicious fetal heart rate changes, a fetal scalp sample can be performed (see Chapter 29).

Sometimes uterine overdistension can predispose to a dysfunctional labour. Oxytocin can be used judiciously if the twins are showing no signs of compromise. Progress should be as for a singleton pregnancy (see Chapter 35).

Because of the possibility of a need to manipulate a second twin after delivery of the first, epidural analgesia is recommended. This is particularly so if the second twin is not cephalic.

The higher risk of postpartum haemorrhage means that blood should be taken early on in the labour for a full blood count and group and save. If the haemoglobin estimation is less than 10 g/dL, blood should be cross-matched.

Delivery

The delivery should be undertaken in a facility where there is easy access to theatre, should the need arise. In some units, delivery in theatre is preferred. The team needed for a twin delivery will include:

- Obstetrician (often two)
- Midwife
- Paediatrician (sometimes two)
- Anaesthetist (especially if an epidural has not been sited previously).

Delivery of the first twin should be accomplished in the normal manner (see Chapter 35), with recourse to instrumental delivery for the normal obstetric reasons (see Chapter 28).

After the first twin is delivered, the lie and presentation of the second twin must be determined. Ultrasound can help. Ultrasound can also help to reposition the fetal heart rate transducer. Continuous monitoring at this point is vital, as the risk of fetal asphyxia secondary to abruption is highest.

If the lie is longitudinal, the second assistant may need to keep the fetus in position until the presenting part engages. At this point, patience is needed to await return of uterine contractions. If contractions have not begun again after 10 minutes, Syntocinon can be started at a normal rate for augmentation (see Chapter 27).

Once the presenting part is beginning to descend into the pelvis, the membranes of the second twin can be ruptured. Pushing should not commence until the presenting part has fully descended and the cervix is fully dilated (often there is some contraction of the cervix between deliveries, especially if there is some delay).

If the lie is not longitudinal, external version can be used to gently turn the fetus to a longitudinal lie. The presentation is less important than the lie. A breech is often as easy to deliver, especially if a foot can be grasped through the membranes before they are ruptured. This is most likely to succeed if the fetuses are of similar weight. If external version is not successful, an internal podalic version can be performed. This will be followed by a breech extraction. This is the only situation in which these manoeuvres are permissible. Internal podalic version involves passing a hand into the uterus to locate and grasp a fetal foot. The foot is then gradually brought down while external pressure on the fetal head encourages the fetus to turn. The breech is then delivered in a similar manner to an assisted breech delivery (see Chapter 7).

If at any time the condition of the second twin gives cause for concern and a vaginal delivery is not yet attainable, recourse to Caesarean section is safest.

It used to be thought that delivery of the second twin should be accomplished within 30 minutes. It is now recognized that with continuous monitoring a longer time is acceptable if all is proceeding well. Undue haste can also lead to problems such as difficult vaginal delivery and cord prolapse.

Third Stage

The incidence of postpartum haemorrhage is much higher in multiple gestations, as a result of uterine atony and a larger placental bed. The third stage must therefore be actively managed. Consideration should be given to continuation of Syntocinon (40 units in 500 mL 5 per cent dextrose solution) for 4–6 hours after delivery, regardless of method of delivery. If heavy bleeding occurs, or if the starting haemoglobin was low, blood transfusion should also be considered.

Postnatal

Caring for twins and triplets is extremely exhausting. Avoiding anaemia is most important in these women, and some will need to continue their iron tablets after delivery, especially if they are breast-feeding.

Many mothers will need extra help after discharge. Other agencies can be of help. These will include:

- Community midwives
- Twins clubs
- Health visitors
- Breast-feeding counsellors.

Financial help can be made available for mothers of triplets and higher order multiples.

Learning Points

- **The degree of risk depends on the chorionicity**
- **The incidence of several complications of pregnancy is markedly increased**
- **There is a need for increased antenatal surveillance**
- **Ultrasound assessment of fetal growth and well-being is central to the antenatal management**
- **The major risk to the fetuses in labour is asphyxia in the second twin**
- **Delivery must be undertaken where easy access to theatre is available**
- **Postpartum haemorrhage is the major maternal risk**

See Also

Large for gestational age (Chapter 13)

Further Reading

Daw E. Triplet pregnancy. In: Studd J, ed. *Progress in Obstetrics and Gynaecology*, vol. 6. Churchill Livingstone, Edinburgh, 1987, pp. 119–32.

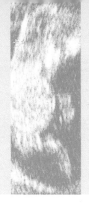

Chapter 15

Previous Caesarean section

Importance

With rising Caesarean section rates, the management of women with a previous Caesarean section is an increasingly common problem. The management of this group of pregnant women is contentious. However, the dictum 'Once a Caesarean section, always a Caesarean section' is not true. Up to 70 per cent of women with a previous Caesarean section can achieve a subsequent vaginal delivery.

Risks and Complications

Hazards

Elective Caesarean section

Increased maternal morbidity such as fever, wound infections
Increased risk of infant respiratory distress – contingent of the Caesarean delivery itself, or preterm delivery following miscalculation of dates
Maternal feeling of guilt/sense of failure and increased postnatal depression

Trial of vaginal delivery

Risk of uterine dehiscence (wound breakdown) or rupture (1–2 per cent)
Maternal fear of an emergency Caesarean section

Clinical Assessment

History

A careful history should be taken at the antenatal booking clinic and it is often helpful to study the previous partogram and operation notes.

Ask about:

The number of Caesarean sections that have been performed
The type of Caesarean section that has been performed
The indication for the previous Caesarean section
The stage at which the Caesarean section was performed
Whether there have been any previous vaginal deliveries
Whether there are any additional pregnancy complications

The risk of uterine rupture in labour increases with the number of previous Caesarean sections. In general, if a woman has had two or more Caesarean sections, a repeat Caesarean section is usually arranged.

The vast majority of Caesarean sections are transverse incisions in the lower segment of the uterus (Figure 15.1). The risk of uterine scar breakdown/rupture is four times greater if the upper segment of the uterus is involved, as in a classical Caesarean section (the thick muscle of the upper uterine segment is incised vertically in the midline); in such cases an elective Caesarean section should be planned. A history of uterine perforation in a previous termination of pregnancy, a previous Caesarean section scar which was torn either laterally or vertically, and a postoperative uterine infection (which may have affected scar healing) are all indications for an elective Caesarean section.

It is important to determine whether the previous Caesarean section was for a 'non-recurrent' cause, such as placenta praevia or a breech presentation, or a cause that is more likely to recur, such as delay in labour. Even when the initial indication was adjudged to be cephalopelvic disproportion, up to 40 per cent of women have been able to deliver vaginally in subsequent pregnancies. In some centres, this is an indication for radiological pelvimetry measurements,

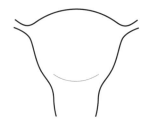

Transverse lower segment incision

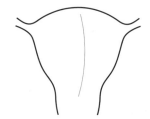

Classical Caesarean section incision

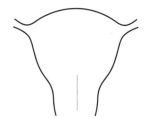

Vertical lower segment incision

Figure 15.1 Uterine incisions for Caesarean section

although several studies have reported that the investigation is of no predictive value.

A Caesarean section performed at full cervical dilatation or following any unsuccessful attempts at delivery using forceps or vacuum extraction is a relative indication for an elective Caesarean section.

Mothers who have had a previous vaginal delivery in addition to their previous Caesarean section are more likely to deliver vaginally after a trial of labour than mothers with no vaginal deliveries, particularly if the vaginal delivery succeeded the Caesarean section.

Examination

Examination findings rarely influence management decisions unless a pregnancy complication such as pre-eclampsia, multiple pregnancy or maternal diabetes is identified; additional complications should lower the threshold to perform a repeat Caesarean

section electively. Unless the pelvis is grossly distorted (e.g. pelvic fractures after a road traffic accident or rickets), clinical pelvimetry measurements are very poor predictors of the success of a trial of vaginal delivery.

Investigation

Radiological pelvimetry measurements are also very poor predictors of the success of a trial of vaginal delivery. Unless the woman has previously delivered a baby vaginally, the only way to accurately determine the size of her pelvis is to see whether a trial of vaginal delivery is successful.

Management

Decide the Mode of Delivery

A provisional plan as to the mode of delivery should be made as early as possible; it can be modified later in pregnancy. The views and expectations of the pregnant woman are of great importance. She may have suffered a long and painful labour that ended in a Caesarean section and may view any possible repeat performance with great trepidation. In contrast, the strong feeling of some parents against Caesarean section is evidenced by the formation of groups such as 'Vaginal Births after Caesareans'.

If the plan is to aim for a vaginal delivery, management should include the detection of any additional indication for an elective Caesarean section. Indications include pregnancy complications such as a breech presentation, pre-eclampsia, fetal growth restriction and placenta praevia.

Any proposed plan must be discussed with the pregnant woman and her partner, and each concern and anxiety should be addressed with care and sensitivity.

Consideration of Induction of Labour

For a vaginal delivery to be achieved, the onset of spontaneous labour is preferable. If the pregnancy is complicated by postmaturity (see Chapter 17), decisions regarding induction of labour are difficult. The available evidence suggests that the use of oxytocin or prostaglandins to induce labour is not associated with a marked increase in scar rupture/dehiscence, but is associated with higher Caesarean section rates.

In the presence of an unfavourable cervix, an elective Caesarean section is probably indicated.

If an elective Caesarean section has been planned, women should be reviewed at approximately 37 weeks' gestation. Delivery in the 39th week of pregnancy should be arranged. Blood should be typed and screened for unexpected antibodies; cross-matching of blood will not usually be required.

Management in Labour

Delivery should be in hospital, with facilities for close monitoring of mother and fetus, and there should be a readily available anaesthetist and operating theatre in order that a Caesarean section can be performed in labour if deemed necessary.

Analgesia

The use of regional (caudal or epidural) analgesia has been questioned because of fears that early signs of scar rupture (pain and tenderness) may be masked. However, these fears do not appear to be justified and regional analgesia is not contraindicated.

Oxytocics

The use of oxytocin for augmentation of labour is controversial, because of speculation that there might be an increased risk of uterine rupture/dehiscence. The limited available data suggest that any increased risks are small; however, any decision to use oxytocics should involve a senior obstetrician. A previous Caesarean section is an indication for intrauterine pressure monitoring in some centres.

Duration of Labour

The maximum duration of labour should depend, to a significant extent, on the woman's previous experience; she may have been traumatized by a long labour which culminated in an emergency Caesarean section. It is clearly preferable to perform a Caesarean section prior to the onset of maternal or fetal distress and, in general, delivery should be within 8–12 hours.

Learning Points

- Up to 70 per cent of women with a previous Caesarean section can achieve a subsequent vaginal delivery
- Decisions regarding mode of delivery depend on the number and type of previous Caesarean sections, the indication for the Caesarean section and the stage at which it was performed, previous vaginal deliveries, additional pregnancy complications and the views of the pregnant woman

See Also

Failure to progress in the first stage (Chapter 27)

Further Reading

Enkin M, Kierse MJNC, Chalmers I. *A Guide to Effective Care in Pregnancy and Childbirth.* Oxford University Press, Oxford, 1989, pp. 247–55.

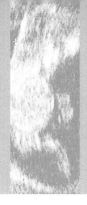

Previous fetal loss

Importance

Any baby born after 24 weeks' gestation, without any sign of life, is classified as a stillbirth. The frequency of stillbirths varies widely throughout the world and depends on the health and physique of the population, allied to the standard and availability of medical care. The perinatal mortality rate (stillbirths + neonatal deaths) ranges from seven to over 100 per 1000 births. The management of a pregnant woman who has suffered a fetal loss in a previous pregnancy requires both diligence and sensitivity.

Causes

Common causes of fetal loss

Premature delivery
Congenital anomaly
Reduced placental perfusion
Asphyxia at delivery
Infection
Haemolytic disease

In many cases more than one aetiological factor is present; in others none can be identified.

Premature delivery is defined as birth occurring before 37 completed weeks, and prematurity remains the leading cause of perinatal morbidity and mortality. Babies born prematurely fall into one of two groups. In the first group, labour begins spontaneously or as a result of prelabour premature rupture of membranes. In the second group, a major complication occurs (such as pre-eclampsia or a placental abruption) and the pregnancy is terminated in the interests of either mother or baby.

Major congenital anomalies complicate approximately 20 per cent of perinatal mortalities. Cardiovascular abnormalities comprise the greatest proportion of these cases, although multiple anomalies are often present. Central nervous system defects (such as spina bifida) occur less frequently now that screening programmes are widespread (see Chapter 10). Chromosome abnormalities are being detected in increasing proportions of perinatal deaths, probably because of increased investigation. However, screening programmes and invasive prenatal tests lead to the termination before viability of a significant proportion of fetuses with Down's syndrome (see Chapter 9).

Reduced placental perfusion leads to intrauterine growth restriction (IUGR, Chapter 21) and pre-eclampsia. These conditions are associated with six-fold to ten-fold increases in perinatal mortality. Maternal conditions associated with reduced placental perfusion, IUGR and pre-eclampsia and increased perinatal mortality include chronic renal disease (Chapter 18), chronic hypertension (Chapter 11), diabetes (Chapter 8) and antiphospholipid syndrome (Chapter 59).

Asphyxia at delivery is often due to antenatal compromise and may be related to reduced placental perfusion before the onset of labour. Occasionally it is clearly the result of an intrapartum event, such as a cord accident (Chapter 26) or shoulder dystocia (Chapter 40). In many centres, the organism most commonly responsible for fetal loss due to infection is group B β-haemolytic *Streptococcus*. This Gram-positive coccus is present in the vagina of 15–20 per cent of pregnant women and may lead to premature labour or premature prelabour rupture of membranes (Chapter 39).

Haemolytic disease is discussed in Chapter 4.

Diagnosis and Clinical Assessment

History

When the woman and her partner attend the antenatal clinic, a careful detailed history of previous pregnancies must be taken. The medical notes from any previous pregnancies should be available for review.

Key questions

Gestational age at time of fetal demise
Infant birthweight
Associated pregnancy complications
Past medical history

The gestational age at the time of the previous pregnancy loss will identify whether the pregnancy was complicated by prematurity; a spontaneous premature delivery should be distinguished from iatrogenic causes of prematurity. Risk factors for prematurity should also be identified. A variety of scoring systems have been devised, with the aim of prospectively identifying pregnancies at increased risk of preterm labour. Several associations with preterm labour are recognized, including poor socioeconomic status, young age and primiparity. However, the scoring systems have had only limited success and the best predictors are probably a previous history of premature labour or mid-trimester loss, or the presence of a multiple pregnancy. A previous history of painless mid-trimester miscarriage or traumatic damage to the cervix may indicate cervical incompetence as an aetiological factor.

Previous infant birthweights will indicate whether previous babies have been small for gestational age (SGA). Birthweight-for-gestational-age charts that have been compiled for the local population should be used. The use of models which correct for confounding variables enables a closer correlation with perinatal morbidity and mortality. The medical notes may indicate whether previous pregnancies were complicated by IUGR, as evidenced by serial ultrasound scans.

A careful history, aided by review of the medical notes, should indicate whether the fetal demise was associated with pregnancy complications or general maternal conditions that led to reduced placental perfusion. Similarly, other pregnancy complications such as Rhesus incompatibility (Chapter 4) should be identified. If the previous fetal loss occurred during labour or shortly after delivery, the intrapartum events and management must be carefully reviewed.

Examination

Examination findings will rarely contribute to the identification of the cause of fetal loss. Occasionally a contributory maternal medical condition (such as an endocrine disorder) may be diagnosed.

Review of Previous Investigations

Postmortem examination results may indicate that the previous pregnancy was complicated by a congenital fetal anomaly. Many stillborn babies show evidence of intrauterine hypoxia at postmortem examination, but this does not explain the cause of death. If a postmortem was not performed, X-rays and photographs may facilitate a diagnosis. Karyotype analysis, performed on samples taken after fetal death, may indicate a chromosomal abnormality.

The placenta should also have been examined histologically; appearances suggestive of a placental abruption or of pre-eclampsia may have been found.

The results of other investigations done following fetal death (Chapter 31), such as those performed to identify an infective or thrombophilic cause, should also be rechecked.

Management

Following any pregnancy that ends tragically with a stillbirth, a second-trimester loss, or a disabled child, the events and possible diagnoses should have been discussed with the couple once the results were available. However, the couple may have further concerns and questions and these should be discussed at an early stage in any subsequent pregnancy. Management should include a sympathetic review of the previous pregnancy.

The psychological trauma that the couple will be experiencing must be taken into account when considering the appropriate management.

Management options may include:

Increased antenatal clinic attendance, especially in the third
    trimester
Serial third-trimester ultrasound scans, for growth and tests
    of fetal well-being
Elective induction of labour, prior to the gestation at which
    the previous pregnancy loss occurred

In many cases no explanation for the previous pregnancy loss is found. However, if the fetal demise was
linked to another pregnancy complication, additional
management should be directed at prevention (or
early detection) of this complication.

Previous Premature Delivery

If the previous pregnancy was complicated by a
spontaneous premature delivery, the pregnant
woman should be educated with regard to the signs
and symptoms of preterm labour. The perception
of contractions, cramp-like pains, low backache and
a 'show' may all prove to be significant and warrant
her attending hospital for assessment in order that
the advantages of tocolytic and corticosteroid therapy
may be obtained (Chapter 38).

If cervical incompetence is suspected, cervical
cerclage can be arranged at 12–14 weeks' gestation.

If there is an infective aetiology of a previous
preterm labour, cervical microbiological swabs should
be taken at 20–24 weeks' gestation. Prophylactic
antibiotic therapy can then be targeted to any infective
agent identified. Randomized trials of prophylactic
antibiotic therapy in the absence of positive swab results
have not shown any benefit. If an infective aetiology
was implicated in the fetal demise (e.g. β-haemolytic
Streptococcus), prophylactic therapy should be given at
the onset of labour.

Other strategies, such as prophylactic administration of tocolytics or corticosteroids, are of unproven
value.

Previous Congenital Abnormality

If there is a previous history of any congenital anomaly,
management should include careful screening for
a structural abnormality (Chapter 10), and prenatal
invasive diagnostic tests may be considered (Chapter 9).

Previous Intrapartum Death

If there is a clear history of intrapartum events
resulting in fetal asphyxia at delivery, a Caesarean
section may be preferable to induced or spontaneous
labour.

Previous Placental Failure

Many of the conditions associated with reduced
placental perfusion (such as pre-eclampsia and
IUGR) have a high recurrence rate in subsequent
pregnancies. There is little evidence that prophylactic
therapies (e.g. low-dose aspirin) reduce the severity
of the disease or the fetal complications. An exception
to this rule is antiphospholipid syndrome; treatment
with low-dose aspirin and heparin has been found
to improve the prognosis for the fetus.

Learning Points

- **Causes of fetal loss include premature delivery,
  congenital anomaly, reduced placental perfusion,
  asphyxia at delivery, infection and haemolytic
  disease**
- **Management may include increased
  antenatal clinic attendance, serial third-
  trimester ultrasound scans, elective induction
  of labour and additional measures directed
  at preventison (or early detection) of any
  complications implicated in the previous
  pregnancy**

See Also

Fetal abnormality: chromosomal (Chapter 9)
Fetal abnormality: structural (Chapter 10)
Small for gestational age (Chapter 21)
Reduced fetal movements (Chapter 20)
Abnormal antibodies: blood group incompatibility
(Chapter 4)
Hypertension (Chapter 11)
Intrauterine fetal death (Chapter 31)
Preterm labour (Chapter 38)

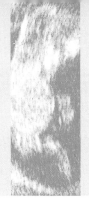

Chapter 17

Prolonged pregnancy

Importance

Between 4 and 12 per cent of deliveries occur at a gestational age greater than or equal to 42 weeks. These pregnancies are termed prolonged. Postmaturity is used as a synonym of prolonged pregnancy, but the term is confusing as it implies the presence of placental insufficiency and a hierarchy of features ranging from loss of subcutaneous fat, through meconium staining and birth asphyxia, to respiratory distress, convulsions and fetal death.

Risks

Prolonged pregnancies are at an increased risk of:

Perinatal mortality
Neonatal seizures
Operative delivery

Perinatal mortality is increased in prolonged pregnancies. This increased perinatal mortality is due to a higher proportion of babies with congenital malformations as compared with babies delivered at term, and an increased risk of intrapartum and neonatal deaths. The risks of antepartum death are not increased. A high prevalence of meconium-stained amniotic fluid is an outstanding feature among the intrapartum and neonatal deaths.

Perinatal morbidity is also increased in prolonged pregnancies, as evidenced by a two-fold to five-fold increase in neonatal seizures, a marker of perinatal asphyxia.

A larger and less mouldable fetal skull leads to an increased risk of poor progress in labour and contributes to the increased incidence of operative deliveries. The prolonged pregnancies of nulliparous women are at a particularly high risk of operative delivery. Induction of labour does not alter the increased risk of operative delivery.

Clinical Assessment

History

The history is rarely crucial to the management. However, it is important to check that there are no risk factors that have been missed. For example, any patient who has had an antepartum haemorrhage or a stillbirth or has essential hypertension and is taking antihypertensive therapy should really have been delivered at 40 weeks' gestation.

Examination

On abdominal examination, the symphysis–fundal height will provide an indication of fetal growth and will determine the degree of engagement of the presenting part. If the symphysis–fundal height measurement leads to investigations that indicate intrauterine growth restriction, induction of labour should be arranged. A pelvic examination will determine whether the cervix is favourable for induction of labour; if the Bishop score is >4, the cervix is considered to be favourable (see Chapter 30).

Investigation

Gestational age is uncertain in approximately 25 per cent of women in reported series due to uncertain menstrual data (poor memory, irregular cycles, lactational amenorrhoea, or last period related to the oral contraceptive pill). An accurate dating scan should be performed in early pregnancy. If the discrepancy between gestational ages calculated from the date of the last menstrual period and from the ultrasound scan is greater than a week, the gestational age should be corrected to that consistent with the ultrasound scan.

Management

Any patient who has not delivered at 41 weeks' gestation should be reviewed in the antenatal clinic. At this visit, the following tasks should be performed:

- the gestational age should be checked;
- a careful history should be taken;
- the abdomen and pelvis should be examined;
- management options should be discussed.

If there are no additional risk factors, the management options are as described below.

Induction of Labour

This can be arranged at 41–42 weeks' gestation (see Chapter 30). If the Bishop score is >4, induction of labour is likely to be successful. There is no justification for induction of labour before 41 weeks' gestation in uncomplicated pregnancies.

Induction of labour can be deferred for a week and the examination repeated in order to determine whether a more favourable Bishop score has been attained. If the cervix is unfavourable, prostaglandin therapy (such as prostaglandin E_2 vaginal gel) to ripen the cervix prior to artificial rupture of membranes should be arranged (Chapter 30).

Conservative Management

If this option is chosen, there should be increased surveillance of fetal well-being (see Chapter 20). Ideally this should include weekly ultrasound measurement of biophysical profile and Doppler umbilical artery waveform analysis. As a minimum, weekly ultrasound estimation of liquor volume and fetal heart rate

tracing should be performed. Most advocates of conservative management would suggest induction of labour after 43 weeks' gestation, when a significant deterioration in perinatal outcome has been reported.

Counselling

There is little evidence to favour any of the above options, and after explaining each option to the woman whose pregnancy is prolonged, a reasonable management plan would seem to be to offer her the choice of routine or selective induction of labour. Patients become anxious as they go past their expected date of delivery. It is important that an accurate gestational age is established at the booking visit, and patients should be warned that they should expect to deliver between 38 and 42 weeks' gestation

Learning Points

- **An accurate gestational age should be established at the antenatal booking clinic**
- **Prolonged pregnancies are at an increased risk of perinatal mortality, neonatal seizures and operative delivery**
- **The evidence in favour of routine versus selective induction of prolonged pregnancies is finely balanced**

See Also

Small for gestational age (Chapter 21)
Induction of labour (Chapter 30)

Further Reading

Royal College of Obstetricians and Gynaecologists. RCOG guideline: Induction of labour. RCOG Press, London, 2001. (Also available at http://www.rcog.org.uk/guidelines/eb_guidelines.html)

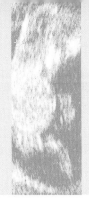

Chapter 18

Proteinuria

Importance

Renal protein excretion increases in normal pregnancy, and proteinuria is not considered abnormal until it exceeds 300 mg/24 hours. Significant proteinuria is associated with increased fetal and maternal risk, and the cause of proteinuria should always be investigated.

Causes

Contamination by vaginal discharge should be excluded by taking a midstream specimen following vulval cleansing and separation of the labia. In the presence of ruptured membranes, it may be necessary to pass a catheter.

Pregnancy predisposes to urinary tract infection, largely because of stasis caused by increased progesterone leading to dilatation of the ureters and renal pelves. The microorganisms generally responsible for urinary tract infections in pregnancy are *Escherichia coli* (responsible for 80 per cent of infections), *Klebsiella*, *Enterobacter* and *Proteus*. Asymptomatic bacteriuria ($>10^5$ organisms/mL) is present in 5–10 per cent of women attending the antenatal booking clinic, and leads to cystitis in 40 per cent and pyelonephritis in 30 per cent of cases.

Proteinuria is a sign of pre-eclampsia. Although the correlation between the degree of proteinuria and the elevation in blood pressure is weak, the magnitude of proteinuria is closely related to the increased fetal risk. Pre-eclampsia is discussed further in Chapter 11.

Acute renal failure associated with proteinuria is rare. Causes include acute tubular or cortical necrosis (secondary to hypovolaemia, septicaemia and shock) and acute glomerulonephritis. Chronic renal insufficiency is more common; causes include chronic pyelonephritis, polycystic kidney disease and chronic glomerulonephritis. Polycystic kidney disease is an autosomal dominant condition which does not present until women are of child-bearing age. Chronic glomerulonephritis may be idiopathic, familial or result from other conditions such as diabetes and systemic lupus erythematosus. Proteinuria may be a temporary phenomenon due to pregnancy-induced renal lesions, or it may be an expression of pre-existing renal disease coinciding with pregnancy. In the first case it should disappear at some time after delivery; in the latter it will remain present.

Antiphospholipid syndrome, an important autoimmune pregnancy complication with a particular tendency to adversely influence pregnancies, is discussed further in Chapters 21 and 59.

Proteinuria may also result from a variety of other conditions once a serious disease stage has been reached (e.g. hyperemesis gravidarum, anaemia or cardiac disease) and is occasionally indicative of rare conditions such as a phaeochromocytoma.

Diagnosis and Clinical Assessment

Screening

An increase in protein output will usually, but not invariably, result in higher concentrations in random urine samples. The volume and concentration of urine will affect protein concentration and may lead to erroneous results of tests on random urine specimens. Screening for proteinuria in antenatal clinics is with reagent strips or 'dipstick' tests that start detecting protein (albumin) concentrations of approximately 50 mg/L. However, dipstick testing of random samples leads to significant false-positive results with a trace/+ reaction.

Careful history, examination and laboratory investigations will usually identify the cause of proteinuria in pregnancy.

History

> **Important features to identify**
>
> Relevant past medical history
> Associated symptoms

A history of recurrent urinary tract infections suggests an underlying predisposition to bacteriuria. Urinary tract infections are also more common in medical conditions such as sickle cell anaemia and diabetes. A history of pre-eclampsia in any previous pregnancy (or of medical conditions predisposing to pre-eclampsia) increases the likelihood that the proteinuria is due to pre-eclampsia. Any history of renal disease is clearly relevant, although the distinction between an exacerbation of pre-existing renal disease and pre-eclampsia may be difficult.

Symptoms of urinary frequency and dysuria, pain in the flank radiating to the loin, and fever, anorexia or vomiting are indicative of a urinary tract infection. Pre-eclampsia is typically asymptomatic.

Examination

A pyrexia and tachycardia indicate a urinary tract infection; loin tenderness is suggestive of pyelonephritis. In general, proteinuria with pregnancy-induced hypertension signifies pre-eclampsia; the signs of pre-eclampsia are discussed in Chapter 11.

Investigation

The relevance of investigations depends on the findings elicited by the history and examination.

> **The following may be indicated:**
>
> 24-hour urine collection
> Tests of renal function
> Urine microscopy
> Urine culture
> Platelet count, liver function tests, clotting screen
> Autoantibody screen – antinuclear and anticardiolipin
>   antibodies, lupus anticoagulant
> Renal ultrasound scan
> Renal biopsy

The definitive test for proteinuria in pregnancy is determination of total protein in a 24-hour urine collection.

Quantitation of proteinuria does not correlate with functional renal impairment; if renal compromise is suspected, tests of renal function must be performed. These include determination of plasma levels of electrolytes, uric acid, urea and creatinine, and measurement of creatinine clearance. An elevation in levels of uric acid indicates tubular damage and this is one of the first parameters to alter in pre-eclampsia. The appropriate investigations if a diagnosis of pre-eclampsia is suspected are discussed in Chapter 11.

Findings of pus cells, red cells and organisms on urine microscopy may allow diagnosis of a urinary tract infection. Hyaline or cellular casts indicate glomerulonephritis. Culture of the urine specimen will identify the organism responsible for any infection and will ensure that antibiotic therapy is appropriate. The presence of an uncommon pathogen and pyuria is suggestive of underlying renal disease. A blood culture is indicated if the infection is severe.

If renal compromise is present, measurement of autoantibodies will exclude antiphospholipid syndrome or may suggest lupus nephritis. A renal ultrasound scan may reveal scarring suggestive of chronic pyelonephritis or may demonstrate pelviceal dilatation. Rarely, a renal biopsy is indicated.

Management

The appropriate management is determined by the diagnosis.

Urinary Tract Infection

Urinary tract infections should be treated by a suitable course of antibiotics (determined by laboratory sensitivity testing). Repeat urine specimens should be cultured after the course of antibiotics and at regular intervals throughout pregnancy.

If the infection recurs, antibiotic prophylaxis (e.g. cephradine 250 mg twice daily) should be prescribed throughout pregnancy. Chronic pyelonephritis develops in approximately one-third of cases in 10–15 years. It is important to investigate these women in the puerperium with an intravenous pyelogram to exclude underlying abnormalities of the urinary tract (such as calculus, hydronephrosis or congenital anomalies).

The management of pre-eclampsia is discussed in Chapter 11.

Renal Disease

The management of renal disease depends on the aetiology and the severity of renal compromise. Certain histological findings (such as glomerulonephritis with crescent formation) are associated with a poor prognosis, as is any renal disease with severely impaired renal function (plasma creatinine >275 μmol/L or urea >10 mmol/L).

Principles of management

Joint management by nephrologists and obstetricians
Preconceptual management of pre-existing renal disease
Close antenatal surveillance to:
- Monitor renal function
- Exclude urinary tract infection
- Detect complications – anaemia, pre-eclampsia
- Monitor fetal well-being
Medical therapy (steroids, azathioprine) if necessary

Occasionally, a grave prognosis for mother and baby leads to the recommendation of termination of pregnancy. Antenatal care should be directed towards the detection of complications; a diagnosis of superimposed pre-eclampsia is often difficult as the features of pre-eclampsia mimic those of chronic renal disease. The timing of delivery will depend on the maternal disease and the fetal growth and well-being.

Learning Points

- Significant proteinuria is associated with increased fetal and maternal risk, and proteinuria should always be investigated
- Causes of proteinuria include contamination, urinary tract infection, pre-eclampsia and renal disease
- Careful history, examination and laboratory investigations will usually identify the cause of proteinuria in pregnancy

See Also

Infections in pregnancy (Chapter 12)
Hypertension (Chapter 11)
Urinary frequency (Chapter 62)

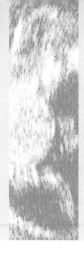

Chapter 19

Pruritus and jaundice in pregnancy

Importance

Severe pruritus (itching) or jaundice in pregnancy may indicate haemolysis, hepatocellular disease or biliary stasis, which merits investigation and treatment. Whilst pruritus is a common symptom of pregnancy, jaundice occurs in about 1 in 1000 pregnancies (this rate varies with patient populations and may be up to 2 per cent).

Causes

Differential diagnosis of jaundice and pruritus

Hepatocellular disease
Viral hepatitis
Chronic liver disease
Severe pre-eclampsia
Acute fatty liver of pregnancy
Obstructive disease
Cholestasis of pregnancy
Cholelithiasis and acute cholecystitis
Haemolytic disease

In addition, severe pruritus can be due to infestations (e.g. scabies), malignancy and generalized skin disorders (eczema, psoriasis). Conditions specific to pregnancy include:

- herpes gestationalis
- pregnancy prurigo.

Viral hepatitis is the most common cause of jaundice in pregnancy. There are three distinct types: A, B and C. Hepatitis A commonly occurs in low socio-economic conditions and in underdeveloped countries. Poor hygiene may predispose to faecal–oral transmission. Pregnancy does not alter the course of the disease and transmission to the fetus is rare. Hepatitis B may lead to chronic disease, a carrier state or transmission to the fetus. Infection occurs via infected blood or other body fluids, and the highest rates are in drug abusers and patients treated with blood products. The maternal mortality rates are not increased in the developed world compared with non-pregnant women. However, in underdeveloped countries, mortality is markedly elevated. In areas of high incidence, such as the Far East, perinatal transmission is a major cause of persistent hepatitis B infection. The clinical presentation and mode of transmission of hepatitis C are similar to those of hepatitis B.

The aetiology of chronic liver disease includes autoimmune disease (chronic active hepatitis), viral hepatitis (B or C) and alcohol abuse. As discussed in Chapter 11, severe pre-eclampsia involves widespread endothelial damage which results in haemolysis and thrombocytopenia.

Acute fatty liver of pregnancy is an extremely rare but commonly fatal disease characterized by a marked fatty infiltration and vacuolization of hepatocytes. Like pre-eclampsia, acute fatty liver of pregnancy is more common in primigravidae and extremely uncommon before the late second trimester.

Cholestasis of pregnancy is due to an oestrogen-sensitivity effect and exhibits a familial tendency. It is frequently recurrent in successive pregnancies (approximately 50 per cent recurrence rate) or if oral contraceptives are prescribed. It is more common in Scandinavian, South American and Mediterranean countries. Perinatal outcome is poor due to an increased risk of preterm delivery (30–50 per cent), placental abruption (10–20 per cent) and a twofold increase in stillbirths. There is also an increased risk of postpartum haemorrhage (due to reduced vitamin K absorption).

Diagnosis and Clinical Assessment

A careful history and examination are the initial steps.

History

Key questions

Duration, severity and onset of jaundice and pruritus
Associated symptoms (epigastric pain, fatigue, nausea, vomiting)

Hepatitis is associated with fatigue, nausea, anorexia and vomiting. Acute fatty liver of pregnancy typically presents with vomiting, abdominal pain and jaundice, and patients may become drowsy or confused. In cholestatic disease, pruritus is the dominant symptom.

Examination

Key features

Jaundice
Abdominal tenderness
Generalized or local skin lesion
Colour of urine and stools

In hepatitis A the jaundice is typically mild and lasts for 10–15 days. The jaundice of acute fatty liver of pregnancy is severe. In cholestasis of pregnancy, the majority of women with the disease have only mild jaundice. Right upper quadrant pain or tenderness is a common feature of hepatitis B/C. Herpes gestationis occurs mainly in the second and third trimesters; crops of papillae become bullous, initially on the trunk and spreading to the limbs. Pregnancy prurigo is characterized by itchy papules, which cover the body.

Cholestatic disease is characterized by the formation of dark urine and pale stools. Signs of pre-eclampsia (Chapter 11) may also be present.

Investigation

Key tests

Full blood count (white cells, platelets)
Bilirubin
Hepatocellular enzymes (e.g. aspartate transaminase or alanine transaminase)
Hepatitis antigen and antibody markers
Bile salts
Autoantibody screen
Renal function (urea and electrolytes, uric acid, creatinine)
Clotting studies
Ultrasound scan of biliary tree

Biochemical tests will help to differentiate between hepatocellular damage and obstructive disease.

Hepatocellular Damage

This is associated with an increase in unconjugated bilirubin and hepatocellular enzymes (aspartate transaminase or alanine transaminase). The diagnosis of hepatitis A is confirmed by finding hepatitis A antibody. Various antibody and antigen markers are useful in the diagnosis and management of hepatitis B. Hepatitis B surface antigen (HbsAg) is commonly found in serum up to 2 weeks prior to the onset and during the clinical disease. The 'e' antigen (HbeAg) is seen early in the disease and is a good index of infectivity and neonatal transmission. The antibody to the core antigen (HbcAb) appears during clinical disease and may persist for years. Confirmation of hepatitis C is more difficult; the development of a positive hepatitis C antibody test may be delayed after the onset of infection, and thus repeated testing is necessary. Laboratory studies in acute fatty liver of pregnancy reveal a significant leucocytosis, moderately disturbed liver function, hypoglycaemia, impaired renal function and often coagulopathy. A positive autoantibody screen would suggest chronic active hepatitis.

Cholestasis (Intrahepatic or Extrahepatic)

This results in a rise in conjugated bilirubin and alkaline phosphatase. Alkaline phosphatase levels rise in pregnancy due to increased placental production, and thus results must be interpreted with caution. In cholestasis of pregnancy, liver enzymes are normal or only mildly elevated. Serum bile salts are elevated and the prothrombin time may be prolonged.

An ultrasound scan may demonstrate dilatation of the biliary tree in cases of extrahepatic obstruction.

Management

Management depends on the diagnosis.

Viral Hepatitis

Hepatitis A is self-limiting, but patients with severe anorexia or vomiting may require hospitalization and fluid replacement. Adequate nutrition and the maintenance of fluid and electrolyte balance are also important in the management of hepatitis B and C. Isolation precautions must be exercised. Hyperimmune serum (HBIG) should be administered to neonates at risk of hepatitis B. There is no known treatment to prevent vertical transmission of hepatitis C infection.

Acute Fatty Liver

Therapy is aimed at symptomatic treatment of hepatic and renal failure. Patients should be placed in intensive care units; intravenous fluids should be administered, together with albumin, dextrose and vitamin K. Coagulation defects may need correction with fresh frozen plasma. The pregnancy should be terminated, usually by emergency Caesarean section.

Cholestasis of Pregnancy

Cholestyramine resin is a theoretically attractive method of reducing symptoms of pruritus (intestinal bile salts are chelated and thus serum bile acids fall).

Patients should also receive parenteral vitamin K supplementation. However, such treatment is rarely satisfactory and antihistamines, skin emollients and ultraviolet radiation are all methods of providing relief from the severe pruritus. Increased monitoring of fetal well-being is indicated, with planned induction of labour at term, or earlier if any fetal compromise is detected. The condition rapidly resolves after pregnancy.

Herpes Gestationalis

Treatment of herpes gestationalis is with oral steroids. Although oral steroids may be necessary to resolve symptoms of pregnancy prurigo, antihistamines and topical steroid cream are often effective.

The management of pre-eclampsia is discussed in Chapter 11.

Learning Points

- Viral hepatitis is the most common cause of jaundice in pregnancy
- Cholecystitis of pregnancy is associated with markedly increased perinatal mortality
- Acute fatty liver of pregnancy is a rare but often fatal condition

See Also

Hypertension (Chapter 11)
Infections in pregnancy (Chapter 12)

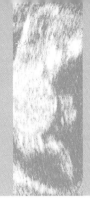

Reduced fetal movements

Importance

One of the most frequent antenatal complaints is of reduced fetal movements. Whilst this is often a perception problem, it should never be ignored. Complete cessation of maternal perception of fetal movement may be a pre-mortem event.

The fetus has periods of activity which last about 40 minutes and passive periods which last about 20 minutes. Fetal activity is increased after the pregnant woman has eaten and when she is resting. Fetuses will usually respond to external stimuli such as palpation of the maternal abdomen.

Screening

Maternal recording of fetal movements is used as a screening test of fetal well-being. The cause of most late fetal deaths is unknown. As these deaths are unpredictable, the extent to which they can be prevented by current forms of antenatal care is limited. Screening by counting fetal movements has theoretical advantages over other screening tests of fetal well-being which are impractical to perform on a daily basis. There are essentially two methods of monitoring fetal movements:

- The pregnant woman begins counting at a set time each day and records the time at which a count of 10 is reached. Advice is sought if there are insufficient movements within a set time limit (Figure 20.1).
- A set time period is used; if the count falls below a set limit, a further time period is used. Advice is sought if the count is again unsatisfactory.

In addition, the woman should seek advice if there is a marked diminution in movements or there are no movements for any 12-hour period.

Randomized trials suggest an equivocal benefit from screening using fetal movements, although the test may increase the stress and anxiety of pregnant women.

Clinical Assessment

If a woman presents with a history of reduced fetal movements, the likelihood of fetal compromise is low. Counts below 10 and above 1000 per 12 hours have been reported for apparently normal fetuses. Maternal perception of fetal movements varies widely; moreover, some normal fetuses are consistently vigorous, while others are consistently sluggish. However, it is important to assess the state of the fetus.

History

Ask about:

Duration of reduced fetal movements
Past obstetric history
Associated symptoms

A poor past obstetric history (previous stillbirth or growth-restricted baby) will increase the clinical suspicion of fetal compromise, as will symptoms of vaginal bleeding or abdominal pain.

Examination

Key features

Maternal well-being
Symphysis–fundal height
Amniotic fluid volume
Auscultation of fetal heart

Maternal conditions associated with an increased risk of fetal compromise, such as pre-eclampsia (see Chapter 11), should be excluded. If the symphysis–fundal height measurement is not consistent with the gestational age, ultrasound measurement of fetal size should be performed (Chapter 21). The abdominal palpation may suggest oligohydramnios, not only by a diminution in the symphysis–fundal height measurement, but also by an inability to ballot the fetus and by the sensation that the uterus is closely wrapped around the fetus. If the fetal heart is not detected on auscultation, urgent ultrasonic confirmation of the fetal heartbeat should be arranged.

Investigations

Investigative options

Electronic fetal heart rate monitoring
Amniotic fluid volume
Measurement of the biophysical profile
Doppler ultrasonography
Biochemical assessment

The use of continuous fetal heart rate monitoring was initially confined to women in labour. However, fetal heart rate patterns can also be assessed in the antenatal period and tracings can be transmitted from outlying centres via telephone lines if there is doubt about the significance of a heart rate pattern. The normal fetal heart rate is between 110 and 160 beats/min (bpm), with a bandwidth variability of 10–20 bpm, no fetal heart rate decelerations, and three accelerations of > 15 bpm for > 15 seconds over a 20-minute period (Figure 20.2).

Amniotic fluid volume is measured ultrasonographically by either (i) the depth of the deepest pocket without cord loops, or (ii) the amniotic fluid index: the sum of the deepest vertical pockets in the four uterine quadrants.

The biophysical profile score is derived from the ultrasonographic measurement of five parameters over 30 minutes, each of which scores 0 or 2 (Table 20.1). A score of 8–10 is normal and no intervention is necessary. If indicated, the test can be repeated in 7 days. A score of 6 is equivocal and either delivery should be considered (particularly if the liquor volume is abnormal or the gestational age is > 37 weeks) or the test should be repeated in 24 hours. A score of 0–4 is abnormal and is an indication for delivery.

Doppler ultrasonography of the umbilical artery provides an estimation of vascular resistance and

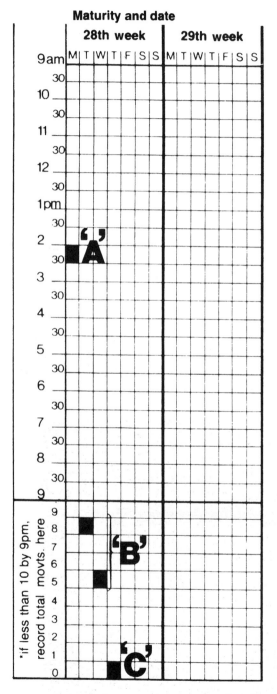

Figure 20.1 A fetal movement or 'kick' chart. A, 10 movements felt by 2.30 pm. B, fewer than 10 movements felt for 2 days in a row. C, no movements for 1 day. Examples B and C should lead to urgent review

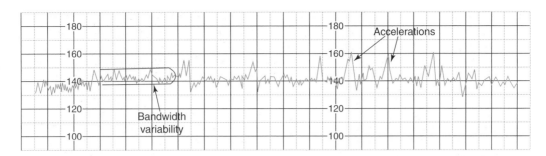

Figure 20.2 Antenatal fetal heart rate tracing with the bandwidth variability and fetal heart rate accelerations indicated

Table 20.1 Biophysical profile

Parameter	Score 2 if present, 0 if absent
Fetal breathing movements	> 1 episode
Body movements	> 4 movements
Fetal tone	Active limb extension/flexion, opening of hand
Liquor volume	One > 3 cm pocket or two >2 cm pockets
Heart rate reactivity	> 2 accelerations with fetal movement

blood flow. An increase in the ratio of flow in systole to that in diastole (S/D ratio) is associated with a risk of fetal compromise. Absent blood flow to the fetus in diastole (Figure 20.3) and flow from the fetus (reversed flow) are both findings of graver significance than an elevated S/D ratio and have been associated with 29 per cent perinatal mortality rates.

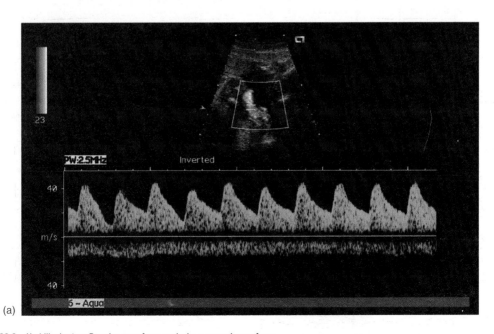

(a)

Figure 20.3 Umbilical artery Doppler waveform analysis: a normal waveform

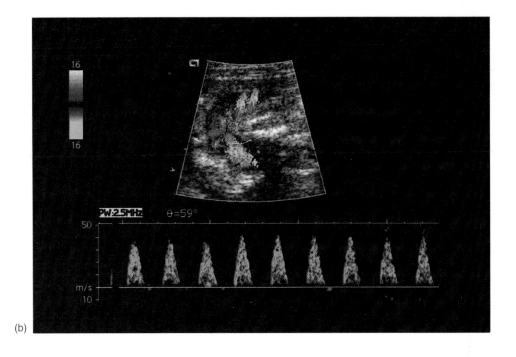

(b)

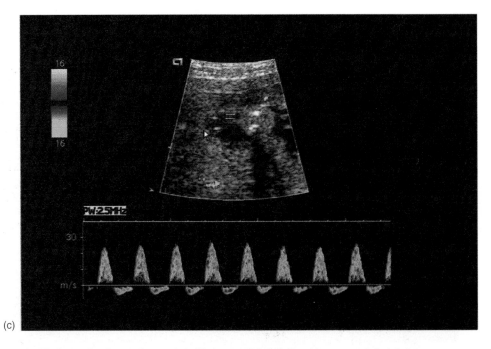

(c)

Figure 20.3 Umbilical artery Doppler waveform analysis: (b) absent end-diastolic flow; (c) reverse end-diastolic flow

Historically, measurement of parameters such as maternal urinary oestriol levels and serum human placental lactogen concentrations were used as a guide to fetal well-being. However, the specificity and sensitivity of these tests is very low and they are now little used.

When used in isolation, each of the tests used to assess fetal well-being has low specificity and sensitivity; management decisions should be based on a combination of all the test results. If reduced fetal movements are reported, the minimum investigation should be an estimation of liquor volume and a fetal heart tracing.

Management

If fetal compromise is suspected on the basis of a combination of the above investigations, the important considerations are the maternal condition and the gestational age. Complications such as pre-eclampsia may necessitate delivery, irrespective of the maturity of the fetus. At gestational ages over 34 weeks, complications resulting from fetal immaturity are relatively uncommon and the threshold for delivery is reduced accordingly.

Learning Points

- **Although reports of reduced fetal movements should not be ignored, the specificity and sensitivity for identifying fetal compromise are low**
- **A combination of the different methods of assessing fetal well-being should be used**

See Also

Previous fetal loss (Chapter 16)
Small for gestational age (Chapter 21)
Intrauterine fetal death (Chapter 31)
Abnormal fetal heart rate patterns in labour (Chapter 29)

Further Reading

Enkin M, Keirse MJNC, Chalmers I. Assessment of fetal wellbeing. In: *A Guide to Effective Care in Pregnancy and Childbirth*. Oxford University Press, Oxford, 1989, pp. 57–66.

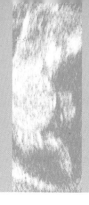

Small for gestational age

Importance

In the second half of pregnancy, the symphysis–fundal height measurements (in cm) should approximate to the gestational age (in weeks). A measurement more than 3 cm below that anticipated from the gestation is 'small for gestational age' and merits investigation. If the pregnancy is found to be complicated by intrauterine growth restrictionfold (IUGR), there is a six-fold to ten-fold increase in the perinatal mortality.

Causes

Factors that influence fetal growth

Maternal size
Ethnic origin
Parity
Infant sex

Maternal booking weight and height independently influence birthweight. In the UK, Asian babies weigh less than Caucasian or African-American babies; moreover, patterns of fetal growth vary – at 34 weeks' gestation, the birthweight of African-American babies is greater than that of Caucasian babies but at term this trend is reversed. The birthweight of second (and subsequent) babies exceeds that of the first child by approximately 100 g. Male fetuses are approximately 150 g heavier than females from 32 weeks' gestation. Ideally, birthweight-for-gestational-age charts that have been compiled for the local population should be used. The use of models which correct for parameters such as maternal size, ethnic origin

and parity and fetal sex enables a closer correlation with perinatal morbidity and mortality.

Causes of Small-for-gestational-age Pregnancies

Common causes

√ Incorrect dates
√ Abnormal lie
√ Oligohydramnios
√ Small-for-gestational-age fetus

If the fetal lie is transverse (see Chapter 23), the symphysis–fundal height will be reduced.

Oligohydramnios is defined as a volume of amniotic fluid below 200 mL or as an amniotic fluid index (an ultrasound measurement of the sum of the largest vertical pockets in the four uterine quadrants) below the normal range for the gestational age. Causes include:

- placental dysfunction in association with IUGR;
- fetal malformations such as absent kidneys or a lower urinary tract obstruction;
- premature rupture of membranes.

The term small for gestational age (SGA) should not be regarded as synonymous with IUGR. SGA is a birthweight below the 10th centile according to the gestational age of infants born in the community concerned (birthweight below the 5th centile or 2 standard deviations below the mean are less commonly used thresholds). IUGR should be defined as a failure of the fetus to achieve its full growth potential antenatally. The difficulty in diagnosing IUGR often leads to SGA infants being described as growth restricted; however, it is important to realize that fetoplacental dysfunction can occur when the infant is not SGA.

Aetiology of IUGR

Fetal abnormality (chromosome or structural anomaly)

Environmental (smoking, alcohol, altitude)

Fetal infection (TORCH syndrome)

Irradiation/cytotoxic agents

Multiple pregnancy

Factors affecting placental perfusion

Fetal structural (Chapter 10) and chromosomal (Chapter 9) anomalies, infections in pregnancy (Chapter 12), substance abuse (Chapter 22) and multiple pregnancy (Chapter 14) are discussed in the chapters stated. The effect of altitude is such that for every 1000 m above sea level there is a 100 g reduction in birthweight.

As detailed in Chapter 11, the pregnancy complication of pre-eclampsia is associated with a failure of the trophoblast cells to invade and convert the maternal spiral arteries to low-resistance vessels. IUGR has a similar pathogenesis, leading to a diminished uteroplacental blood supply. Other maternal conditions associated with diminished placental perfusion include renal disease, essential hypertension (especially if treated with antihypertensive agents) and antiphospholipid syndrome.

Diagnosis and Clinical Assessment

The cause of the small symphysis–fundal height measurement should be established.

History

Ask about:

Date of last menstrual period

Past obstetric history

Past medical history

Fetal movements

The gestational age should be checked, i.e. that the dates from the last menstrual period are consistent with ultrasound dating. Birthweights of any babies will indicate whether there is a past history of IUGR; if so, the risk of IUGR is increased by five-fold to ten-fold. As detailed above, the past obstetric and past medical histories may indicate conditions associated with decreased placental perfusion. Fetal movements provide an indication of fetal well-being (Chapter 20).

Examination

Key findings

General maternal well-being

Fetal lie

Amniotic fluid volume

The general examination should exclude maternal conditions associated with poor fetal growth such as pre-eclampsia. If the fetal lie is transverse, the symphysis–fundal height will be reduced. An inability to ballot the fetus and the sensation that the uterus is closely wrapped around the fetus may suggest oligohydramnios.

Investigation

The relevant investigation is an ultrasound measurement of fetal size. The fetal parameters most commonly measured are the abdominal circumference and the biparietal diameter or the head circumference.

Fetal abdominal circumference predicts IUGR because it reflects the size of the small liver and the thin layer of subcutaneous tissue that are associated with IUGR. The most accurate measurement is the smallest one obtained between fetal respirations at the level of the hepatic vein, as the smallest perimeter will be that closest to the plane perpendicular to the spine.

The head circumference is less susceptible to extrinsic alteration than the biparietal diameter and facilitates a differentiation of cases of IUGR into those which are symmetrical (both head and abdominal circumferences are reduced) and the majority of cases which are asymmetrical (the abdominal circumference is reduced to a greater extent than the head circumference).

Although IUGR can be suspected after a single scan demonstrates abnormally low measurements, it can only be diagnosed with conviction after serial scans (Figure 21.1).

Management

If IUGR is diagnosed, the appropriate management depends on:

The gestational age

The pattern of growth restriction

The severity of growth restriction

Assessment of fetal well-being

Early-onset or symmetrical IUGR

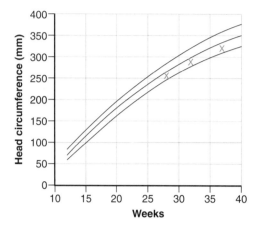

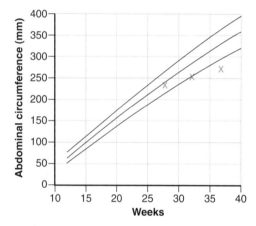

Figure 21.1 Serial ultrasound measurements of fetal size. Normal head circumference growth is seen, but abdominal growth is diminished. This is an example of asymmetrical intrauterine growth restriction

If IUGR is identified before 32 weeks' gestation, or the pattern of IUGR is symmetrical, i.e. both head and abdominal circumferences are reduced, the likelihood of a fetal anomaly or infection is increased.

Management options

Detailed ultrasound scan to exclude a structural anomaly
Placental biopsy to karyotype the fetus
Fetal blood sampling to identify any viral infection and
    determine the acid–base status
Assessment of fetal well-being
Steroid administration

If a mid-trimester detailed scan has not been performed, an ultrasound scan to exclude a structural

anomaly should be arranged. Karyotyping should be considered (preferably from a placental biopsy in order to obtain a rapid response). About 20 per cent of cases of early-onset or symmetrical IUGR will be associated with a chromosomal disorder. Diagnosis of a major structural fetal anomaly or a chromosomal abnormality incompatible with life may affect the management of the pregnancy and the mode of delivery.

The role of fetal blood sampling to identify any viral infection and assess fetal acid–base status is controversial. In about 20 per cent of cases, the cordocentesis procedure induces a fetal bradycardia; if the test has any place, it is within a tertiary referral centre.

Steroids should be administered in order to accelerate fetal lung maturity in case early delivery is necessary. If delivery is deemed necessary, the mode of delivery will usually be by Caesarean section.

Late-onset IUGR

The usual cause of IUGR identified after 32 weeks' gestation is uteroplacental dysfunction, and the pattern of IUGR is characteristically asymmetrical.

Assessment of fetal well-being

Electronic fetal heart rate monitoring
Ultrasound measurement of amniotic fluid volume
Ultrasound determination of biophysical profile score
Doppler umbilical artery waveform analysis
Biochemical methods

Once a pregnancy has been identified as complicated by late-onset IUGR, fetal well-being should be assessed (see Chapter 20). If the gestation is > 36 weeks, labour should be induced unless a vaginal delivery is contraindicated. If there is evidence of fetal compromise, delivery should be planned; the mode of delivery will depend on the gestation and the degree of fetal compromise. If there is no evidence of compromise and the gestation is < 36 weeks, there should be repeated assessment of fetal well-being.

Learning Points

- **Birthweight is affected by maternal size, ethnic origin, parity and infant sex**

- **Small for gestational age (SGA) should not be regarded as synonymous with IUGR IUGR should be defined as a failure of the fetus to achieve its full growth potential**
- **The appropriate management of IUGR depends on the gestational age, the pattern and severity of growth restriction and assessment of fetal well-being**

See Also

Large for gestational age (Chapter 13)
Reduced fetal movements (Chapter 20)
Fetal abnormality: chromosomal (Chapter 9)
Hypertension (Chapter 11)
Infections in pregnancy (Chapter 12)
Substance abuse (Chapter 22)
Multiple pregnancy (Chapter 14)

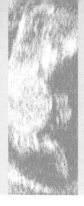

Chapter 22

Substance abuse

Importance

The use of a variety of potentially harmful substances, both legal and illegal, has increased markedly in recent years. The abuse of these substances can have profound effects on the mother and baby. The complications of substance abuse are difficult to quantify, as various social problems, often inadequate antenatal care and poor nutrition compound them.

Risks

Legal Substances

Smoking

Approximately 33 per cent of pregnant women smoke, despite public education programmes that explain the risks to the smoker (such as heart disease and cancer) and to the fetus. In addition, young women are smoking at increasingly earlier ages. Complications of maternal smoking result from the effects of carbon monoxide and from decreased placental perfusion consequent upon nicotine vasoconstriction. Risks increase with the number of cigarettes smoked.

> **Pregnant smokers place the baby at increased risks of:**
>
> Intrauterine growth restriction (IUGR)
> Preterm delivery and premature prelabour rupture of membranes (PPROM)
> Placental abruption
> Possible long-term developmental abnormalities

Alcohol

Alcohol crosses both the placenta and the blood–brain barrier freely. The toxic effects of alcohol are due to direct effects and the effects of metabolites such as aldehyde. After genetic causes, alcohol ingestion in pregnancy is the most common cause of mental retardation. Toxicity is dose related and is maximal in the first trimester.

Whilst the occasional drink of alcohol during pregnancy carries no known risk, regular consumption conveys a risk of 'fetal alcohol effects' (IUGR or subtle behavioural or developmental abnormalities). Consumption of six or more units of alcohol/day (1 glass wine = 1 unit) carries a risk of 'fetal alcohol syndrome' developing.

> **Fetal alcohol syndrome**
>
> Mental retardation
> Intrauterine and postnatal growth restriction
> Congenital abnormalities – particularly brain, cardiac and spinal defects
> Craniofacial abnormalities – including a flattened nasal bridge, absent or hypoplastic philtrum, and a short nose

Illegal Substances

The direct effects of illegal substance abuse are often eclipsed by lifestyle problems associated with drug dependence: poor diet and hygiene, physical and emotional violence, and sexual promiscuity or prostitution (leading to sexually transmitted diseases).

Cocaine

Cocaine is a potent stimulant of the central nervous system with marked vasoconstrictive effects. There is great potential for addiction and abuse. Cocaine abuse is a cause of rare maternal cardiac events, including myocardial infarction, aortic rupture and cerebrovascular accidents.

Congenital anomalies – especially heart and central nervous
system
Placental abruption
Preterm labour and PPROM
IUGR
Vascular lesions – fetal bowel and limb infarction

Survivors are at an increased risk of sudden infant
death syndrome (SIDS), learning difficulties and
behavioural problems.

Marijuana

Although no documented effects of marijuana have
been noted in human pregnancy, the active ingredi-
ent (9-tetrahydrocannabinol) has been found to have
teratogenic effects in animal studies.

Opiates

The risks of opiates such as heroin include three-fold
to seven-fold increases in the incidence of stillbirths,
preterm delivery and neonatal death. However, these
risks relate to the lifestyle associated with heroin
intake, rather than to direct effects of the drug.

The potentially fatal newborn withdrawal syndrome occurs in approximately 66 per cent of cases
and is characterized by a high-pitched cry, poor feeding, hypertonicity, tremor, hyperirritability, sneezing,
diarrhoea and seizures. The syndrome usually occurs
within 2 days after delivery but may present up to 10
days of age.

Hallucinogens

There is no good evidence of untoward pregnancy
outcomes with lysergic acid diethylamide (LSD) or
other hallucinogens.

Diagnosis

History

Accurate identification of the substances that have
been, or are being, ingested is an essential prerequisite of effective risk assessment. Some women will be
referred via drug and alcohol misuse support agencies; a careful, detailed and non-judgmental history
at the time of the antenatal booking clinic will elicit a
history from other women. However, substance abuse
is consistently under-reported and some women will
not present until complications have ensued.

Management

Legal Substances

Pregnancy presents a unique opportunity to cease or
reduce maternal cigarette ingestion, a possibility that
is aided by the decreased appetite and nausea of pregnancy. Smokers and alcohol drinkers should be carefully counselled at the booking visit and encouraged
to stop or reduce intake at this and subsequent visits.
Discontinuation of smoking during pregnancy has
been shown to reduce the risks of complications.
Similarly, reduction of heavy alcohol ingestion, even
in mid-pregnancy, can benefit the infant. However,
smoking/alcohol cessation programmes must be
used with understanding, sensitivity and compassion. Much anti-smoking/alcohol 'advice' merely
induces guilt and anxiety.

Illegal Substances

Management principles

Multidisciplinary approach
Detection of other health problems
Cessation or substitution programme
Appropriate antenatal care
Establish an interpartum and postnatal plan

The management of illegal substance addiction during
pregnancy requires a host of social, nutritional,
educational, medical and psychiatric interventions,
and these women are best managed in specialized
programmes. Social workers may need to assist with
complex social problems before and after delivery.
Drug and alcohol misuse support agencies will be
involved in efforts to stop or substitute the drug of
misuse. Ideally, obstetricians, paediatricians and
anaesthetists will be involved in the management
plans. Compliance and attendance are often poor,
and 'drug liaison' midwives have proved effective in
enhancing attendance and coordination of antenatal
care.

Detection of other health problems is particularly
pertinent in women whose drug dependency exposes
them to risks related to sexually transmitted infections
(STIs) and poor nutrition. Women should be
specifically counselled regarding their risk of exposure
to human immunodeficiency virus (HIV) and offered
an HIV test if this is appropriate. Medical treatment

and avoidance of breast-feeding reduce vertical transmission to the baby.

Methadone substitution improves the pregnancy outcome in cases of opiate addiction. The advantage of methadone is that it can be taken orally, is long-acting and constant blood levels are achieved. In addition, by prescribing the drug in a controlled fashion, it is hoped that the problems associated with street use and the accompanying high-risk sexual behaviour are reduced. Methadone is the only drug available to treat opioid-addicted women. The easiest way to determine the optimal dose of methadone (to avoid both intoxication and withdrawal symptoms) is to admit the pregnant addict to a drug dependency unit. If a dose below 20 mg/day can be achieved, only a minority of babies will develop signs of withdrawal. Manipulation of the dose of methadone should be avoided in the third trimester because of an association with increased fetal problems attributable to fetal withdrawal *in utero*.

Antenatal care should be tailored to the needs of the individual. A detailed mid-trimester ultrasound scan to detect fetal anomalies should usually be performed. Serial ultrasound scans to assess fetal growth may be deemed appropriate. Every effort to enhance compliance should be made; attendance is often better at afternoon rather than morning clinics! Despite the frustrations of caring for this group of women, pregnant addicts have very genuine needs, and effective antenatal care can improve outcomes.

Interpartum and postnatal management plans should be discussed at antenatal clinic visits. Again, individualized plans should be made. Opiate addiction is not a contraindication to opiate analgesia in labour, but larger doses than normal will be necessary. If congenital abnormalities or the risk of newborn withdrawal syndrome necessitate admission to the special care baby unit, this should be discussed before delivery. Decisions regarding breast-feeding will depend on HIV status and the dose and nature of the substance of abuse; again, it is preferable to discuss this subject before delivery.

Learning Points

- Social problems, inadequate antenatal care and poor nutrition compound the complications of substance abuse
- Abuse of both legal and illegal substances has adverse effects on pregnancies
- Risks often relate to the lifestyle associated with substance abuse, rather than to direct effects
- Management of substance abuse in pregnancy should be multidisciplinary

See Also

Small for gestational age (Chapter 21)

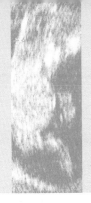

Chapter 23

Unstable or transverse lie

Importance

A lie is described as unstable when the lie and presentation repeatedly change after 37 weeks' gestation. The incidence of an unstable lie is < 1 per cent, and that of a transverse lie in labour is < 0.5 per cent. If the fetal lie is transverse at the time of labour, there are risks of cord prolapse and a compound presentation (which ultimately leads to fetal death and uterine rupture).

Causes

Predisposing factors

Multiparity
Polyhydramnios
Multiple pregnancy
Placenta praevia or pelvic tumours
Fetal anomaly (e.g. hydrocephalus) or uterine anomaly
Fetal macrosomia or contracted maternal pelvis

All forms of malpresentation are associated with a higher incidence of fetal abnormality. In order for the vertex to engage, the head must be flexed and the fetus must have normal movements and tone to allow movement into the correct position. Any disorder that affects the ability of the head to engage or the fetus to move will increase the incidence of malpresentation. Also, increased liquor volume can allow the fetus to be more mobile and thus not to engage. This is associated with a number of fetal abnormalities (see Chapter 10).

Some maternal factors will also have an impact on the fetal lie. The commonest of these are uterine abnormalities, which prevent the fetus from turning as term approaches. Other maternal causes occur when the fetal head cannot engage because of a mass within the pelvis, such as an ovarian cyst or fibroid, or more rarely a very small pelvic inlet. In many cases, the presentation will still be cephalic, but the fetal head will be high. Importantly, a placenta praevia can be the cause of a transverse lie or high presenting part. A very lax maternal abdomen, such as is seen in some grandmultipara, can predispose to an unstable lie, where the fetal presentation changes frequently as the pregnancy reaches term.

Diagnosis and Clinical Assessment

Unless obscuring factors are present (such as multiple pregnancy, placental abruption, obesity), the diagnosis of a transverse lie is straightforward.

History

The key features in the history are similar to those relevant to a breech presentation (see Chapter 7).

Examination

Key findings

Laterally expanded general contour
Reduced symphysis–fundal height
No fetal pole in fundus/lower uterus
Rounded, hard ballottable fetal head in one or other flank
Back palpable across the abdomen: above/below the umbilicus

A vaginal examination should be performed in order to exclude a pelvic tumour or a grossly contracted pelvis. This should not be performed if there is any suggestion of placenta praevia (such as antepartum haemorrhage of uncertain origin).

Investigations

Ultrasound scan is used to confirm the presentation and exclude significant fetal anomalies, pelvic tumours and placenta praevia.

Management

If the examination findings identify an unstable or a transverse lie, the pregnant woman should be admitted to hospital from 37 weeks' gestation. This enables daily observation of fetal lie and presentation, and immediate clinical assistance if membranes rupture or labour begins. If the fetal lie resolves and stabilizes as a longitudinal lie for 24–48 hours, the woman can be discharged home to await the onset of labour.

If the unstable/transverse lie persists, there are three options:

- external cephalic version (ECV), as above, then spontaneous labour is awaited;
- ECV followed by induction of labour;
- elective Caesarean section – the lie should be corrected to longitudinal at operation and a lower segment incision rather than a classical incision should be performed.

Management in Labour

Persistent transverse lie incompatible with vaginal delivery (except in extreme prematurity) and labour carries a risk of cord prolapse when membranes rupture. Caesarean section is thus the preferred option. This can usually be accomplished through a lower segment incision, but if the fetal back is down, a vertical upper segment incision may need to be used to facilitate delivery. This is called a classical incision. In all subsequent pregnancies, the mother will need to be delivered by Caesarean section, as the risk of uterine rupture in labour is 2–5 per cent.

Learning Points

- **Pelvic tumours, fetal abnormalities and placenta praevia should be excluded in cases of unstable lie**
- **Transverse lie is associated with an increased risk of cord prolapse**

See Also

Breech presentation (Chapter 7)

Section 3

On the delivery suite

24. Abdominal pain in pregnancy 99
25. Antepartum haemorrhage 102
26. Cord prolapse 106
27. Failure to progress in the first stage 108
28. Failure to progress in the second stage 112
29. Abnormal fetal heart rate patterns in labour 115
30. Induction of labour 123
31. Intrauterine fetal death 126
32. Maternal collapse 130
33. Meconium 137
34. Neonatal resuscitation 139
35. Normal labour 142
36. Pain relief in labour 148
37. Postpartum haemorrhage 151
38. Preterm labour 155
39. Rupture of membranes while not in labour 159
40. Shoulder dystocia 163

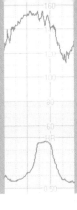

Abdominal pain in pregnancy

Importance

Abdominal pain is the presenting complaint in a large proportion of antenatal admissions. A clear diagnosis will be made in a substantial proportion of cases; in others, no diagnosis will be made despite investigation. As the possible causes of abdominal pain include several conditions associated with significant maternal and perinatal morbidity and mortality, every case warrants careful evaluation.

Causes

Differential diagnosis

- Onset of labour or spurious (false) labour
- Urinary tract infection – cystitis or pyelonephritis
- Appendicitis
- Cholecystitis
- Placental abruption
- Round ligament pain
- Red degeneration of a fibroid

Spurious or false labour can often be distinguished from true labour by a failure of the contractions to increase progressively in strength and duration, and by the absence of a show. Women may be greatly distressed by the contractions and backache is often present.

Acute appendicitis is the commonest surgical condition to accompany pregnancy (1 in 2000 pregnancies). The incidence approximates to that of non-pregnant women. The maternal risks of peritonitis and sepsis, and the fetal risks of premature labour and fetal demise are greatest in cases of perforation. The difficulty in making a diagnosis of appendicitis in

pregnancy increases the risk of perforation. When perforation occurs, maternal and fetal mortality rates of 17 and 43 per cent have been reported.

The differential diagnosis of abdominal pain in pregnancy includes a <u>placental abruption</u>; this is defined as separation of a placenta which is implanted normally in the upper segment of the uterus after 24 weeks' gestation. The resulting bleeding may be revealed or may be entirely concealed. Only small placental abruptions, where abdominal pain is the predominant symptom, will be considered in this chapter; placental abruptions associated with significant antepartum haemorrhage are discussed in Chapter 25.

The round ligaments enlarge markedly in pregnancy. Round ligament pain results from stretching, causing spasm of the hypertrophied muscle ligament.

Red degeneration is a common complication of large fibroids in pregnancy. The pain is caused by ischaemic necrosis within the fibroid that has outgrown its blood supply. Urinary tract infections and cholecystitis are discussed in Chapters 18 and 19, respectively.

Diagnosis and Clinical Assessment

History

Ask about:

Gestational age
Characteristics of the pain
Associated symptoms
Relevant previous history

An accurate history is essential in making a diagnosis.

The likelihood of true or spurious labour increases with advancing gestational age. Appendicitis, urinary tract infections and cholecystitis can occur at any gestation. Round ligament pain is uncommon after 30 weeks' gestation.

In true or spurious labour, the abdominal pain reflects rhythmical, regular contractions, with pain-free intervals. In true labour, the episodic abdominal pain increases in amplitude and frequency. Following a small placental abruption, a cramping pain may be experienced, or perhaps only a mild ache. The abdominal pain in cystitis tends to be suprapubic, whereas pyelonephritis is associated with loin or back pain. The distortion of the abdominal anatomy by the gravid uterus generally leads to a displacement of the appendix upwards and to the right with advancing gestation (Figure 24.1). However, in some cases the appendix remains in the right lower quadrant or in the vicinity of the right kidney, and hence the location of maximal pain in appendicitis is very variable. In cholecystitis, the pain is maximal in the right upper quadrant and may radiate to the back. Round ligament pain is often initiated or exacerbated by sudden movement and is described as an aching, dragging pain, often more severe on the right side of the abdomen, just lateral to the uterus. Red degeneration of a fibroid causes severe constant abdominal pain.

Symptoms of frequency and dysuria are typical of a urinary tract infection. A history of a 'show' of mucus and blood, or of rupture of membranes,

suggests the onset of labour. Antepartum haemorrhage suggests a placental abruption. Nausea and vomiting may be associated with a urinary tract infection, cholecystitis and appendicitis.

A history of urinary tract infections indicates an underlying predisposition to recurrent infections. Urinary tract infections are also more common in medical conditions such as sickle cell anaemia and diabetes. Clearly, a previous history of an appendicectomy will exclude appendicitis. A previous history of uterine fibroids (more common in older women) increases the likelihood of the pain being due to red degeneration.

Examination

> **Check for:**
>
> Tachycardia
> Pyrexia
> Site of maximal tenderness
> Uterine contractions
> Cervical dilatation

On general examination, characteristic features of appendicitis include foetid breath, pyrexia and a tachycardia. A pyrexia and tachycardia are also associated with a urinary tract infection and cholecystitis.

On abdominal examination, loin tenderness is suggestive of pyelonephritis, and right upper quadrant tenderness is typical of cholecystitis. As discussed above, the site of the appendix varies, and thus the location of maximal tenderness is equally variable in appendicitis. Following a small placental abruption, there may be tenderness over the uterus, and the uterus may be more irritable than normal. In round ligament pain, there is unilateral tenderness over the round ligament. Palpable fibroids, with tenderness over the fibroid, are suggestive of a diagnosis of red degeneration. Fibroids may also cause a malpresentation.

On vaginal examination, a finding of progressive dilatation and effacement of the cervix is diagnostic of the onset of labour.

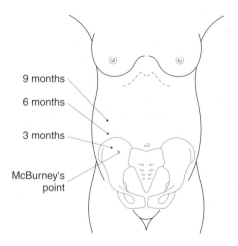

9 months
6 months
3 months
McBurney's point

Figure 24.1   Position of the appendix during pregnancy, which alters with advancing gestation; the site of an appendectomy incision must also alter

Investigations

The choice of appropriate investigations depends on the history and examination findings.

Relevant investigations

Urine microscopy and culture
White blood cell count
Serum amylase level
Kleihauer test
Ultrasound scan

Findings of pus cells, red cells and organisms on urine microscopy may allow diagnosis of a urinary tract infection. Culture of the urine specimen will identify the organism responsible for any infection.

Normal pregnant women may have a mildly elevated white blood cell count; however, a marked elevation is consistent with appendicitis. As in non-pregnant women, a normal amylase level suggests that intraperitoneal inflammation is unlikely, whereas a very high level is indicative of pancreatitis. A Kleihauer test of maternal blood may detect a fetomaternal haemorrhage (fetal cells are resistant to an acid pH) that is consistent with a placental abruption.

The diagnosis of uterine fibroids can usually be confirmed by ultrasound scan. The ultrasound examination of the uterus may indicate a placental abruption, but the absence of positive ultrasound findings does not exclude an abruption. Gallstones may also be demonstrated on an ultrasound scan.

Management

The appropriate management is wholly dependent on the diagnosis. In a substantial number of antenatal women admitted with abdominal pain, no aetiology of the pain is identified, despite thorough investigation. The outcomes of these pregnancies does not differ from those of uncomplicated pregnancies.

Appendicitis

The greatest risk is that delayed diagnosis leads to delayed treatment, i.e. appendicectomy. After the first trimester, a high incision over the site of maximal tenderness should be performed. Tocolytic therapy reduces the risk of preterm labour.

Cholecystitis

This is treated conservatively (antibiotics, intravenous fluids and analgesia).

Placental Abruption

A small placental abruption is managed by bed rest until the pain and any bleeding have resolved. If tests of fetal well-being (see Chapter 20) are satisfactory, the woman can be discharged home and kept under regular surveillance until delivery. An antepartum haemorrhage at term is an indication for delivery. Anti-D gamma globulin should be administered to Rhesus-negative women. The management of larger placental abruptions with significant antepartum haemorrhage is discussed further in Chapter 25.

Round Ligament Pain

Treatment of round ligament pain is with rest and paracetamol analgesia. The condition usually resolves in 2–3 weeks.

Red Degeneration

The pain of red degeneration should be treated with analgesics. Myomectomy is virtually never indicated.

Other Causes of Abdominal Pain

The management of labour and of urinary tract infections is discussed in Chapters 35 and 18, respectively.

Learning Points

- **The differential diagnosis of abdominal pain in pregnancy includes the onset of labour, urinary tract infection, appendicitis, cholecystitis, placental abruption, round ligament pain, red degeneration of a fibroid**
- **The site of the appendix varies in pregnancy. This can delay a diagnosis of appendicitis and lead to increased perinatal and maternal mortality**

See Also

Proteinuria (Chapter 18)
Pruritus and jaundice in pregnancy (Chapter 19)
Antepartum haemorrhage (Chapter 25)
Normal labour (Chapter 35)
Pain relief in labour (Chapter 36)

Chapter 25

Antepartum haemorrhage

Definition

Any vaginal bleeding in pregnancy after 24 weeks and before the onset of labour.

Importance

Pregnancies complicated by antepartum haemorrhage (APH) have an increased risk of perinatal mortality, preterm labour and growth restriction.

Causes

Causes of APH

Main causes
- Placenta praevia
- Placental abruption

Others
- Marginal bleeding from the placenta
- 'Show'
- Local infections of the cervix and vagina
- Tumours
- Varicosities
- Vasa praevia

In placenta praevia the bleeding is predominantly maternal. Growth restriction can occur with repeated small bleeds, but is not generally a feature. Placenta praevia is associated with a doubling in the rate of congenital abnormality. It is more common in women who have had previous Caesarean sections. Placenta praevia can be divided into minor (grades I and II) and major (grades III and IV) cases (see Figure 25.1).

With placental abruption the fetal condition becomes compromised as the placenta shears off the uterine wall. Abruptions severe enough to cause fetal compromise can lead to a consumptive coagulopathy in 30 per cent of women. This is a dangerous condition for mothers and carries a maternal mortality rate of 1 per cent. A combination of coagulopathy and hypotension can lead to renal failure.

Growth restriction is common and probably reflects a poor placenta. This condition also carries an increased risk of congenital fetal malformation. This is more common in women who smoke.

Placenta praevia and abruptions account for 50 per cent of bleeding and represent the greatest threat to the fetus and mother. Although other causes of bleeding appear to be less significant (vasa praevia when a fetal vessel ruptures being the exception), they carry an increased perinatal mortality of at least 3 per cent. They must therefore represent a group of pathological conditions, and thus all APH must be taken seriously.

Diagnosis and Clinical Assessment

Some APHs are life threatening to the mother and fetus. A rapid assessment of the condition of both is a vital first step. If either mother or fetus is compromised, management must be to resuscitate and deliver if necessary.

Fortunately most APHs are moderate or small and permit a full assessment of mother and fetus, with time to establish a diagnosis if possible.

History

Ask about:

Gestation

Amount of bleeding

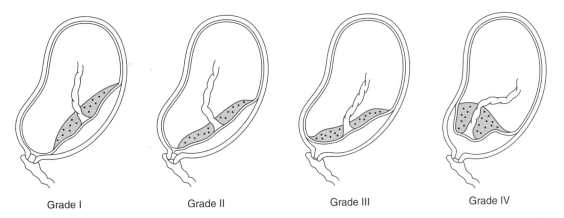

Grade I Grade II Grade III Grade IV

Figure 25.1 Placenta praevia. Grade I: placenta does not reach the internal os. Grade II: lower margin of the placenta reaches (but does not cover) the os. Grade III: placenta covers os when closed but does not cover dilated os. Grade IV: placenta lies centrally over the os

Associated or initiating factors
- Abdominal pain
- Coitus
- Trauma
Leakage of fluid
Previous bleeding
Position of the placenta if known
Previous Caesarean sections
Fetal movements
Smoking
Maternal blood group

Many women will have had an ultrasound prior to admission with bleeding, as fetal anomaly scanning at 18–22 weeks is routine in many obstetric units. This may provide an initial assessment of the placental site.

Placenta praevia usually presents with painless bleeding. Often a small bleed will precede a much larger one. Placental abruption presents with bleeding and pain. The pain can precede the bleeding.

Smoking increases the risk of placenta praevia, placental abruption and marginal bleeding. This is a dose-dependent effect. Even after an APH, women who are still smoking find it very difficult to stop. Pregnant women cannot use nicotine patches and thus are more difficult to help. Intervention at this stage of pregnancy is generally unsuccessful.

Fetal growth restriction is associated with both marginal placental bleeding (from the edge of the placenta) and placental abruption. The mother may have noticed that her baby has been less active.

Immediate Assessment and Management

Immediate assessment of maternal and fetal status is mandatory. Women with significant bleeding will need full resuscitation and consideration for delivery (see below).

Maternal examination

Pulse and blood pressure
Abdominal palpation
- Uterine size
- Tenderness
- Contractions
- Presentation
- Degree of engagement of the presenting part

Vaginal examination

Assess the degree of bleeding
Ascertain cervical changes, which may be indicative of labour
Look for local causes of bleeding
Take bacteriological samples if infection is suspected

A vaginal examination is only performed once a placenta praevia has been excluded.

In placenta praevia the presenting part is usually high, being prevented from engaging by the placenta lying in the lower segment. The fetal condition remains good until the maternal blood loss causes compromise.

In abruption, the maternal and fetal condition may be worse than the blood loss would suggest, as the bleeding is often concealed behind the placenta

(Figure 25.2). Contractions may follow and are often of high frequency. On palpation, the uterus feels tense and tender. Fetal parts are difficult to feel. The uterus may contract readily when manipulated.

Initial fetal assessment will include palpation of size, lie and presentation, auscultation of the fetal heart, and fetal heart rate recording.

Careful history-taking and examination can elucidate the other causes of bleeding. Marginal bleeding from the edge of the placenta can precipitate labour. This type of loss is often recurrent. Vasa praevia leads to fetal exsanguination and acute fetal compromise is seen.

Investigations

Relevant investigations

Full blood count

Group and save with blood cross-matched

Clotting screen

Ultrasound

Kleihauer test

Ultrasound examination has a number of uses. It can be used to establish fetal well-being in conjunction with cardiotocography (CTG), by using the biophysical profile (see Chapter 21) and umbilical artery Doppler velocimetry. It can locate the placenta in relation to the internal cervical os and measure fetal size (the abdominal circumference and head circumference are the most useful measurements). Ultrasound is *not* helpful in diagnosing abruptions

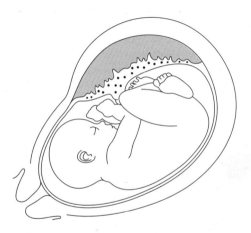

Figure 25.2 Concealed placental abruption

and can only be useful in ascertaining the site of bleeding if a placenta praevia is confirmed.

Magnetic resonance imaging can be helpful in localizing the placenta.

If the source of bleeding is fetal, the fetus is usually quickly compromised. Very rarely, an Apt's test, which relies on fetal haemoglobin being resistant to denaturization by acid, can help if fetal blood loss is suspected.

A Kleihauer test is mandatory for all Rhesus-negative women. All RhD-negative women will require 500 IU anti-D (unless they are already sensitized). The Kleihauer test will tell whether there has been a large fetomaternal haemorrhage, in which case more anti-D will be needed. This is not a useful test in other circumstances, as fetal cells may appear in the maternal circulation in as many as 15 per cent of women at some time in pregnancy, and a lack of fetal cells in the maternal circulation does not rule out an abruption.

Management

Delivery must be expedited if the maternal condition is compromised. If the fetus is compromised, the decision to deliver will be based on the gestational age. In most cases, delivery will be indicated. The method of delivery will be determined by the cause and severity of the bleeding, the fetal gestation and status.

Resuscitation

A team approach should be adopted to resuscitate and safely deliver women with massive obstetric haemorrhage (see Chapter 37). This team will include:

- The obstetric team
- An anaesthetic team
- Senior midwives
- Haematologists
- Paediatricians.

All women with significant bleeding need intravenous access with a large cannula (12 or 14 G).

Placenta Praevia

Women with significant bleeding from a placenta praevia will need delivery by Caesarean section. In cases of acute bleeding, a general anaesthetic should be administered. These women may bleed heavily both during the section and afterwards. The lower segment does not contract efficiently and can lead to severe postpartum haemorrhage. If the placenta praevia is as a result of a previous Caesarean section, there is a risk of the placenta being morbidly adherent to the scar (placenta accreta). In some cases, this may only be safely managed by Caesarean hysterectomy.

If bleeding from a placenta praevia appears to be settling, then delivery can be deferred to achieve fetal maturity. Steroids should be given to enhance fetal lung maturity if the gestation is less than 34 weeks. These women should be admitted and delivered at 37–38 weeks.

Placental Abruption

Placental abruption causing maternal or fetal compromise necessitates delivery. If the fetus is already dead, vaginal delivery after stabilization of the mother is usually the safest option. However, if the bleeding continues and the mother's condition cannot be stabilized, delivery should be achieved by the quickest method, which may be Caesarean section. Coagulopathy will only begin to resolve once the placenta is delivered, but may be severe enough to warrant replacement with fresh frozen plasma, cryoprecipitate and platelets. These women usually labour very quickly. Epidural or spinal anaesthesia must not be used if the clotting studies are abnormal. Central venous pressure lines can be useful but should be sited through an antecubital long line, and not sited or removed until clotting is normal.

During and after delivery it is vital to keep:

- urine output above 30 mL/hour;
- haematocrit above 30 per cent;
- systolic pressure above 100 mmHg.

It may be necessary to admit to the intensive therapy unit if there has been a severe abruption with disseminated intravascular coagulopathy, for intensive monitoring.

Women with a lesser degree of abruption require intravenous access, admission and full fetal assessment as above. Steroids should be given to mature the fetal lungs. Women should remain in hospital whilst bleeding continues or the uterus remains irritable or tender. If any evidence of fetal compromise develops, delivery should be expedited.

Ongoing Pregnancy

Principles

No bleeding, however light, should be dismissed without full investigation

Once APH has occurred, that pregnancy becomes high risk, and a management plan for ongoing fetal surveillance must be formulated and discussed with the mother

Women must be advised to watch for warning signs such as a decrease in the frequency of fetal movements, further bleeding or pain, and should be assessed again should any of these occur

If bleeding settles and the mother is discharged, it is vital that a plan for pregnancy is made. Even if the cause is thought to be minor, extra fetal surveillance is needed as a higher fetal mortality rate is seen. Fetal surveillance for growth and well-being should be instituted at least monthly. If all remains well, induction of labour at term is not needed, but the degree of surveillance after the due date may need to be increased.

Learning Points

- **APH presents a significant risk to mother and fetus**
- **Placenta praevia is the commonest cause**
- **Never perform a vaginal examination until the placental site is known**

See Also

Abdominal pain in pregnancy (Chapter 24)
Postpartum haemorrhage (Chapter 37)

Cord prolapse

Definition

Prolapse of the umbilical cord through the cervix.

Importance

Blood flow to the fetus is jeopardized by compression of the cord or by vasoconstriction of the umbilical arteries due to cold. This leads to critical fetal compromise in a short time.

Causes

In order for the cord to pass through the cervix, the presenting part must not be occluding the outlet. Therefore, any condition in which this occurs may predispose to cord prolapse.

> **Factors which may predispose to cord prolapse**
>
> Malpresentation such as footling breech or transverse lie
> Multiparity
> Hydramnios
> Artificial rupture of membranes with a high presenting part

Because malpresentation is commoner in preterm delivery, cord prolapse is also commoner in these cases. Multiparity is a risk factor only because the head may not engage until late, and the probability of malpresentation is higher. Hydramnios is only a risk if the presenting part has not engaged. The excessive volume of liquor can wash down the cord as the membranes rupture. Iatrogenic cord prolapse can occur if the membranes are artificially ruptured when the presenting part is not engaged.

Diagnosis

The diagnosis is usually made in two ways:

- the cord is felt on vaginal examination;
- the fetal heart rate undergoes a profound and prolonged deceleration.

Management

This is an obstetric emergency.

> **Priorities**
>
> Deliver the baby as soon as possible
> Attempt to minimize cord cooling and compression until delivery can be accomplished

If the cervix is fully dilated, vaginal delivery can be undertaken, if this is thought to be achievable. Otherwise, delivery must be by emergency Caesarean section.

Whilst preparation for delivery is being made, there are various methods which can prevent pressure of the presenting part on the cord:

- The examiner's hand keeps upward pressure on the presenting part vaginally. This is only feasible for a short time and as long as the mother does not have to be transported far for delivery.
- Instilling 500 mL fluid via a Foley catheter into the maternal bladder. This expands the bladder and pushes the presenting part out of the pelvis.
- Placing the mother in the knee–chest position (Figure 26.1). This is only effective if there are no contractions, relying on gravity to keep the presenting part out of the pelvis.

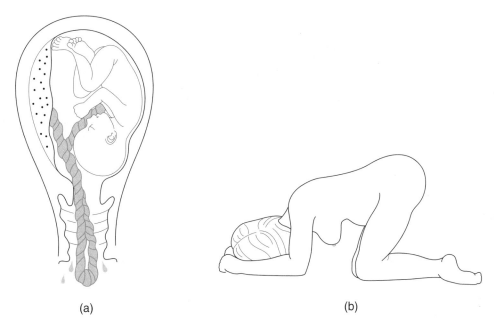

Figure 26.1 (a) Cord prolapse. (b) The knee–chest position

The fetal heart rate should be continuously monitored. As long as the cord is neither cold nor compressed, the fetus should not be compromised. Delivery should be accomplished as soon as possible. Delays of even an hour with good outcomes have been reported if the compression is removed.

Learning Points

- Cord prolapse is an obstetric emergency
- The only treatment is delivery
- This should be accomplished as soon as possible

See Also

Unstable or transverse lie (Chapter 23)
Abnormal fetal heart rate patterns in labour (Chapter 29)

Failure to progress in the first stage

Definition

Failure of labour to proceed at a defined rate. The definition devised by Freidman is the most widely used. This takes progress of dilatation of the cervix at 1 cm/hour to be normal. This may be an overestimate, as the data are not normally distributed.

Importance

Delay in the first stage of labour may present a risk to both the mother and the fetus. Fetuses become gradually more hypoxic as labour progresses. Long labours are associated with a higher incidence of fetal infection. Maternal morbidity in terms of difficult vaginal or Caesarean delivery becomes more likely. In the developing world, prolonged labour due to obstruction leads to pressure necrosis and fistula formation, if the woman survives at all.

Causes

Whilst descent and rotation of the head are important, it is cervical dilatation which mainly defines progress. There are three recognized patterns of failure to progress in the first stage. These are all easily recognizable on partographic representation (Figure 27.1).

Prolonged Latent Phase

The mean length of latent phase is 8.6 hours, with a standard deviation (SD) of 6 hours in nulliparae; in

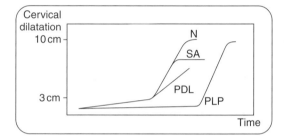

Figure 27.1 Partograms showing patterns of failure to progress in labour. PLP, prolonged latent phase; PDL, primary dysfunctional labour; SA, secondary arrest; N, normal

multiparae the corresponding figures are 5.3 hours and 4 hours. Failure of cervical remodelling appears to be the cause in many women. A persistent occipito-posterior position may also cause this.

Primary Dysfunctional Labour

This affects 26 per cent of nulliparae and 8 per cent of multiparae; 85 per cent of women respond to Syntocinon augmentation, but the rates of instrumental delivery are high. This suggests a combination of ineffective uterine activity with some true or positional obstruction.

Secondary Arrest

This is a particularly dangerous situation, especially in multiparae. It affects 6 per cent of nulliparae and 2 per cent of multiparae. This condition is more likely to be due to a true mechanical problem.

Clinical Assessment

If labour does not appear to be progressing at the expected rate, it is vital to assess the mother and fetus to try to establish a cause. No solution to failure to progress in the first stage can be offered without a full assessment of the mother and fetus.

There are three key factors to consider:

- the powers
- the passages
- the passenger.

Powers

Are the Contractions Adequate (Strong Enough or Frequent Enough)?

The contraction frequency does not normally need to be more than three to four in every 10 minutes. Contraction strength is much more difficult to identify. Intrauterine pressure catheters can be used, but are often unhelpful. A normal pressure is 60 mmHg, but many women will progress adequately on much lower pressures.

Passages

Is the Cervix Compliant?

In order for labour to progress normally, the cervix must have undergone remodelling, which causes softening. Throughout the whole of pregnancy, the cervix must retain the pregnancy. At term, under the influence of oestrogen and relaxin, this must change to allow the cervix to efface and dilate. Sometimes this process does not occur. This is especially common in labours that are induced before this process is complete (see Chapter 30).

Is the Pelvis of Normal Shape and Size?

The bony pelvis is usually shaped to allow descent and rotation of the fetal head (see Chapter 35). The shape and size of the pelvis can be critical. An android pelvis is more likely to cause slowing of labour, as it does not easily allow rotation of the fetal head. The shape of the pelvis can sometimes be felt by careful vaginal examination. More often than not, vaginal examination of the pelvis is unhelpful. Maternal height is the best indicator of pelvic capacity.

Passenger

Is the Baby Too Big?

Size can be estimated clinically, by ultrasound scan and by asking the mother's opinion, if she has had children before.

Factors known to increase fetal size
Maternal diabetes
Maternal obesity
Previous large babies
Prolonged pregnancy

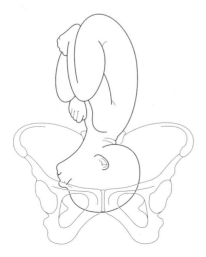 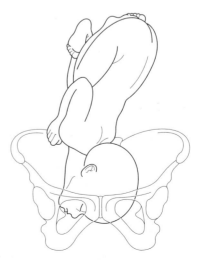

Figure 27.2 Brow presentation – conversion to either face or vertex presentation may occur during labour

Is There a Problem with the Fit of the Presenting Part?

The presentation is critical. Malpresentation such as a brow (Figure 27.2) presents a diameter to the pelvis of 13.5 cm. This is not compatible with vaginal delivery.

A malposition, which is defined as a fetal head that does not follow the normal pattern of rotation from occipitotransverse to occipitoanterior, may also present a larger diameter, as the fetal head is egg-shaped, not spherical. Occipitoposterior positions are the most common malpresentation and present a diameter of 12.5 cm (Figure 27.3).

> **Signs that the head is not fitting well through the pelvis**
>
> Failure of dilatation on repeated vaginal examination
> Failure of descent (on abdominal palpation)
> Moulding, where the mobile bones of the skull meet, obliterating the fontanelles and eventually overriding each other
> Caput, which is oedema of the scalp

The condition of the fetus should be assessed by review of the fetal heart rate recording and fetal blood scalp sampling if indicated (see Chapter 29).

Management

After a full assessment, the treatment can be addressed. This will be directed at the pattern of delay. There are additional considerations in the management of women who have had a previous Caesarean section or where there is a malpresentation (see Chapter 15). Evidence of fetal compromise will usually be an indication for delivery by Caesarean section. When Syntocinon is used, there should be continuous monitoring of the fetal heart rate.

Prolonged Latent Phase

Augmentation with oxytocin does not improve outcome. This leads to increased Caesarean section rates and low neonatal Apgar scores. The mainstays of management are:

- sympathy
- patience
- making the mother comfortable
- avoiding intervention except where fetal compromise is suspected.

Primary Dysfunctional Labour

The mainstay of management is careful Syntocinon augmentation with regular assessment to ensure progress.

Secondary Arrest

This condition is more likely to be due to a true mechanical problem. Before augmentation of uterine

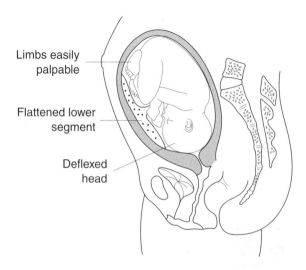

Limbs easily palpable

Flattened lower segment

Deflexed head

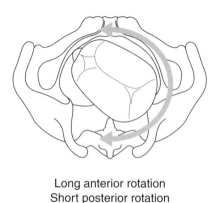

Long anterior rotation
Short posterior rotation

Figure 27.3 Clinical findings associated with occipitoposterior position

activity is undertaken, it is vital to establish that there are no signs of obstruction.

If it can be established that there is no sign of obstruction and that uterine inertia appears to be the cause, Syntocinon augmentation can be used. Progress will improve in 65 per cent of women, but the Caesarean section rate is ten times that of the background rate, even in those women who appear to progress.

If there are signs of obstruction or if there continues to be failure to progress with Syntocinon, delivery should be by Caesarean section.

Multiparae who are contracting well do not undergo secondary arrest unless there is a good reason. Syntocinon augmentation in these women can lead to rupture of the uterus and fetal (and even maternal) death.

Learning Points

- **Prolonged latent phase should not be augmented**
- **Syntocinon is usually appropriate in primary dysfunctional labour**
- **Secondary arrest is a dangerous condition in multiparae**
- **Never augment without making a diagnosis of the cause of the delay**

See Also

Previous Caesarean section (Chapter 15)
Abnormal fetal heart rate patterns in labour (Chapter 29)
Normal labour (Chapter 35)
Failure to progress in the second stage (Chapter 28)

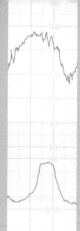

Failure to progress in the second stage

Definition

Failure to achieve a spontaneous vaginal delivery after a defined duration of active pushing.

The point at which spontaneous delivery becomes unlikely is difficult to define. In multiparous women, 95 per cent will have delivered within an hour. After 2 hours, spontaneous delivery is very unlikely. In nulliparous women, there is no time at which a distinction can be drawn. Most women are exhausted after an hour of active pushing, and so many units use this as a cut-off for intervention.

Importance

Pushing reduces uterine blood flow. Prolonged pushing can lead to fetal hypoxia. Delay may be indicative of a pathological process. The rate of instrumental delivery varies between units. In many areas, the liberal use of epidural analgesia has led to an increase in the numbers of women who experience delay.

Causes

The same factors need to be assessed in the second stage as in the first stage of labour (see Chapter 27).

> Causes for delay in the second stage
>
> Inadequate contractions
> Fetal size
> Narrow pelvic outlet

Malpresentation
Malposition

During the transition phase, as labour moves from the first to the second stage, the contractions are normally boosted by the Ferguson reflex (see Chapter 35). Epidural analgesia abolishes or reduces this.

The cervical component of delay in the first stage is not important here. The bony pelvis is very important and may contribute to failure of the presenting part to descend or rotate.

The size of the fetus can be critical. Sometimes cephalopelvic disproportion only becomes apparent in the second stage. More often, it is preceded by a primary dysfunctional labour or secondary arrest. It must be particularly suspected where a primary dysfunctional labour has not been corrected by Syntocinon. The position of the presenting part is also critical. Malpositions or malpresentations can present a larger diameter to the pelvis and result in failure to deliver.

Diagnosis and Clinical Assessment

This is made if, after active directed pushing, there is no sign of impending delivery, after a set time period (usually 1–2 hours).

History

> Ask about:
>
> Is this a first labour?
> Any history of difficult deliveries or large babies?

Are there any risk factors for fetal macrosomia (see
   Chapter 13)?
How tall is the mother?
Has progress in the first stage been normal (see
   Chapter 27)?
Is the epidural too effective for efficient pushing?

Examination

Abdominal palpation

Contraction frequency and strength
Fetal size
Fetal position (where is the fetal back?)
Whether any fetal head is still palpable in the abdomen

Vaginal examination

Shape and size of the bony pelvis
Level of the presenting part in relation to the ischial spines
Position of the presenting part
Degree of moulding and caput

The mother's general condition should be assessed as she may be too anxious, frightened or exhausted to push effectively. After a full assessment has been performed, it may be possible to elucidate why delivery has not occurred. Fetal condition should be assessed for any signs of fetal intolerance to maternal pushing (see Chapter 29).

Management

The treatment is to deliver the baby by the safest means for both baby and mother. The options are:

- continue pushing
- augment contractions
- assisted vaginal delivery
- Caesarean section.

If progress is still occurring and the fetus appears to be tolerating labour, a further period of pushing can be allowed. If contractions are not regular or strong, consideration may be given to using Syntocinon in the second stage for a short time (usually 0.5–1 hour).

If there is no sign of progress, contractions are good, or if maternal or fetal condition is causing concern, then delivery should be promptly undertaken.

Assisted Vaginal Delivery

Before an assisted vaginal delivery is begun, certain requirements must be met.

Requirements for assisted vaginal delivery

Rupture of membranes
Fully dilated cervix
Cephalic presentation
Knowledge of the position of the fetal head
Adequate pelvis by clinical pelvimetry
Fetal head one-fifth or less palpable abdominally

If these requirements are not met, Caesarean section may be a safer method of delivery. If there are features suggesting that vaginal delivery may be difficult, such as poor progress in the first stage of labour or the presence of caput or moulding on vaginal examination, instrumental delivery should be performed in theatre.

Two methods exist for assisting vaginal delivery: forceps and ventouse. Adequate analgesia is essential. A ventouse delivery may be accomplished with perineal infiltration of local anaesthetic or an additional pudendal block, which provides anaesthesia to sacral nerve roots 2, 3 and 4. Forceps deliveries can be more uncomfortable. A pudendal block is the minimum analgesia for a non-rotational forceps, but epidural or spinal analgesia is preferred.

Progress must be made with each pull for both methods. The attempt is abandoned in favour of Caesarean section if progress is not made. Delivery should be accomplished after four contractions.

Forceps Delivery

Forceps are designed to cradle the head of the fetus and provide traction around the head to assist delivery. There are many types, but the two most commonly used are as follows:

- Neville–Barnes forceps – these have a pelvic and cephalic curve (Figure 28.1) and are designed to deliver a fetus in a direct occipitoanterior position;
- Kielland's forceps – these have a cephalic curve, but a very minimal sacral curve. They are used for rotational deliveries, where the fetal head is occipitotransverse or occipitoposterior (Figure 28.2).

The blades are positioned to lie over the parietal eminence. Traction occurs in the line of the pelvis, with contractions. An episiotomy is usually performed.

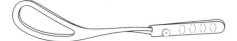

Figure 28.1 Neville–Barnes forceps

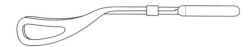

Figure 28.2 Kielland's forceps

Ventouse

The ventouse or vacuum aids delivery by utilizing a metal or Silastic cup, which fixes to the fetal head under vacuum, allowing traction on it. Using the correct cup, delivery can be accomplished in most cases, even when rotation is required. The cup is applied over the fetal occiput and an initial vacuum of 20 kPa is achieved. A check is performed to ensure no maternal tissue is trapped and that the cup is correctly positioned. The vacuum is then increased to 80 kPa. Traction occurs in the line of the maternal pelvis with contractions and good maternal effort. An episiotomy is not always necessary, as the cup does not increase the fetal head diameter.

What are the Risks to the Mother and Baby?

The maternal risks relate mainly to perineal trauma. The risk of third-degree or fourth-degree tears is four to ten times that with spontaneous delivery. This is higher in units that use midline episiotomy. Deliveries where the fetal head is still high carry the highest risk of maternal trauma and should not be attempted. Ventouse deliveries are associated with less maternal trauma, but are more likely to fail (up to 27 per cent will fail, especially if there is marked caput, a big baby or an occipitoposterior position). Ninety per cent of forceps deliveries should be successful.

The risks to the fetus are also primarily of trauma. Ventouse deliveries carry a higher risk of minor trauma such as cephalohaematoma (8 per cent vs. 3 per cent for forceps), bruising and abrasions, and a small risk of the more severe subgaleal haemorrhage.

Forceps deliveries are associated with facial nerve injury, which usually resolves spontaneously, bruising to the fetal face and, rarely, intracranial haemorrhage. More difficult deliveries carry a higher risk to the fetus.

It must be noted that fetuses delivered by Caesarean section may also sustain injury, and a second stage Caesarean section is not without risk to the mother. Long-term follow-up studies have shown no difference between infants delivered spontaneously or by assisted vaginal delivery.

Following an assisted vaginal delivery for delay in the second stage, there is a higher risk of postpartum haemorrhage. This is from two areas: perineal trauma and uterine inertia. Prompt perineal repair and liberal use of additional Syntocinon infusions help to minimize this.

Learning Points

- Delay in the second stage must be correctly diagnosed
- Assisted vaginal delivery is only one remedy. The others include improved contractions, more time and Caesarean section

See Also

Normal labour (Chapter 35)
Failure to progress in the first stage (Chapter 27)
Shoulder dystocia (Chapter 40)

Abnormal fetal heart rate patterns in labour

Definitions

The cardiotocograph (CTG) is made up of a recording of the fetal heart rate (FHR) and uterine contractions (tocograph). The heart rate is determined by electronic fetal monitoring (EFM) either by using external Doppler ultrasound to detect the movement of the fetal heart or by measuring the interval between QRS complexes using a fetal scalp electrode (FSE) attached to the presenting part.

The *baseline* is the mean FHR in beats/minute (bpm). *Variability* is the term used to describe (in bpm) the small deviations from the baseline lasting less than 15 seconds. *Accelerations* are an increase in the FHR of more than 15 bpm for more than 15 seconds. *Decelerations* are falls in FHR of more than 15 bpm for more than 15 seconds.

Importance

Electronic fetal monitoring is now the most common method used for fetal assessment during labour in the UK. It is a monitoring technique that is not without problems. The major limitation is that it has a poor specificity for detecting fetal compromise. It has a place in the monitoring of fetuses which are identified as being at increased risk, but randomized controlled trials have not demonstrated that electronic monitoring is superior to intermittent auscultation in problem-free pregnancies. Whilst it is recognized that a fetus which shows a normal heart rate pattern during labour is likely to have a good outcome, most fetuses which demonstrate FHR abnormalities during labour will also have a good outcome. Defining which fetuses are truly compromised represents one of the most difficult aspects of intrapartum management. An understanding of the physiology of FHR changes is helpful.

Factors Affecting Fetal Response to Labour

The normal FHR pattern represents a balance of the sympathetic and parasympathetic nervous systems of the fetus. Thus for a FHR pattern to be normal, an intact central nervous system (CNS) is required. Damage to the CNS of the developing fetus will impact upon the FHR pattern. A number of physiological and pathological factors will alter this pattern, usually in fairly well-defined ways.

The ability of the fetus to tolerate labour will be determined by fetal reserve, placental perfusion, duration of labour, frequency of contractions and maternal condition. Factors that will influence or reflect fetal ability to tolerate labour may be obvious at the onset of the labour or occur as labour progresses. Recognition of these is an important aspect in determining further management when FHR abnormalities arise (Table 29.1). The presence of one or more of these factors is an indication for continuous EFM.

The presence of meconium may increase the index of suspicion that the fetus is compromised (see Chapter 33). Placental gas transfer only occurs during uterine relaxation. If contractions are too frequent, the ability of the fetus to clear carbon dioxide can be impaired, producing firstly a respiratory acidosis, and

Table 29.1 Risk factors for impaired fetal ability to cope with labour

Pre-existing maternal problems	Pre-existing fetal problems	Intrapartum events
Pre-eclampsia	Fetal growth restriction	Use of oxytocin
Post-term pregnancy	Prematurity	Epidural analgesia
Prolonged rupture of membranes	Oligohydramnios	Vaginal bleeding
Diabetes	Multiple pregnancy	Maternal pyrexia
Antepartum haemorrhage	Breech presentation	Meconium
Maternal medical problems	Abnormal Dopplers	FHR of < 100 or > 160

eventually, if not resolved, hypoxia and metabolic acidosis. If a placenta is unhealthy, even normal uterine contractions may be enough to impair gas transfer. However, excessive uterine activity, as can occur when oxytocin is used, can compromise placental gas exchange even across a healthy placenta.

Conditions such as repeated small abruptions and pre-eclampsia can affect the placental efficiency in gas exchange. A large number of other conditions can also produce pathological changes in the placenta, but these are the two most commonly encountered. A poorly functioning placenta may also be reflected as effects on fetal growth, liquor volume and umbilical artery Doppler waveform.

CTG Classification

Cardiotocographs are classified as normal, suspicious or pathological (abnormal) (Table 29.2) by four key features: baseline FHR, variability, accelerations and decelerations (Table 29.3).

Table 29.2 Cardiotocograph classification

Category	Definition
Normal	All four features on the CTG are in the reassuring category
Suspicious	Any one non-reassuring feature on the CTG
Pathological	Any one abnormal feature or two or more non-reassuring features

Table 29.3 Categorization of fetal heart rate features

Feature	Reassuring	Non-reassuring	Abnormal
Baseline	110–160 bpm	100–109 or 161–180 bpm	< 100 or > 180 bpm
Variability	5 bpm	< 5 bpm for > 40 minutes	< 5 bpm for > 90 minutes
Accelerations	Present	Uncertain significance if absent when CTG is otherwise normal	Uncertain significance if absent when CTG is otherwise normal
Decelerations	None	Early or variable Single prolonged deceleration up to 3 minutes	Late, variable with abnormal features Single prolonged deceleration > 3 minutes

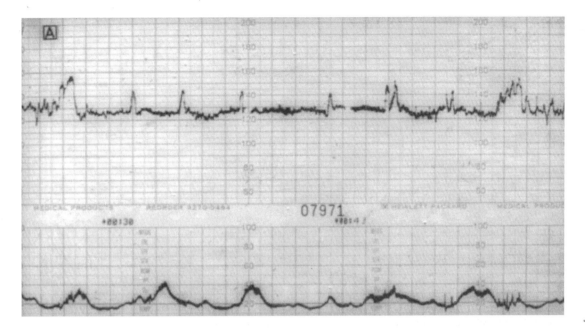

Figure 29.1 An intrapartum cardiotocograph showing a normal fetal heart rate pattern

Reassuring Heart Rate Features (Figure 29.1)

Baseline Rate

The baseline should be between 110 and 160 bpm. The baseline rate is susceptible to a number of determinants. The resting heart rate will be affected by maternal temperature, and a rise in baseline is seen as maternal temperature increases. The fetus will also show a rise in baseline FHR in response to gradually developing hypoxia and acidosis. This is one of the very few coping mechanisms the fetus has, as it is unable to increase its stroke volume.

Variability

The variability, which is the bandwidth in the quiet state, is normally between 5 and 25 bpm. The baseline variability is the balance of the parasympathetic and sympathetic nervous systems.

Accelerations

A normal CTG should include at least two accelerations in 20 minutes. Accelerations are associated with fetal movement, and in labour may be seen with contractions, as sympathetic drive is activated. They are signs of fetal health and demonstrate a normal response to a physiological event. The absence of accelerations with an otherwise normal CTG is of uncertain significance.

Tocograph

The final part of the CTG to evaluate is the tocograph. This is a readout of the contraction frequency and duration. It is most usually measured via a pressure transducer strapped to the maternal abdomen. Very occasionally, an intrauterine pressure catheter is used. If this is the case, the tocograph can also provide data on contraction strength. The abdominal transducer cannot do this, the peak being associated only with the tightness of the belt around the abdomen. An assessment of contraction frequency and duration (with strength if available) forms a vital part of the assessment of an abnormal CTG.

Non-reassuring and Abnormal Fetal Heart Rate Patterns

Bradycardia

This is a drop from the baseline of more than 15 bpm for greater than 3 minutes. The causes include:

- severe fetal hypoxia
- maternal hypotension
- prolonged cord compression.

The fetus cannot sustain a bradycardia for long. In general, if a bradycardia persists for 9 minutes, the fetus should be delivered without delay. During this time, it is imperative that causes such as hypotension

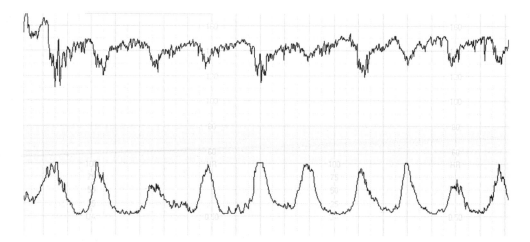

Figure 29.2   Early decelerations on the cardiotocograph

are corrected, as doing so will also resuscitate the fetus. Occasionally a long-lasting or intermittent bradycardia can be due to fetal heart block. This is uncommon, and if fetal compromise is suspected, erring on the side of caution is safest.

Tachycardia

This is a prolonged rise in baseline above the normal rate (160 bpm). The causes will include:

- pyrexia
- fetal compromise (usually gradual-onset hypoxia)

- drug effects (especially beta-sympathomimetics used to suppress preterm labour).

Loss of Variability

This is a loss of variation (bandwidth) of the FHR about the baseline rate. A variability of less than 5 bpm is considered non-reassuring if it persists for more than 40 minutes and abnormal if it continues for more than 90 minutes. (Table 29.3). Loss of normal variability is seen when the balance between the parasympathetic and sympathetic systems is affected.

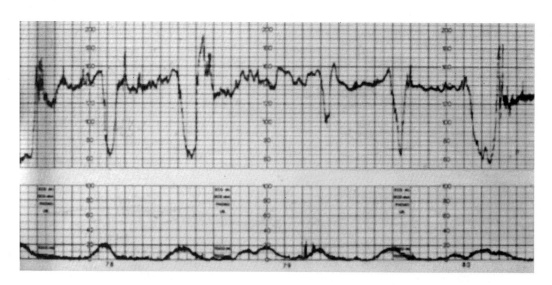

Figure 29.3   Variable decelerations on the cardiotocograph

Early Decelerations

These start with the onset of the contraction, reach a nadir at the contraction's height and resolve as it wanes (Figure 29.2). They are thought to be due to head compression, producing an increase in vagal output, slowing heart rate temporarily until the compression is relieved. They are very uncommon.

Variable Decelerations

As the name implies, these may be variable in timing, shape and duration (Figure 29.3). They often have a characteristic overshoot before and after the contraction. They are usually due to umbilical cord compression. Their characteristic shape is produced because the umbilical vein is more compressible than the umbilical artery. This leads to an initial reduction in fetal blood pressure, as venous return is impeded. A rise in heart rate occurs to compensate. As the arteries become compressed, the heart rate falls. This is relieved as the arteries decompress, and an overshoot is seen just before the vein decompresses. Variable decelerations are seen in 20 per cent of all labours. If they are prolonged or repetitive, they can lead to hypoxia, as the fetal reserves are depleted. They are more commonly seen when the liquor volume is reduced, as the cord becomes more easily compressed against the uterine wall.

Variable decelerations are described as atypical when they are slow to recover or there is a loss of variability during the deceleration.

Late Decelerations (Figure 29.4)

These are the most worrying type of deceleration. They reach a nadir after the low point of the contraction. They represent deficiencies of placental gas transfer and may indicate developing hypoxia.

Diagnosis and Clinical Assessment

When FHR abnormalities are seen on the CTG, it is important to examine the case as a whole, before trying to decide how best to proceed.

As we have seen, the causes of changes in the CTG are many and varied. The CTG represents the effect of a combination of events on the FHR. In order to under-

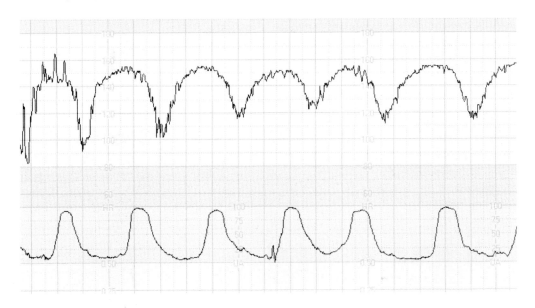

Figure 29.4 Late decelerations on the cardiotocograph

stand what the changes mean, it is vital to try to piece together why these may be happening. Even in cases of bradycardia, a search for the cause is important, as this may be easily remediable (e.g. supine hypotension).

History

Ask about:

Use of prostaglandins or oxytocin
Presentation
Time of rupture of membranes and colour of the liquor
Frequency and duration of contractions
Progress (dilatation and descent)
Type of analgesia (pethidine, recent siting or top-up of epidural)
Recent vaginal examination, vomiting or use of bedpan

Whenever possible, it is important to obtain a history of the pregnancy and labour. This will provide clues to help interpret the CTG. The important features relating to the pregnancy will include an accurate estimate of gestation, details of any past history of adverse pregnancy outcome or small babies and any problems encountered in this pregnancy. Relevant antenatal problems will include a history of antepartum haemorrhage, hypertension, intrauterine growth restriction and diabetes.

Examination

When CTG changes are seen, a full reassessment of the mother can often yield important information.

Check:

Maternal condition for:
- Signs of dehydration (ketosis, dry tongue etc.)
- Tachycardia
- Hypotension
- Pyrexia
Vaginal examination for:
- Progress (dilatation, descent)
- Moulding and caput
- Colour of the liquor/bleeding
- Prolapsed cord

Once all the available information has been accrued, it is important to try to make a diagnosis. CTG changes in themselves are not a diagnosis, but only a sign of a problem that is reflected in the changes seen.

Management

Management is determined by the diagnosis and CTG classification. Whilst sometimes it is not possible to make a diagnosis, there will always be features of the history and examination which help to define the management.

Suspicious CTG

Priorities

Ensure that the quality of the CTG is adequate
Assess the mother to establish possible causes
Remedy any reversible causes
Continue to observe CTG for further suspicious features

If the quality of the CTG does not allow interpretation, this may be due to poor contact with an external transducer or the scalp electrode becoming detached. Check the maternal pulse and establish the true FHR by auscultation using a Pinnard's fetal stethoscope. If monitoring externally, consider changing to FSE or, if already using this, check the position of the transducer.

CTG abnormalities may be seen in response to changes in maternal condition. The commonest are bradycardia secondary to hypotension, tachycardia secondary to maternal pyrexia, or tachycardia and variable decelerations secondary to uterine hyperstimulation with oxytocin.

Hypotension
This may be caused by:

- epidural anaesthesia (the uterine blood flow falls in response to vasodilatation in the legs);
- supine position (aortocaval compression);
- vasovagal stimulus (vomiting etc.).

Shifting the maternal position to left lateral, giving a bolus of 500 mL i.v. fluid or antiemetics can alleviate most of these causes and return the uterine perfusion to normal, allowing fetal resuscitation. Hypotension due to blood loss will usually necessitate delivery.

Pyrexia/Tachycardia
Pyrexia can be due to infection or prolonged epidural anaesthesia (impaired maternal heat exchange). Administration of antibiotics and antipyretics can produce a normalization in the temperature and FHR. When infection is suspected (pyrexia of $> 37.8°C$ on

two occasions an hour apart), antibiotics must be given in high dose as group B streptococcal infection may be the cause and can be potentially life threatening for both fetus and mother. Other causes of maternal tachycardia include dehydration and use of tocolytics (Chapter 38) and should respond to giving additional fluids and reducing the rate of tocolytic infusion, respectively.

Uterine Hyperstimulation

This is a common scenario in many induced or augmented labours. Placental gas exchange only occurs during uterine relaxation, and thus prolonged hyperstimulation can lead to gradual fetal compromise. The CTG findings will usually be contractions of frequency of more than four every 10 minutes. FHR changes may show a gradual increase in heart rate, as the fetus adapts to developing hypoxia, a loss in variability, also with increasing hypoxia, and variable decelerations, usually caused by cord compression.

Reducing or stopping the oxytocin infusion may produce a complete resolution in these changes, as fetal gas transfer is restored to normal. If uterine hypercontractility persists, tocolysis may be necessary (see Chapter 38). If this then means that progress in labour is halted, consideration of Caesarean section may be required.

In all these cases, if the CTG returns to normal, no further assessment of fetal well-being is required. If the CTG remains suspicious, monitoring should be continued to detect any further suspicious features, taking into account the overall clinical situation.

Pathological CTG

> **Priorities**
>
> Move mother into left lateral position
> Assess the mother to establish possible causes as above
> Remedy any reversible causes as above
> Decide if fetal blood sampling or other means of assessing fetal status are indicated
> Expedite delivery

Deciding if Fetal Blood Sampling (FBS) is Indicated

The most common scenario is that a cause is suspected or discovered which cannot be remedied (e.g. mild growth restriction) and in order for the labour to be allowed to continue, a further assessment of fetal well-being is required. CTG changes are poor indicators of true hypoxia and acidosis. Even in the presence of the worst changes, only 50 per cent of fetuses will be acidotic. Therefore, another method of identifying truly compromised fetuses must be used. The aim is to identify fetuses that are becoming acidotic due to impaired gas transfer, anaerobic glycolysis and lactic acidosis. The most commonly used method is fetal scalp blood sampling.

However, delivery of the baby will be the preferred option when the changes on the CTG are pathological and the immediate well-being of the baby is thought to be compromised. This is more likely when there is a history of growth restriction, hypertension, prematurity, postmaturity or meconium. If there is evidence of significant abruption (see Chapter 25), cord prolapse (see Chapter 26) or scar dehiscence (Chapter 15) on examination, immediate delivery is mandatory. In these cases, the CTG may show a bradycardia, a tachycardia or prolonged late decelerations. Delivery will also be the preferred option when a CTG is pathological but other means of establishing fetal well-being are not feasible, such as in very early labour, or are contraindicated.

> **Contraindication to FBS**
>
> Maternal infection (HIV, herpes simplex, hepatitis)
> Fetal bleeding disorders
> Prematurity (< 34 weeks)
> Prolonged bradycardia

Fetal Scalp Blood Sampling

This is performed by inserting a small endoscope *per vaginum*, which allows visualization of the fetal scalp. The patient should be in the left lateral position. A small puncture is then made and a capillary sample of fetal blood taken.

The normal fetal pH is 7.2–7.45. If scalp pH is 7.25 or more, FBS should be repeated if the FHR abnormality persists. In labour, pH levels of 7.21–7.24 require close surveillance with repeat sampling within a short time (30 minutes) to detect a trend. Additional information such as the base deficit, which gives information about the degree of compensation occurring (normal is > -8 mEq/L), and the oxygen and carbon dioxide levels, which can help to differentiate respiratory from metabolic acidosis, can be very valuable.

Both the absolute pH and trend help in deciding whether the labour can be allowed to continue. A pH of < 7.2 should lead to immediate delivery of the fetus. Continuing CTG abnormalities in the presence of a normal pH and base deficit will necessitate further sampling. Performing two samples can demonstrate a trend that can then be used to decide on the likelihood of achieving a vaginal delivery. Judgement must be used to weigh up all the factors in labour before a decision can be made on the best management.

Whilst it is recognized that fetuses with a low pH are vulnerable, most will be delivered in good condition with normal Apgar scores. The pH shows little correlation with fetal outcome, except for the extremely low values (< 7.0). The inability of both CTG and pH values to predict outcome is probably related to the fact that many events in labour are anteceded by events in pregnancy, which go undetected. Pathological changes on the CTG and inability to tolerate labour may simply be the end stage of a long-lasting prelabour pathological state. The introduction of CTG monitoring onto all labour wards in the UK has not reduced the rate of cerebral palsy.

Other methods of fetal evaluation have included fetal stimulation by methods such as vibroacoustic stimulus. A fetus which shows accelerations following stimulation is thought to be healthy and not in need of immediate delivery. These methods are not commonly used in units that have access to pH sampling, but have been shown to be of use when this is not available.

Expedite Delivery

Where fetal compromise is suspected or confirmed, delivery should occur as soon as possible, consistent with maternal safety. Ideally this should be within 30 minutes. The mode of delivery will depend on the stage of labour, although Caesarean section may be the preferred option in the second stage if a difficult rotational instrumental delivery is anticipated.

After Delivery

Umbilical artery acid–base status should be assessed by taking paired blood samples from the umbilical artery and vein.

Learning Points

- **The CTG is a tool for assessing fetal status that cannot be used in isolation. Factors relating to the pregnancy and labour are important in evaluating an abnormal CTG**
- **A normal CTG is very reassuring, but abnormalities do not mean the fetus is truly compromised**
- **Other methods of evaluation of fetal status can be used to give further information**
- **CTG changes can reflect antepartum events that may have long-lasting effects on outcome**
- **The CTG is most useful in detecting gradual changes in labour in at-risk fetuses**

See Also

Reduced fetal movements (Chapter 20)
Meconium (Chapter 33)
Normal labour (Chapter 35)

Further Reading

National Institute for Clinical Excellence. *The Use of Electronic Fetal Monitoring. Inherited Clinical Guideline C.* National Institute for Clinical Excellence, London, 2001.

Induction of labour

Importance

Induction is an important technique to initiate labour when there is sufficient fetal or maternal need. Induction rates vary widely between units and over time but are typically around 20 per cent in the UK. Whilst the technique may be viewed by women as desirable to end a pregnancy, it is generally not without risk, and these risks must be carefully balanced against the indications before embarking on an induction of labour.

Indications

> **The most common indications**
>
> Prolonged pregnancy
> Fetal growth restriction
> Maternal hypertension
> Antepartum haemorrhage at term
> Maternal request

Once a pregnancy reaches 40 weeks +10 days, the risks of induction of labour are balanced by the problems of prolonged pregnancy (see Chapter 17). At gestations of less than this, induction of labour results in a higher Caesarean section rate. In other circumstances where there is fetal or maternal disease, the risks of continuing the pregnancy must be balanced against the likelihood of success. In conditions where there is a need for urgent delivery, and the chances of a successful induction are small, Caesarean section is a better option.

Maternal request is a common reason given for induction of labour. Whilst this may be successful where the cervix is favourable, even in a multipara it is not without risk and should not be undertaken lightly.

Risks

> **Fetal risks**
>
> Uterine hyperstimulation
> Fetal hypoxia
> Cord prolapse

Fetal risks will be related to the process of induction, or the indication for induction, which may indicate a poorly functioning placenta. The fetus is only oxygenated during uterine relaxation. How long a fetus copes with overcontraction will be related to the placental and fetal condition. Often it is those pregnancies that have encountered problems, such as intrauterine growth restriction (IUGR) or pre-eclampsia, which need to be induced. Cord prolapse can occur with artificial rupture of the membranes (ARM) if the presenting part is not fixed in the pelvis. This is more of a problem with multiparae.

> **Maternal risks**
>
> Prolonged labour
> Failure to establish in labour
> Instrumental vaginal delivery
> Caesarean section
> Postpartum haemorrhage
> Uterine rupture

Maternal risks relate in the main to a failure to labour efficiently and problems of the fetal response. Both of these lead to a higher incidence of operative vaginal delivery. Prostaglandins occasionally produce profound uterine hypertonus, necessitating urgent Caesarean section. Multiparous women are particularly sensitive to Syntocinon, and its use can cause hyperstimulation and uterine rupture in a small number of women. Primary postpartum haemorrhage is more common after induction with Syntocinon.

In addition, prolonged labour and repeated vaginal examinations can lead to an increased incidence of postpartum endometritis and secondary postpartum haemorrhage.

Clinical Assessment

History

The reason for induction should be reviewed. If the indication for induction is prolonged pregnancy, the dates must be calculated and confirmed. The history and notes should be reviewed for any contraindications to induction.

Contraindications to induction

Absolute contraindications
- Known or suspected placenta praevia
- Multiple previous Caesarean sections
- Transverse lie

Relative contraindications
- Previous single Caesarean section
- Breech presentation

Examination

This will include an assessment of blood pressure, pulse and temperature, and the noting of any problems (hypertension, other maternal medical disease). Abdominal palpation should be performed to determine the size (with symphysis–fundal height measurement), lie, presentation, engagement and liquor volume.

A pelvic examination will determine whether the cervix is favourable for induction of labour. The Bishop's score is derived from an assessment of cervical dilatation, length, station, consistency and position (Table 30.1). This is used to decide how to conduct the induction. The findings on vaginal examination are taken in conjunction with the abdominal findings, especially the degree of engagement.

Investigations

An admission cardiotocograph should be performed to establish immediate fetal well-being (see Chapter 29).

Management

The aim of induction of labour is to achieve a vaginal delivery of a healthy baby within a reasonable time period, with minimal maternal problems. Because of the risks to mother and fetus, induction at the request of the mother must only be undertaken after full counselling and when the expectation of vaginal delivery is high. These decisions can only be made on an individual basis.

Before arranging formal induction, women should be offered membrane sweeping. This involves inserting a finger through the cervix and making a circular sweeping movement to separate the membranes from the cervix. This increases the chance of labour occurring spontaneously in the

Table 30.1 Modified Bishop's score for cervical status

	Score			
	0	**1**	**2**	**3**
Dilatation (cm)	0	1–2	3–4	5+
Length of cervix (cm)	>4	2–4	1–2	<1
Station[a]	−3	−2	−1, 0	+1, +2
Consistency	Firm	Medium	Soft	–
Position	Posterior	Mid/anterior	–	–

[a]Measured in cm relative to the ischial spines.

following 48 hours but may be associated with some discomfort and bleeding.

Methods of Induction of Labour

The method of induction will be determined in the main by whether the membranes are still intact.

Intravaginal Prostglandins

This is the method of choice when the membranes are intact, but can also be used after rupture of the membranes. The most commonly used method is to insert prostaglandin E_2 into the posterior fornix of the vagina. These preparations come in gel and tablet form. Nulliparous women with an unfavourable cervix (Bishop's score of less than 5) are given an initial dose of 2 mg, and multiparous women and nulliparae with a Bishop's score of more than 4 are given an initial dose of 1 mg. This method can be repeated after 6 hours until labour is established or the membranes are ruptured and the induction continued with oxytocin. The maximum dose is 4 mg in nulliparous women with an unfavourable cervix and 3 mg for all others.

Oxytocin Infusion

Oxytocin (Syntocinon) infusion is a suitable alternative to prostaglandins after rupture of the membranes. This may occur spontaneously or by forewater amniotomy (ARM). This is usually accomplished using a specifically designed amniotomy hook. Following this, oxytocin can be given at a controlled rate, titrated against contraction frequency. Early introduction of oxytocin reduces the number of women undelivered at 24 hours.

Oxytocin infusions start at a low rate of 1–4 mU/min and increase incrementally to a maximum of 32 mU/min. Most women will progress normally with doses of up to 12 mU/min. The dose is increased every 30 minutes until adequate contractions occur.

Monitoring

The degree of maternal monitoring will be guided by the mother's condition and the analgesia she chooses. At the very least, pulse temperature and blood pressure should be measured hourly once labour is established.

Induction of labour is a high-risk state for the fetus. Once labour is established, most fetuses will need to be continuously monitored.

Failure to Induce Labour

This is defined as failure of the cervix to dilate beyond 3 cm despite appropriate methods and a reasonable period of time. It may be that the cervix never reaches a dilatation at which an ARM is possible, or that dilatation does not occur following ARM and 4–8 hours of oxytocin. This occurs in 5 per cent of women when prostaglandin is needed for a low Bishop's score. When this occurs, Caesarean section is the only method of accomplishing delivery. If the induction is being performed for postmaturity, some would advocate a full fetal assessment and waiting for a few days if the fetus appears healthy, with a repeat attempt then. This can only be performed if the forewaters are still intact. It is not feasible when the indication for induction is fetal or maternal compromise.

Learning Points

- **Induction of labour carries risks to the fetus and mother**
- **The indication for induction must outweigh the potential risks**
- **Two common methods utilize prostaglandins and oxytocin**

See Also

Prolonged pregnancy (Chapter 17)
Cord prolapse (Chapter 26)
Abnormal fetal heart rate patterns in labour (Chapter 29)

Further Reading

National Institute for Clinical Excellence. *Induction of Labour. Inherited Clinical Guideline.* National Institute for Clinical Excellence, London, 2001.

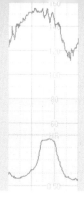

Chapter 31

Intrauterine fetal death

Definition

Intrauterine fetal death (IUFD) refers to the death of a fetus of 24 weeks' gestation or more, prior to delivery. Losses can be divided into antenatal, occurring before labour, and intrapartum, in which the fetus dies during labour. This distinction is important, as the underlying aetiology may be very different.

Importance

Nearly 1 per cent of women suffer the loss of their baby in the last half of pregnancy. This not only poses a huge psychological burden, but may also be a risk to immediate maternal health. Rigorous and sympathetic management is vital at this vulnerable time. This chapter will deal with IUFD before labour. Intrapartum IUFD may be as a result of an antenatal event, many of which are covered here. Where this occurs in a viable fetus, unrecognized problems are common. The problems of cardiotocograph (CTG) analysis are covered in Chapter 29.

Causes

Common causes of IUFD

Abruption
Pre-eclampsia
Chorioamnionitis or other fetal infection
Chronic fetal hypoxia
Fetal abnormality
Obstetric cholestasis
Fetal macrosomia
Fetomaternal haemorrhage

The causes of IUFD may be obvious at presentation, such as abruption (see Chapter 25), whilst others may not be immediately apparent and require careful investigation before they can be identified.

This list is not exhaustive, and other rare causes of fetal death can be found. It is important to direct investigation towards the suspected cause.

Diagnosis

Initial Diagnosis

The diagnosis of an IUFD may be suspected very soon after admission, when the fetal heart is not heard on auscultation. Very occasionally, the diagnosis is made incidentally at routine ultrasound scan. When the diagnosis is suspected, it is important that someone skilled in ultrasound is available to confirm it and look for other signs which may have an impact on further management, such as overriding of skull bones, which may suggest death of a few days' duration, fetal hydrops (swelling) or a very large fetus. The information must be conveyed to the parents with the minimum delay, and the opportunity for them to spend some time alone to come to terms with their loss is then important.

History

A history must be carefully taken. This must be done in a sensitive manner. Some details such as smoking or drug abuse are important, but it is important to avoid attaching any guilt to this. Many mothers feel that they must be to blame in some way. In general this is not true. Even with factors that are known to be associated with problems such as smoking, IUFD is a rare outcome.

Bleeding or pain

Leakage of fluid

Reduced fetal movements

Flu-like illness, or rashes (or an affected child at home)

Previous poor pregnancy outcome

Personal or family history of thrombosis

Symptoms of pre-eclampsia (see Chapter 11)

Itching

Examination

Check for:

Hypertension

Proteinuria

Uterine tenderness

Uterine activity

Fundal height

Pulse rate

Temperature

Pre-eclampsia may become apparent. Symptoms and signs are covered in Chapter 11. Abruption significant enough to cause an IUFD will present with pain, maternal hypotension or collapse, and usually bleeding. Chorioamnionitis is discussed in Chapter 39.

Other clinical signs include a fundus that is small or large for dates. Scratch marks may be indicative of severe itching in cases of obstetric cholestasis.

Investigations

Relevant investigations

Maternal HbA1c

Kleihauer test

Karyotype

C-reactive protein (CRP)/vaginal and cervical swabs for bacteriology

Placental swabs

Thrombophilia screen

Lupus anticoagulant and anticardiolipin antibodies

TORCH screen

Parvovirus B19 serology

Maternal and paternal chromosome analysis

Maternal urine toxicology screen

These must be tailored to the suspected cause. There are some tests that can be useful, but they must be performed early.

Maternal glucose metabolism returns to normal very soon after IUFD. HbA1c gives a slightly longer-term measure. This can be useful in cases of macrosomia, although it is recognized that glucose metabolism may be normal in cases of macrosomia, and the actual reason for the higher rate of IUFD in macrosomic fetuses is not well understood.

Fetal cells in the maternal circulation are quickly broken down, especially if they are of an incompatible ABO group. Fetomaternal haemorrhage can be missed if this test is not performed early on.

It is difficult to obtain a karyotype from fetuses that are very macerated. This is a vital piece of information, as even in the non-dysmorphic (normal-looking) fetus a significant number will have karyotypic abnormalities. Placenta, fetal skin and blood, and fetal iliac crest samples can all be sent. Chondrocytes are the longest surviving cells and may give a result when all others fail to grow.

Postmortem examination of the placenta should be undertaken in every case.

Conditions for which examination of the placenta is of value

Pre-eclampsia

IUGR

Abruption

Infection

Fetomaternal haemorrhage

Postmortem examination of the fetus should be discussed at the appropriate time with all parents. Whilst it is the parents' right to decline postmortem examination of the fetus, every effort should be made to explain this process to the grieving parents, to offer a limited postmortem if appropriate, or to consider X-rays and needle biopsies at the very least. Forty per cent of fetuses will have the diagnosis materially altered by a postmortem examination. This information can be vital in advising parents about future pregnancies. Parents should be told that they can see and hold their baby after the postmortem examination. Many parents will consent to postmortem and gain valuable information from it if they are counselled at the appropriate time by a senior member of staff.

Chorioamnionitis may be the cause of fetal demise or a late stage of a prolonged labour process in an already dead fetus. Swabs, CRP and post-mortem can all point to this diagnosis.

It is becoming more apparent that a significant number of IUFDs are secondary to placental vascular disease with an underlying thrombophilia. Treatment can be offered in subsequent pregnancies if this is shown to be the cause.

Infection can lead to fetal hydrops. This is usually apparent at birth. Parvovirus leads to fetal anaemia and myocarditis. Cytomegalovirus causes thrombo-cytopenia, hepatitis and intracranial lesions.

Parental chromosome analysis is useful if the karyotype from the fetus fails to grow. Urine toxi-cology must be undertaken with care. Drug abuse is fairly common and may be an incidental finding. Cocaine can cause sudden IUFD, and maternal hyper-tension can be seen in association. Postmortem may reveal fetal intracranial infarcts.

Management

The management of abruption is discussed in Chapter 25.

Delivery

Fetal maceration can lead to disseminated intra-vascular coagulation (DIC) in the mother. If clotting is abnormal, delivery must be expedited. Otherwise, the mother can be offered the choice to go home and return for delivery the following day. This period of adaptation, with time to tell the family, is often appreciated.

Delivery must be achieved by the safest route for the mother. Many women are horrified at the thought of having to go through labour. Explanation that this will lead to a safe delivery and quick recovery and return home must be given. The parents need the full support of a midwife during this time.

Labour can be induced by a combination of:

* mifepristone (antiprogesterone)
* misoprostol (a synthetic prostaglandin)
* prostaglandins E$_2$, or gemeprost (see Chapter 30)
* Syntocinon (see Chapter 30).

After 24 weeks, care must be taken not to cause excessive uterine contraction, as this can lead to uterine rupture. Analgesic options can include epidural (if clotting studies are normal), morphine or pethidine.

After Delivery

The baby must be weighed, examined and wrapped. The weight is important as it may hold the clue to growth restriction, and if postmortem is declined this is the only opportunity to gain this information. The placenta must be examined and sent for postmortem.

Parents may wish to see and hold their baby. Even if there are significant fetal abnormalities, the oppor-tunity to do this is important. Parents' fears are often far greater than the reality.

Photographs are useful. Some parents will return for these even years after the event. Arrangements for burial, cremation or disposal of the stillborn baby are best undertaken by a bereavement team, who can fol-low up the family, ensure that the birth is registered (if after 24 weeks) and provide support.

Guidance about lactation should be given. Gen-erally, all that is required is a supportive brassiere. A single dose of the dopamine agonist Cabergoline is effective. This must not be used in women with pre-eclampsia.

Follow-up

Bereavement counselling is vital. Many couples feel very vulnerable on their return home. Other support groups such as SANDS (Stillbirth and Neonatal Death Support Group) can be useful contacts.

An appointment to go through the findings should be offered. This can be arranged away from the unit where the infant was delivered if parents prefer.

Learning Points

- **Sensitive and sympathetic handling of parents is vital**
- **Investigation should be as thorough as possible. Bereaved parents usually want answers**
- **Choice should be offered at all times wherever possible**

See Also

Previous fetal loss (Chapter 16)
Reduced fetal movements (Chapter 20)
Induction of labour (Chapter 30)

Maternal collapse

Importance

The unexpected collapse of a woman on the labour ward is a frightening event for all concerned. The causes are sometimes, but not always, obvious. The situation is often life threatening for both the mother and, if undelivered, the fetus. Prior to delivery, the risks to the mother are exacerbated by the high oxygen demand of the fetoplacental unit, which means that hypoxia is often severe and of much more rapid onset than in the non-pregnant woman. Additionally in the supine position, the uterus can cause severe enough aortocaval compression to reduce cardiac return by 30–40 per cent. In a cardiac arrest this is significant and can impair the likelihood of success unless relieved.

Causes

> **Causes of maternal collapse**
>
> Haemorrhage
> Vasovagal episodes (faints)
> Eclamptic fits
> Rupture of the uterus
> Amniotic fluid embolism
> Cerebrovascular accident
> Uterine inversion
> Myocardial infarction

Haemorrhage from the placenta/placental bed is the most common cause of obstetric collapse. This chapter discusses the thought process and approach to management of obstetric collapse encountered on the labour ward, with the exception of antepartum and postpartum haemorrhages, which are covered in Chapters 25 and 37.

Fits in pregnancy or the puerperium may be caused by a number of different disease states. The outcomes for these are very different and, as such, it is vital for the correct diagnosis and management to be undertaken.

> **Conditions which can cause fits in pregnancy**
>
> Eclampsia
> Epilepsy
> Infection (encephalitis/meningitis)
> Cerebral tumours
> Cerebrovascular accident or cerebral sinus thrombosis
> Drug withdrawal/abuse
> Metabolic disturbance (especially hypoglycaemia, if diabetic)

Epilepsy and eclampsia are the two most common causes. Epilepsy affects 1 in 150 pregnant women. Fits may become more common in pregnancy for a number of reasons, including poor drug compliance because of anxiety about the effects on the fetus, reduced drug levels due to increased free drug clearance and, in the puerperium, lack of sleep, which is known to exacerbate fits. New-onset epilepsy in pregnancy is very uncommon.

Eclampsia is the severest end of the pre-eclampsia–eclampsia spectrum. By definition, this only occurs between 20 weeks' gestation and 10 days postpartum. New-onset fits in pregnancy are eclampsia, until proven otherwise. Eclamptic seizures affect 1 in 2000 women in the UK. Epileptic women can develop eclampsia. If features of pre-eclampsia are apparent, this must be considered.

The other causes, though rare, do occasionally occur in pregnancy and must be considered if findings are atypical. Not uncommonly, faints happen in pregnancy. Some shaking movement is often seen. Women who faint do not have a postictal period.

Cerebral oedema
Cerebrovascular accident/cerebral ischaemia
Renal failure
Liver dysfunction
Adult respiratory distress syndrome (ARDS)

Amniotic fluid embolism is a poorly understood, catastrophic and rare event. It has an incidence of 1–3.3 per 100 000 pregnancies. It is fatal in at least 61 per cent of cases, and some women sustain permanent neurological damage. The pathophysiology is of an anaphylactoid reaction, resulting in huge disseminated intravascular coagulation (DIC), triggered by the high concentrations of phospholipids in amniotic fluid.

Previously associated factors were thought to be precipitate labour, oxytocin use and multiparity, but these associations are now less clear. Of fetuses *in utero* at the time of amniotic fluid embolism, only 40 per cent will survive.

Amniotic fluid embolism

70 per cent occurs during labour
11 per cent occurs after vaginal delivery
19 per cent occurs during or after Caesarean section

Cerebrovascular accidents do occur in pregnancy. They can broadly be divided into:

- subarachnoid haemorrhage (1–5 per 10 000 pregnancies);
- non-haemorrhagic strokes (4 per 100 000 pregnancies).

Eclampsia accounts for 47 per cent of cases of non-haemorrhage strokes and 44 per cent of haemorrhages.

Causes of non-haemorrhagic stroke include extracranial vertebral artery dissection, postpartum cerebral angiopathy, thrombophilias and DIC associated with cerebral vascular accident. Intraparenchymal haemorrhages are associated with rupture of a cerebral vascular malformation (usually aneurysm or arteriovenous malformation) in 37 per cent of cases.

Uterine rupture occurs often in association with one of the following features:

- previous uterine surgery (Caesarean section, myomectomy, perforation at termination of pregnancy);
- Syntocinon use in a multiparous patient (especially if the reason for commencement of Syntocinon was a secondary arrest);
- difficult instrumental delivery (especially rotational delivery using Kielland's forceps).

Cardiac arrest as a result of myocardial infarction is an uncommon event in women of child-bearing age, but carries a 20 per cent mortality, especially if occurring around the time of delivery.

Initial Assessment

A rapid assessment must be performed whilst resuscitation is taking place. Considering the list of differential diagnoses above, a number of factors need to be sought.

Ask about:

The events surrounding the collapse
Antepartum risk factors
Problems in previous pregnancies

The case notes may be vital in cases where there are no accompanying relatives. If the patient is fitting, ask about previous fits and medication. If there is a history of epilepsy, try to establish previous fit frequency and reasons why this may have changed, such as not taking medication etc.

The symptoms of pre-eclampsia must be sought, even if pre-existing epilepsy is noted.

Symptoms of pre-eclampsia

Headache
Upper abdominal pain
Visual disturbance
Nausea or vomiting

There may be a note of recent hypertension or proteinuria.

Examination

Check:

Blood pressure
Pulse
Obvious bleeding
Abdominal examination

If the patient is diabetic, a rapid blood sugar will differentiate hypoglycaemia from hyperglycaemia.

Diagnosis and Management

Priorities

Summon help
Establish an airway – ABC
Secure breathing – ABC
Gain circulatory access
Rapid assessment
Resuscitate and deal with the cause

The mother is the primary patient and her life must not be put at risk unnecessarily to save the fetus.

Resuscitation

Establishing an Airway

As mentioned above, the pregnant woman is very vulnerable to hypoxia. In addition, because of uterine distension and the effects of progesterone on the gastric sphincter mechanisms, aspiration is much more likely. In the unconscious woman, intubation should be performed and a cuffed endotracheal (ET) tube placed. This should be accomplished by an experienced person, as failed intubation is a dangerous situation and pregnant women are often very difficult to intubate.

Breathing

The high oxygen demands of pregnancy mean that 100 per cent oxygen should be used in the short term for resuscitation.

Circulation

A wide-bore cannula should be placed in each antecubital fossa, and blood taken for urgent full blood count, cross-match and clotting screen. If bleeding is suspected, large amounts of fluid and blood will be needed (see Chapter 25). Also, in order to reduce aortocaval compression due to a gravid uterus, the patient must be tilted to an angle of at least 15° (Figure 32.1). This is best accomplished with a firm board rather than a wedge, because if cardiac massage is required, a firm surface is needed.

Once these basic life-saving measures have been taken, the progress and further management will be determined by the cause of the collapse.

Haemorrhage is discussed in the chapters on antepartum and postpartum haemorrhage (Chapters 25 and 37).

Vasovagal Episodes

These are not uncommon, especially after delivery, and may be associated with vomiting. They are usually self-limiting, requiring only the positioning of the mother in a head-down position with a tilt, if still undelivered, and facial oxygen through a conventional facial mask. A rapid return of blood pressure, with a resolution of

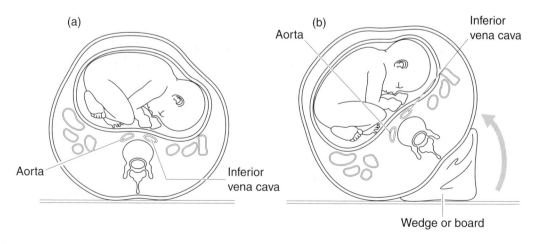

Figure 32.1 Avoiding aortocaval compression. (a) Before tilt. (b) After tilt, using a wedge or board.

the maternal bradycardia to normal within a few minutes, is the norm. Antepartum, there is usually evidence of fetal bradycardia, which resolves as blood pressure is restored.

If there is any doubt, or delayed recovery, the normal ABC principles must be followed and another cause sought.

The Fitting Patient

When presented with a fitting patient, the immediate management must be to ensure the safety of the woman. During the tonic–clonic phase, the patient must be protected from harming herself by moving any hard objects away, and prevention of falling and head injury. The tonic–clonic phase usually lasts only 2–3 minutes. During the tonic phase, it is impossible to insert anything into the mouth and this should not be attempted. Facial oxygen may be administered, the woman should be placed on her side and the head tilted back (the recovery position). Epileptic fits are generally self-limiting (less than 3 minutes) and it is not usually necessary to give any drugs; these can cause excessive drowsiness and compromise the airway in the postictal phase.

If the tonic–clonic phase lasts more than 3–4 minutes or rapidly recurs, it must be terminated. Traditionally 5–10 mg of i.v. diazepam are used, but if the cause is thought to be eclampsia, it is better to give a bolus of 4 g magnesium sulphate.

The airway must be secured and severe hypertension (>160/100 mmHg) must be controlled with a bolus of hydralazine or labetalol.

There is usually a profound fetal bradycardia associated with the maternal hypoxia during the fit. Monitoring the fetal heart at this stage can be deleterious, as it can lead to action that may be inappropriate and jeopardize maternal well-being. The quickest way to resuscitate the fetus is to resuscitate the mother.

Once the mother is stable then a full history (usually from relatives) and examination must be performed.

Examination

Carry out the following:

A general assessment of condition, noting any
- Facial oedema
- Petechiae/rashes
- Jaundice
- Needle marks

Cardiovascular examination
Blood pressure
Abdominal examination
Fetal size, lie and presentation
Epigastric tenderness
Neurological examination
Focal neurological signs
Fundoscopy (papilloedema, retinal haemorrhages)
Hyperreflexia/clonus

Investigations

Check:

Urinalysis for proteinuria
Full blood count
Clotting screen
Urea, creatinine, electrolytes
Liver function tests
Glucose

These mainly centre on the diagnosis of eclampsia. Derangements of haematological, renal and liver indices point to eclampsia as a diagnosis. The degree of hypertension may not be marked or may come on after the fit. Heavy proteinuria is usually present.

If the fits are new in onset, and eclampsia is not suspected, cerebral imaging to look for other causes must be undertaken. Magnetic resonance imaging (MRI) is completely safe in pregnancy. Computerized tomography (CT) scanning can also be performed with almost no fetal risk.

Management

If the fit is deemed to be of epileptic origin, then once a full maternal recovery has been made, the aim is to try to modify drug treatment to prevent further fits if possible. Education of the patient and ensuring compliance are important. Serum drug levels can be helpful, particularly to ensure compliance. Follow-up by a team experienced in the management of epilepsy in pregnancy can be helpful.

Eclampsia entails careful multidisciplinary management in a high-dependency setting. The team should include:

- Consultant obstetrician
- Consultant anaesthetist
- Senior midwife
- Haematologist.

The aim is to stabilize the maternal condition, deliver and carefully monitor until the disease process resolves.

Prevention of Further Fits

The treatment of choice is magnesium sulphate. This has been shown to reduce the recurrence of fits. It is given as an initial bolus, with a maintenance infusion to follow. A serum level of 2–3 mmol/L is ideal.

> **Signs of magnesium sulphate overdose**
>
> Loss of reflexes
> Drowsiness
> Respiratory depression
> Cardiac arrest

Loss of reflexes is the first sign. In units where magnesium assays are not available, this can be used. When reflexes are lost, the infusion should be stopped.

Control of Hypertension

Hypertension poses a risk to the maternal cerebral vasculature. The aim is to reduce the blood pressure to 140/90 mmHg. Levels persistently above 160/100 should be treated. Bolus doses of hydralazine (2.5–5 mg) or labetalol 20 mg are best. Oral antihypertensives may be needed once the disease process is reversed. These must be gradually stopped, as rebound hypertension is not uncommon.

Management of Fluid Balance

The underlying pathology in eclampsia is endothelial damage. Capillaries easily leak fluid into the extravascular compartment, leading to cerebral and pulmonary oedema. Careful fluid balance is critical. No more than 100 mL/hour of i.v. fluid should be given. Urine output must be measured hourly (site a Foley catheter). If the urine output is less than 100 mL over 4 hours, then consideration is given to central monitoring. Central venous pressure monitoring can be misleading. Pulmonary capillary wedge pressures are more helpful, but require intensive care monitoring.

Blood loss at delivery should be replaced.

Delivery

Once the mother is stable, she should be delivered. Delivery is the only cure for the condition. Delivery should be accomplished by the quickest and safest method. If the pregnancy is 34 weeks or more and the cervix is very favourable, consideration can be given to vaginal delivery. This is often the safest for the mother.

The fetus will be vulnerable because of poor placental function and should be continuously monitored.

> **Remember that:**
>
> Syntocinon is antidiuretic and must be administered in small volumes of fluid
> Magnesium is a tocolytic, and Syntocinon may be needed in increased doses
> Only a short trial of labour should be allowed
> Blood loss should be replaced with blood
> Epidural anaesthesia must not be given if there is abnormal clotting

After Delivery

All biochemical and haematological parameters must be checked 4- to 6-hourly until there is evidence of continuing improvement. Regular assessment of clinical condition must be performed, especially lung fields, as pulmonary oedema can occur rapidly.

Magnesium must be continued for 24 hours after the last fit. Only when the mother's condition has been stable without magnesium may she be transferred out of the high-dependency setting. Antihypertensive medication may be needed for a prolonged period of time and should be stopped only gradually. If the hypertension does not settle, investigation for underlying pathology must be undertaken in the postnatal period.

Ruptured Uterus

> **Signs of uterine rupture**
>
> Sudden drop in blood pressure
> Abdominal pain
> Fetal bradycardia
> Vaginal bleeding
> Upward movement of the presenting part (as the fetus is pushed out of the uterus into the abdomen)

The treatment will require full resuscitation as for major obstetric haemorrhage (Chapter 25). Crystalloids first and blood, when available, are the most appropriate replacements. These must be rapidly infused and blood should be warmed if possible. If 6 units are transfused, fresh frozen plasma may also be needed.

The mainstay of management is to stop the bleeding. This requires urgent laparotomy. General anaesthesia is usually preferred, as peripheral vasodilatation associated with regional anaesthesia may further compromise the mother and surgery may need to be extensive.

If the uterus is scarred, the rupture is almost always through the scar, although it may extend to involve vessels on the lateral walls of the uterus. In an unscarred uterus, the tear is usually in the upper segment and bleeding is usually torrential. Saving the life of the mother is the most important objective and, if bleeding is heavy, hysterectomy is usually the safest and quickest option.

Splenic artery aneurysm often presents in a similar way, with collapse, fetal bradycardia or death, and at laparotomy the peritoneal cavity is full of blood. These need to be dealt with in association with the surgeon. Pressure on the bleeding aneurysm to prevent bleeding is needed until help arrives.

Amniotic Fluid Embolism (AFE)

Signs of AFE

Transient pulmonary hypertension followed by severe systemic hypotension

Profound hypoxia leading to collapse

Left ventricular failure

Secondary coagulopathy

Treatment of AFE is directed towards three goals:

- improved oxygenation;
- maintenance of both cardiac output and blood pressure;
- correction of coagulopathy.

Fetal distress is universal with amniotic fluid embolism. These mothers require intensive monitoring if they survive the event. The intensive therapy unit is the place most suited to the high level of input needed.

Cerebrovascular Accident

Intracranial haemorrhage is more common in the pregnant than in the non-pregnant woman and presents with:

- headache
- seizures
- neurological deficit.

Occlusive events usually cause neurological deficit as the presenting symptom. Collapse due to cerebro-vascular accident carries a very high mortality. Full resuscitation and investigation once stable are the mainstays of management.

Cardiac Arrest

The management is the same as for the non-pregnant woman, with some special considerations. If there is no cardiac output (feel the carotid pulse), chest compressions must be started straight away:

- Call the arrest team.
- Tilt the mother, if undelivered.
- ABC.

If the mother is intubated, the ratio is five compressions to one breath. If there is no ET tube, the ratio is 15 to two. A femoral pulse must be felt for. If this cannot be felt, but a carotid pulse is present, the degree of tilt is not enough. Occasionally an unsuccessful arrest resuscitation will require delivery of the fetus. This can decrease aortocaval compression, reduce the oxygen demand of the uteroplacental unit, and increase the chances of success. If the fetus is viable, there may also be the chance of fetal survival.

After the Acute Event

With any significant cause of maternal collapse, there will be a need for further intensive monitoring and care. Ventilatory support can usually only be provided within an intensive therapy setting, but most labour wards have a high-dependency area where post-operative surgical cases can be adequately cared for.

All women will require monitoring of:

- blood pressure
- respiratory rate
- oxygen saturation.

Further intensive monitoring may be needed for some women. Decisions regarding how and where to care for each woman must be made on an individual basis.

Following any collapse, it is very important that a full explanation is given to the relatives. If the outcome is successful, once the patient is fully recovered she will also need careful counselling of the events, with guidance on further management and any possible recurrence risks. Some staff will find collapse situations disturbing, especially if the outcome is not good. Support should be available for all who need it.

Learning Points

- **Resuscitating the mother is the most efficient way of resuscitating the fetus**
- **New-onset fits in pregnancy are eclampsia until proven otherwise**
- **Fits which do not resolve in 2–3 minutes should be terminated with diazepam or magnesium sulphate depending on the cause**
- **Eclampsia is treated by stabilization of the mother and delivery**

See Also

Antepartum haemorrhage (Chapter 25)
Postpartum haemorrhage (Chapter 37)

Chapter 33

Meconium

Importance

Thick meconium may suggest oligohydramnios and a poorly functioning placenta. This indicates a fetus that may already have undergone processes associated with poor placental function. Fetuses with little reserve do not tolerate labour well and are more likely to become hypoxic.

Meconium plus hypoxia can lead to meconium aspiration syndrome (MAS).

Meconium aspiration syndrome

Meconium below the vocal cords at delivery

Respiratory compromise which may be mild, moderate or
severe

Some infants also demonstrate signs of
hypoxaemic–ischaemic encephalopathy

This condition has a 40 per cent mortality rate

Meconium alone does not lead to MAS. There also needs to be an added hypoxic insult.

Causes

Passage of meconium into the amniotic fluid is a normal event in fetuses that progress beyond term (50 per cent at 42 weeks' gestation). It is probably a physiological process at these late gestations, as the fetus matures. In approximately 10 per cent of pregnancies, meconium is found at rupture of membranes. One in 20 of these will go on to have significant problems.

The association between the passage of meconium and fetal hypoxia has been recognized. It is thought likely that this relates to chronic events during pregnancy. Meconium is graded as thin or thick. The importance of this is that thick meconium is undiluted by amniotic fluid. For this to occur there must be an underlying pathological process leading to the oligohydramnios, or lack of amniotic fluid. Hypoxia is a well-recognized cause of oligohydramnios. This is a chronic condition where, as the placental function becomes poorer, the fetus adapts by redistributing blood to vital organs (the brain, heart and adrenal glands). As a result, the kidneys become poorly perfused and the urinary output, which becomes the amniotic fluid, decreases.

Diagnosis and Clinical Assessment

Identification of which fetuses are truly at risk and delivery before hypoxia occurs are vital in avoiding MAS. Even then, some fetuses will be affected, as MAS can occur before the onset of labour.

Ultrasound scanning is not helpful in determining the presence of meconium. Vernix (the waxy substance covering babies before term) produces identical findings. Ultrasound examination is useful in identifying fetuses with poor growth, decreased liquor volume and abnormal umbilical artery Doppler waveforms. These fetuses are at higher risk of MAS if labour is complicated by meconium.

Fetuses with normal heart rate tracings are not at increased risk of MAS.

Management

Monitoring of Fetal Well-being in Labour

The oligohydramnios associated with meconium leads to a higher rate of variable decelerations due to cord compression (see Chapter 29). Fetuses with less reserve may be less tolerant to these decelerations than healthy fetuses. Continuous heart rate monitoring is vital. Fetal blood sampling may be helpful in deciding which fetuses require delivery. If the cardiotocograph is pathological (see Chapter 29), consideration is given to delivery without delay.

Amnio-infusion

Amnio-infusion, where saline is infused under gravity into the amniotic cavity, has been shown to reduce variable decelerations. It appears to have some protective effect against meconium aspiration. It probably works by reducing the hypoxia produced by recurrent or prolonged cord compression. However, it does not have any effect on those fetuses that sustain damage prior to labour.

At Delivery

It has always been thought that meconium enters the lungs at the first breath. This has been recently shown to be false, and that gasping *in utero* leads to meconium aspiration. The value of pharyngeal and tracheal suction is therefore unknown. Certainly the lower Apgar scores seen in some babies who have meconium-stained liquor are due to vigorous suction, which can delay the onset of respiration and produce bronchospasm. In general, meconium should be cleared from the upper airway. If the meconium is thick, examination of the cords has been accepted management, with aspiration of meconium through a large-bore suction catheter if there is meconium present.

Learning Points

- Thick meconium implies oligohydramnios and the potential for long-standing placental dysfunction
- Thick meconium plus fetal heart rate abnormalities increase the risk of fetal hypoxia
- Delivery or further fetal assessment (by fetal blood sampling) must be undertaken
- Prompt delivery does not always prevent MAS. In some babies, this is a sign of a chronic pathological process

See Also

Abnormal fetal heart rate patterns in labour (Chapter 29)
Intrauterine fetal death (Chapter 31)

Chapter 34

Neonatal resuscitation

Definition

Neonatal resuscitation relates to the immediate care after delivery of an infant who has poor tone, a low heart rate and makes little or no respiratory effort (sometimes described as the 'flat baby').

Importance

About 1 per cent of low-risk babies will require help to commence respiration after birth. To some extent, this can be predicted from the clinical history or labour events. However, of low-risk babies, about 1 in 5 of those who need resuscitation at birth cannot be predicted from such at-risk scenarios. Skilled help must therefore be immediately available at delivery, but an understanding of how to deal with an unexpectedly flat baby is important.

Causes

Common causes of poor condition at birth

Intrapartum hypoxia
Antenatal hypoxia
Drugs
Infection
Fetal abnormality

Intrapartum hypoxia occurs when there is insufficient placental transfer of oxygen and carbon dioxide during labour, leading to a gradual or acute hypoxia in the fetus. Uterine hyperstimulation with oxytocics can lead to gradual hypoxia, as placental gas transfer only occurs during uterine relaxation. If the placenta is functioning poorly as a result of a disease process such as pre-eclampsia or significant postmaturity, the contractions of normal labour may be enough to compromise the fetus. Acute situations such as placental abruption lead to sudden loss of gas exchange and acute hypoxia.

Antenatal events can have a profound effect on the neonate. Severe antenatal hypoxia can lead to brain damage that may be evident at birth with a baby that is in unexpectedly poor condition. Evaluation of the umbilical artery pH may reveal a normal or slightly low result out of keeping with the condition of the baby.

Drugs such as pethidine and diazepam have a depressive effect on the fetus and neonate. The fetal heart rate pattern changes, with poor variability. After delivery, the neonate may have a normal heart rate but makes no respiratory effort.

Infection with organisms such as group B *Streptococcus* can occur both prior to and during labour. Neonates may present with an overwhelming infection and in very poor condition at birth. They can also be acidotic as a result of the infective process.

Occasionally fetal abnormality will present with a neonate who is difficult to resuscitate. Some conditions such as congenital myotonic dystrophy may not be diagnosed until delivery.

Clinical Assessment

History

Prior to delivery, there may be some clues that an infant may be born in poor condition.

Maternal hypertension
Known growth restriction
Known fetal abnormality
Maternal drug abuse

Events during labour

Cardiotocograph changes
Drug administration during labour
Maternal pyrexia and fetal tachycardia
Acute events such as abruption or uterine rupture
Meconium-stained liquor

Meconium-stained liquor increases the risk that a baby will be hypoxic at birth. It also presents separate additional risks to the neonate. These are discussed in Chapter 33.

Examination

The Apgar score is the standard method of assessing the neonate at delivery (Table 34.1). The first two factors are the most important and guide the rest of the management. The test was not designed to give prognostic information, and indeed cannot, but was designed to help establish which babies require resuscitation.

The Apgar score is first assessed at 1 minute. This allows time for drying and stimulating the infant before resuscitative measures are undertaken.

Management

The first priority after birth is drying of the baby and wrapping to prevent heat loss. Particular attention must be given to drying the head, which may present a large exposed area for evaporative heat loss. This may be particularly important for the tiny infant who has reduced energy reserves and high transepidermal water (and heat) losses.

Babies with poor respiratory effort or a heart rate of <100 at 1 minute require further resuscitation.

Resuscitation

There are three levels of resuscitation:

• bag and mask ventilation
• intubation and ventilation
• full cardiopulmonary resuscitation.

Bag and Mask

Eighty per cent of infants born in a poor condition will be adequately resuscitated by bag and mask ventilation. Two to six long breaths of 30 cmH$_2$O are given initially to assist the child in the formation of a functional residual capacity (FRC). The majority of the inflation pressure is still likely to be provided by the child taking the first gasp and developing high negative intrathoracic pressures.

Following establishment of FRC, smaller breaths are appropriate to inflate the expanded lungs, unless the baby has commenced spontaneous respiration.

One hundred per cent oxygen has been recommended for use in resuscitation. However, infants requiring help with the initiation of the first breath need only stimulation or chest inflation, such that most term babies can be effectively resuscitated with air.

Intubation and Ventilation

If the baby is responding poorly to bag and mask ventilation, the heart rate is less than 60 beats/minute (bpm) or inflation is difficult to achieve, intubation should be undertaken. The same procedure for initial breaths is undertaken, followed by

Table 34.1 The Apgar score

Score	0	1	2
Heart rate	Absent	< 100 bpm	> 100 bpm
Respiratory effort	None	Slow, irregular	Good, crying
Muscle tone	Flaccid	Some limb flexion	Active motion
Reflex irritability	No response	Cry	Vigorous cry
Colour	Blue, pale	Body pink	Pink body and limbs

40–60 breaths /minute. Ventilation is continued until spontaneous respiration is established. Once extubated, the baby must be closely observed. During prolonged and difficult resuscitation, it is important to achieve well-oxygenated blood as soon as possible and oxygen concentrations of 100 per cent are required.

Cardiopulmonary Resuscitation

Full cardiopulmonary resuscitation must be started when the heart rate is <60 bpm. Chest compressions are commenced until palpable cardiac output >80–100 bpm is achieved. Two techniques have been described:

- Two handed – where the chest is encircled with both hands so that the fingers lie behind the baby and the thumbs are opposed over the mid-sternum 1 cm below the inter-nipple line;
- One handed – two fingers are used over the mid-sternum 1 cm below the inter-nipple line.

Cardiac output is higher in the two-handed technique and is preferred. Where cardiorespiratory support is provided by one individual, the one-handed technique is technically easier. A rate of 120 bpm with a ratio of 3:1 or 5:1 compressions to lung inflations is optimal. Once the heart rate is above 80–100 bpm, cardiac massage can be stopped.

Reversal of Respiratory Depression

When the mother has received opiate analgesia, respiratory depression can occur. Reversal of this can be achieved with naloxone. Naloxone is used at a dose of 100 μg/kg (British Resuscitation Guidelines). It should only be given to infants whose mothers have received opiate analgesia more frequently than 3-hourly or within 4 hours of delivery, and to those who, once the airway is secure and ventilation is established, are pink and have a good heart rate but poor respiratory drive.

Naloxone must not be given to infants of mothers who have been misusing opiates, as it can precipitate neonatal convulsions.

Treatment of Infection

Infection may be suspected as a result of the presence of:

- maternal pyrexia
- fetal tachycardia
- prolonged rupture of membranes.

Fetal and neonatal infection increases the metabolic rate of the infant, making it more prone to hypoxia and acidosis. Full resuscitation must be undertaken in cases of suspected infection, with aggressive management of low blood pressure and antibiotic therapy.

Follow-up

Any infant who has required more than bag and mask resuscitation may be at risk of hypoglycaemia, and early feeding is given where appropriate. Those infants who required extensive resuscitation should be admitted to the neonatal intensive care unit for observation. Parents should be adequately counselled when their infant requires resuscitation, as this can be an extremely distressing time. They may need extra help and reassurance before being discharged home with their baby.

Learning Points

- Even after low-risk labours, infants can be born in poor condition
- Antenatal and intrapartum events contribute to the infant's condition at birth
- Recognition of risk factors should be used to alert paediatric staff
- All labour ward staff should be practised in basic neonatal resuscitation

See Also

Substance abuse (Chapter 22)
Meconium (Chapter 33)
Abnormal fetal heart rate patterns in labour (Chapter 29)

Normal labour

Definitions

Labour is the process by which the fetus is expelled from the uterus. It is defined as the onset of regular, painful contractions with progressive cervical efface-ment and dilatation of the cervix accompanied by descent of the presenting part.

> ### Three stages of labour
>
> First stage – from the onset of labour until the cervix reaches full dilatation
> Second stage – during which the fetus is expelled
> Third stage – delivery of the placenta and membranes

Progress in the first stage of labour tends to follow an S-shaped curve and can also be divided into three phases:

- latent
- active
- decelerative.

These definitions are used to divide labour into identifiable stages, so that deviations from what is 'normal' can be identified and remedied. You will see that one of the problems facing professionals caring for women in labour is the lack of scientific evidence on which the normal values are based, and the diffi-culties identifying changes from this. Each definition will be discussed in more detail below.

Importance

An understanding of the processes of normal labour is important, as it is only from this that problems will be identified and correctly dealt with. As many as 50 per cent of first-time mothers will need some help during labour and can be said to have deviated from what can be viewed as 'normal'. Keeping fetal and maternal morbidity to a minimum is the aim of the management of labour.

Normal Physiology

Onset of Labour

As pregnancy advances, contraction frequency and strength increase. The onset of labour when con-tractions become regular, and in most cases painful, may thus be extremely difficult to identify. Many women will be admitted with 'false alarms' before they are truly in labour. The hallmark of the labour is change in the cervix.

Other signs such as rupture of membranes or a show may help in some cases, but not all women who exhibit these will be in labour (see Chapter 39).

Latent Phase

During the latent phase, little cervical dilatation occurs, but the cervix is effacing (shortening) in preparation for the active phase. A normal latent phase is 8 hours in nulliparae and 6 hours in multi-parae. Once the cervix reaches 3 cm dilatation, the latent phase finishes and the woman moves into the active phase.

Active Phase

The average rate of dilatation during the active phase is 1 cm/hour in both nulliparae and multiparae. However, the curve is S-shaped and slowest at the

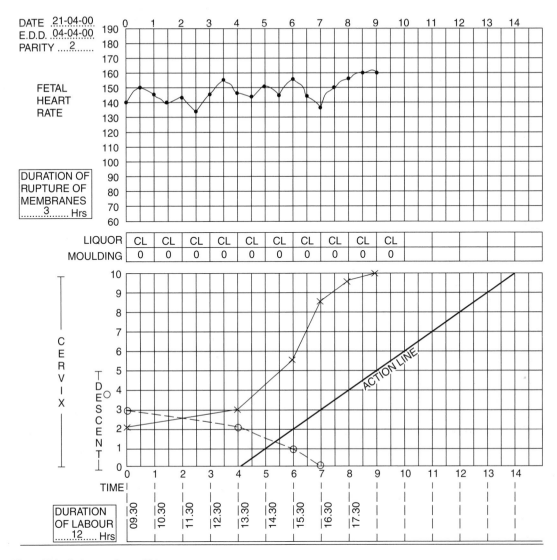

Figure 35.1 Partogram of normal labour

take-off (or accelerative phase) and decelerative phase as full dilatation is reached (Figure 35.1). The maximum slope is what is usually used to define progress during the active phase of labour.

As with all measurements, the 'average' rate of progress is exactly that, and thus 50 per cent of the population will progress at or below this rate. Drawing a distinction between what is acceptable progress and what becomes problematic is one of the most difficult dilemmas we have in modern obstetrics. Augmentation is not without problems, but prolonged labour also carries risks (see Chapter 27). The World Health Organization recommends an action line placed 3 hours behind the ideal progress line, set at 1 cm/hour (Figure 35.1). Whilst this is not perfect, it represents a reasonable compromise.

During the first stage, the fetal head, which normally presents to the pelvic brim in the occipito-lateral position, flexes and undergoes rotation through the pelvis to reach the outlet in the occipitoanterior position. This is termed internal rotation.

Second Stage

This is the stage of expulsion of the fetus and begins once the cervix is fully dilated (or 10 cm by traditional definition). This means that no part of the cervix can be felt over the fetal head. As the presenting part descends, women experience a strong urge to bear down. This is assisted by the Ferguson reflex, where stretching of the cervix and upper vagina in late first and second stages feeds back to the pituitary via the pelvic nerves and produces an increase in the release of endogenous oxytocin. Contractions become more frequent and strong and expulsive efforts are enhanced. This reflex can be eliminated by the use of epidural anaesthesia. Because of the widespread use of epidural anaesthesia (see Chapter 36), the second stage can be divided into passive and active components. The passive stage allows further descent and rotation of the fetal head. The active phase is entered once bearing down efforts occur.

The second stage is normally less than an hour. This is an arbitrary limit and in nulliparae is not predictive of lack of successful spontaneous delivery. As long as the fetus is healthy, the mother is coping and progress is being made, she should be allowed to continue to push. In multiparae, however, if after an hour of pushing the baby remains undelivered and delivery is not close, then help may be required.

As the head is delivered it extends over the perineum and then rotates to its normal position with respect to the fetal shoulders. This is termed restitution. The shoulders rotate into the anteroposterior plane (external rotation), and with gentle downward traction the anterior shoulder is delivered first, followed by the posterior shoulder and the rest of the baby. The cord is clamped and divided and the baby passed to the mother.

Third Stage

The placenta is usually delivered within 30 minutes. A physiological third stage awaits spontaneous separation of the placenta, without the administration of exogenous oxytocics. This is favoured by some women and is the norm in countries where oxytocics are unavailable, but carries the risk of heavier bleeding. The average blood loss for a physiological third stage is 500 mL. Most units recommend Syntocinon 10 units or Syntometrine (500 μg ergometrine plus 5 units Syntocinon) to limit postpartum loss. These definitely reduce loss, but have a few side-effects, of which nausea and vomiting are the most troublesome.

Perineal trauma, either a tear to the vagina and/or perineal tissue or a deliberately placed incision (episiotomy), are common in first labours. They are repaired after delivery of the placenta. Synthetic polyglycolic acid sutures are the best at minimizing short-term discomfort.

Cinical Assessment

On admission to the delivery ward, maternal and fetal assessments are made.

Maternal Assessment

On arrival on the delivery ward, full assessment of the pregnancy will be made, and any risk factors that could have a bearing on labour are identified.

Check:

Blood pressure
Temperature
Pulse
Urinalysis for protein, blood and ketones
Contraction frequency

The findings are recorded on the partogram. During labour the maternal assessment should be repeated at least 2-hourly. A full discussion of the wishes of the mother should be undertaken and any birth plan explored.

Fetal Assessment

Key features

Assessment of fetal size
Engagement of the presenting part
Fetal lie
Fetal well-being

Assessment of fetal size is generally performed by palpation, sometimes with additional symphysis–fundal height measurement. The aim is to detect small and large fetuses.

Degree of engagement of the fetal head is determine by palpation and measured in fifths of the head palpable abdominally. Thus, 5/5 means that the whole of the head is still palpable and the head unengaged. This is plotted on the partogram.

Fetal lie can be felt by palpation of the fetal back and limbs. It is useful information to be gained prior to vaginal examination, as it will aid definition of position.

Many units utilize an admission fetal heart rate tracing to assess immediate fetal well-being (see Chapter 29). In the presence of a normal admission trace in an uncomplicated pregnancy, intermittent fetal heart rate monitoring may be used for ongoing monitoring in labour. The fetal heart rate is recorded on the partogram.

Vaginal Examination

Once the fetal and maternal conditions have been appraised, a vaginal examination is performed to assess the progress of labour.

Key features

Cervical dilatation, effacement, consistency and degree of application to the fetal head
The presence or absence of membranes over the head
The position of the fetal head
The station in relation to the ischial spines
Evaluation of moulding and caput
Colour of the liquor

These features should be recorded on the partogram.

Position is defined by the relationship between the denominator and the maternal pelvis. In the case of a vertex presentation, the denominator is the occiput. (In a breech presentation, the denominator is the sacrum, and in a face presentation, the chin or mentum.)

The station is an estimation of the relationship between the presenting part and the ischial spines, measured in centimetres above or below the spines. Because the fetal head may become distorted during labour, abdominal palpation is more important than measuring descent vaginally.

Moulding is the degree of overlap of the fetal skull bones. This important sign may be a feature of obstructed or poorly progressing labours. Caput, which is oedema of the fetal scalp, is less important, but often found in prolonged labour.

Clear liquor is seen in uncomplicated labours. The presence of meconium-stained liquor, or of no liquor at all, increases the possibility of fetal hypoxia.

Management During Labour

Now that you understand the principles of normal labour, as far as can be defined, there are some prin-ciples of management which help to ensure that all runs smoothly and that problems are identified as soon as possible, without submitting large numbers of women to inappropriate interventions.

Principles of management of labour

Observation and appropriate and timely intervention to prevent fetal or maternal morbidity
Support of the mother, with provision of pain relief, nutrition where appropriate, and emotional support
Respect for the wishes of the parents

The Role of the Primary Carer

Recent randomized controlled trials have also shown that women cared for in labour by midwives with whom they are familiar, and who provide continuous care in labour, have improved outcomes in terms of the need for pharmacological pain relief, the incidence of episiotomy and perception of labour. Few other interventions in labour can be shown to improve outcomes in this way.

Nutrition in Labour

The risk of emergency Caesarean section under general anaesthesia, with the possibility of aspiration of gastric contents, is much lower in modern obstetrics. It is thus recognized that women assessed as low risk in labour should be allowed to eat and drink a restricted diet. This excludes fats and fizzy drinks, but allows a choice which many women find valuable.

Mobility

Women should be allowed to mobilize and adopt a comfortable position for labour as far as possible. The use of continuous fetal monitoring and epidural anaesthesia limits this, but even here advances are being made to encourage more mobility, with portable monitors and less motor blockade during analgesia. In some units, women may even walk under supervision with epidural anaesthesia. This is important for the following reasons:

- Demands for pharmacological methods of pain relief appear to be reduced if women are not confined to the bed.
- Freedom to move and adopt a range of positions heightens emotional well-being and ability to cope.

- When women are not restricted, they tend to naturally favour upright postures and will instinctively squat, kneel, sit, walk or go on their hands on knees ('all fours').

Assessment of Progress

In order to assess the progress of labour, it is normal for the vaginal examination to be performed at least 4-hourly. There is a margin for error in examinations, and where possible these should be performed by the same person.

The progress of labour is represented graphically. If progress falls behind the action line, then intervention may be required. There are three key elements in the documentation of progress in labour:

- cervical effacement
- cervical dilatation
- descent of the presenting part.

In order to represent these easily, the last two are charted graphically on a document called a partogram. This will also carry other important information, such as contraction frequency and maternal and fetal observations. This will make identification of the stages of labour easier and allow rapid transfer of complex information between professionals.

Fetal Monitoring

If the fetal heart rate on admission was normal, and no risk factors that may increase the possibility of fetal susceptibility to hypoxia are present, two options are available for monitoring the fetus:

- intermittent monitoring with a Pinard's stethoscope, hand-held Doppler or fetal heart rate monitor;
- continuous electronic fetal heart rate monitoring.

The advantages of the former are that the mother may be mobile and will feel less restricted. The disadvantages are that this should be performed every 15 minutes during the first stage and every 5 minutes in the second stage, thus making it labour intensive. Continuous fetal monitoring has the advantage of prompt identification of minor changes that may be difficult to hear and does not require such a high level of attendance. The disadvantages are that it restricts the mobility of the mother and may lead to intervention for clinically unimportant fetal heart rate changes. Continuous monitoring is of proven benefit in high-risk (see Chapter 29) or poorly progressing labours. It does not confer any advantage in mothers who are identified as low risk and who are labouring normally.

Prior to either type of monitoring, the maternal pulse should be palpated at the same time as listening to the fetal heart sounds to differentiate between maternal and fetal heart rates.

Second Stage

Most women have an uncontrollable urge to push once the second stage commences. This is not so when epidural analgesia is used. It is therefore important in these women to allow the analgesia to wear off to such an extent that they have some urge to push but are not suddenly incapacitated with pain. The mother should adopt a position in which she feels comfortable to push. As long as the mother and fetus are well and progress is being made, the second stage may be allowed to continue. Intervention should be advised if the mother becomes exhausted, the fetus appears to be compromised or, in multiparae without epidural, an hour has elapsed.

Various techniques have been adopted to deliver the fetal head. These generally involve encouraging flexion of the head as it delivers to minimize perineal damage. This is of unproven benefit. Episiotomies are made in far fewer women in modern obstetrics, as two facts have been established:

- Tears heal as well as, if not better than, episiotomies.
- An episiotomy does not prevent third-degree tear.

If an episiotomy is to be cut, the mother should be informed.

Third Stage

Oxytocics reduce blood loss and are administered with the delivery of the anterior shoulder. Lengthening of the cord, contraction of the uterus and sometimes a short brisk blood loss herald separation of the placenta. The left hand is used to palpate the abdomen above the symphysis pubis, to ensure the fundus stays above this level. The placenta is delivered by gentle cord contraction. Maternal

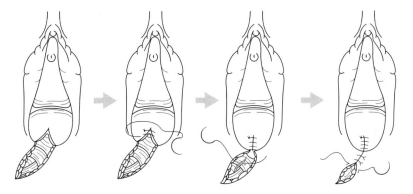

Figure 35.2 Perineal repair

effort can help this process if the placenta is difficult to deliver or the cord snaps.

The placenta is inspected to ensure it is complete, and a vaginal examination is performed to identify any perineal trauma.

Repair of Perineal Trauma

Tears and episiotomies tend to involve the vaginal skin, skin of the perineum, the perineal body, transverse perinei and bulbocavernosus muscles.

The repair is undertaken with good lighting and adequate analgesia (either a topped-up epidural or infiltrated local anaesthetic). It can be accomplished with polyglycolic acid sutures throughout, which cause less short-term pain. The vaginal skin is closed first, followed by approximation of the perineal muscles (see Figure 35.2). The perineal skin can be left open as long as it is approximated to 0.5 cm and there is good haemostasis. This causes less long-term discomfort.

Following delivery, the mother and baby should be placed skin to skin and breast-feeding encouraged.

Many babies will spontaneously move towards the nipple if placed on the mother's abdomen after delivery. Couples appreciate this time with their new baby and this should be a priority for all newly delivered mothers.

Learning Points

- **Normal labour is difficult to define**
- **Minimizing fetal and maternal morbidity is the key aim**
- **Modern obstetrics allows many things that were previously prohibited, such as feeding in labour**
- **Respect for mother's wishes is paramount**

See Also

Abnormal fetal heart rate patterns in labour (Chapter 29)

Pain relief in labour (Chapter 36)

Pain relief in labour

Importance

Pain during labour exceeds the expectations of women in at least 30 per cent of cases. Efforts to relieve this have been documented in cultures as far back as the Ancient Egyptians.

Labour pain is unpredictable, and total pain relief that does not interfere with the labour process or the mother's consciousness is difficult to achieve. Women need to be provided with information about available options in the antenatal period, when they can assess them for themselves and decide which pathways of pain relief they would wish to follow. All women, even those who have laboured before, should be encouraged to keep an open mind and not to perceive an unexpected need for pain relief as a failure.

Assessment

When a woman is admitted in early labour, part of the initial assessment will be to ask about her preferred choices for pain relief. Many women will prefer to climb the pain control ladder, moving on to a more efficacious method as labour advances. Some women know that they wish as much pain relief as possible early on and will request epidural analgesia once labour is confirmed. Some factors can be recognized as increasing the need for greater levels of pain relief.

Factors influencing level of pain relief needed

Prolonged labour
Augmentation or induction of labour
Fear/anxiety
Decreased mobility

Management

Principles of pain relief in labour

Provide information about the forms of pain relief available
Encourage women to keep an open mind
Discuss views on pain relief on admission in labour
Be realistic about the limitations of each method
Be aware of the effects of analgesia on the labour process, which may lead to maternal complications
Know which analgesics have fetal effects, and how these may be monitored

The carer has a vital role in labour, as the mother's ability to cope is improved if a practitioner provides continuous support. In fact, this is the only intervention in labour that has been shown not only to reduce the need for pharmacological pain relief, but also to improve neonatal and maternal outcomes.

Antenatal Education

Ideally, discussion should take place before labour, so that the woman is well informed about the options available to her in labour. It is important that during pregnancy women are made aware of options for pain relief and understand both their advantages and disadvantages.

On admission in labour, a full discussion can take place. Factors that may influence the labour will be more apparent and the needs of the mother will be easier to ascertain. A written birth plan can help to facilitate communication when a woman is admitted in established labour, when verbal communication may be hampered.

During labour, it is common for women to progress from one form of pain relief to the next. It is important that they are given accurate information with which to make these choices and do not feel that they have failed if they find their chosen method is inadequate for their needs.

Pain relief options

Simple measures

Transcutaneous nerve stimulation (TENS)

Inhalation analgesia

Opiates

Regional analgesia

Simple Measures

These will include having someone to rub the back, using a TENS machine or immersing in warm water. TENS has been utilized for many types of pain, including joint pains, especially back pain, and is popular with women who are keen to avoid pharmacological forms of pain relief in labour. TENS machines are often available for hire. There is no compelling evidence that TENS has an analgesic effect and it is likely that it carries no significant advantages over simple back rubbing.

The use of warm water during the first stage of labour as a form of pain relief has been practised for many years. The availability of large pools enables better and more prolonged immersion. This encourages relaxation, thus enabling the body to produce its own endogenous opiates in response to painful stimuli. Whilst objective testing of water immersion has not been shown to provide relief of pain, it gives physical support of body weight, encourages an upright or squatting position and, most importantly, gives great satisfaction to mothers, with no side-effects if limited to use in the first stage.

Advantages/disadvantages of simple measures

Advantages
- Easy and cheap
- TENS and back rubbing are safe for the fetus
- Mobility is encouraged, which can aid descent and rotation of the fetal head

Disadvantages
- These simple measures provide only limited analgesia
- There have been cases of water inhalation in babies born underwater
- Overheating of the fetus during maternal immersion increases oxygen requirements and is potentially harmful (this is avoided if the water temperature is kept at 34 °C)

Inhalation Analgesia

Nitrous oxide is available in a mixture containing 50 per cent oxygen and 50 per cent nitrous oxide (Entonox). When inhaled, the nitrous oxide is analgesic in sub-anaesthetic concentrations and, because of its low solubility in blood, rapidly achieves analgesic concentration in the brain after five to six breaths. This effect rapidly reverses between contractions. As a method of pain relief, it is not very effective. It has problems in that it takes five to six breaths to reach analgesic concentrations.

Advantages/disadvantages of inhalation analgesia

Advantages
- Easy to administer
- Controlled by the mother

Disadvantages
- Only 30 per cent report real analgesic effects
- Nausea and sedation occur if continued after contraction ceases
- Dehydration after prolonged use
- Hyperventilation can lead to decreased oxygen delivery to the fetus (respiratory alkalosis shifts the maternal oxygen dissociation curve to the left, reducing oxygen availability to the fetus)

Opiate Analgesia

The most commonly prescribed opiate for pain relief in labour is pethidine. Other opiates, including morphine, are occasionally used. Although opiates are widely used, they do not produce good analgesia to cope with labour pains, which are episodic. In order to overcome the acute pain of contractions, large doses of opiates may be needed and side-effects can be problematic.

Advantages/disadvantages of opiate analgesia

Advantages
- Easy to give
- Licensed for midwifery administration without prescription

Disadvantages
- Only 25–30 per cent of women report good analgesia
- Nausea – due to both a central effect and delayed gastric emptying
- Sedation – especially if repeated doses
- Decreased respiratory drive
- Loss of feelings of being in control

Significant fetal sedation may lead to difficulties in classifying the cardiotocogram (CTG) (see Chapter 29) and neonatal respiratory depression is fairly common (see Chapter 34).

Regional Analgesia

This is the only method of analgesia in labour that can be said to produce true pain relief. Two modes of delivery are possible, which can be combined: (i) infusion of local anaesthetics (usually Marcain) into the epidural space through a fine catheter (epidural analgesia); and (ii) single injection of a lower dose into the cerebrospinal fluid (spinal anaesthesia).

The addition of small quantities of opiates reduces the need for large doses of local anaesthetic and may help to preserve mobility in women who chose epidural analgesia. Epidural analgesia is designed to provide continuous analgesia, either by infusion or by intermittent top-ups during labour. Spinal anaesthesia produces a quicker acting block, but is a single dose, and thus the effects will wear off after a few hours. It is ideal when a good anaesthetic effect is required for a short time, such as to facilitate an instrumental delivery or Caesarean section. Some units combine the approaches, giving combined spinal/epidural anaesthesia to improve to onset of action, but provide ongoing analgesia.

Advantages/disadvantages of regional anaesthesia

Advantages
- Degree of pain relief
- Little or no neonatal depression due to drug effects
- No maternal sedation
- Reduced need for general anaesthesia
- Very high levels of maternal satisfaction

Disadvantages
- Increased instrumental delivery rate
- Peripheral vasodilatation
- Reduced uterine blood flow
- Risk of headache
- Incomplete block

The major advantage of regional anaesthesia and analgesia is its ability to provide true relief of labour pains. It is much safer if Caesarean section is required, markedly reducing the need for general anaesthesia and its attendant risks.

However, there are some profound disadvantages, which must be fully understood by mothers before use.

Regional analgesia reduces maternal ability to push and in primigravidae increases the need for instrumental operative delivery and perineal trauma accompanying this. The Ferguson reflex is abolished, as labour approaches the second stage, and Syntocinon augmentation is more commonly needed. Loss of mobility reduces the opportunity for gravity to aid descent.

Sympathetic blockade leads to vasodilatation of the legs, redistributing blood flow, which may lead to fetal compromise if placental perfusion is borderline. Even if hypotension does not occur, significant changes in uterine blood flow are seen. Prolonged epidural usage prevents maternal heat dissipation, leading to pyrexia, fetal tachycardia and increased oxygen demand.

Very occasionally, dural puncture will occur with the epidural needle. This can lead to significant headache and require further treatment. If unrecognized and normal doses of Marcain are given, widespread spinal blockage can ensue, with respiratory and cardiac arrest. Rarely, severe complications such as epidural haematomas occur, leading to paralysis. Epidural analgesia cannot be used in women with clotting abnormalities or low platelets.

A patchy or incomplete block occurs in up to 30 per cent of women. If expectations are high, this leads to significant dissatisfaction.

Despite the disadvantages, epidural analgesia is the most common method used by primigravidae in many units in the UK.

Learning Points

- **The provision of one-to-one care in labour reduces the requirements for pharmacological pain relief**
- **Women need to be encouraged to keep an open mind, especially in a first labour**
- **Antenatal education is vital to provide information about pain relief in a fully informed way**
- **Only regional analgesia has been shown to provide true pain relief in labour**
- **Regional analgesia is associated with some effects which may compromise maternal and fetal outcomes**

See Also

Normal labour (Chapter 35)

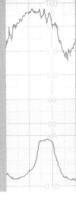

Postpartum haemorrhage

Definition

Postpartum haemorrhage (PPH) can be divided into both primary and secondary categories. Primary PPH is blood loss exceeding 500 mL in the first 24 hours following delivery. Secondary PPH is more difficult to define, but encompasses any excessive bleeding after 24 hours.

Importance

Postpartum haemorrhage can be a life-threatening event (6.4 per million maternities in the UK, 1991–1993). The morbidity is also high. Blood transfusion following delivery may be needed, and many women will be discharged with a low haemoglobin, which takes a few weeks to become normal.

Causes

Causes of PPH

Uterine atony
Genital tract trauma
Placental site bleeding
Uterine rupture or inversion
Clotting disorders

Uterine atony is the commonest cause of significant PPH. It is most likely to occur if the uterus has been overworked or overdistended. These conditions occur in prolonged labour (especially if augmented with Syntocinon), multiple pregnancy, polyhydramnios and large babies.

It is also more common in grand multiparae. Recent studies have shown that the mean blood loss for expectant management of the third stage is 500 mL. An actively managed third stage reduces the PPH rate by two-thirds.

Genital tract trauma may be perineal, vaginal or cervical. Typically, the uterus feels well contracted and the bleeding continues in a steady fashion. If large vessels are involved, the bleeding may be heavy. Prolonged labour is associated with a greater risk of genital tract bleeding, as there is a higher incidence of perineal oedema and instrumental delivery with subsequent perineal trauma.

Placental site bleeding is most likely to cause problems in association with three specific pathological conditions:

- *Retained placenta* prevents the uterus from adequately contracting. Often the placenta has already detached, but is still completely or partially within the cavity of the uterus.
- *Placenta accreta* occurs when the trophoblast invades beyond the decidua basalis. Further invasion into or through the myometrium is termed increta and percreta. Morbidly adherent placenta is more common in women who have had surgery on the uterus, including previous Caesarean section, myomectomy, septostomy or even sometimes just a rather aggressive dilatation and curettage. Bleeding is most severe when the placenta is partially removed, as the vessel thus uncovered cannot contract in the normal way.
- *Placenta praevia* (see Chapter 26) leads to PPH because the lower segment of the uterus does not contain the thick layer of myometrium, which causes vessel constriction. The large venous sinuses that supplied the placental bed thus continue to bleed.

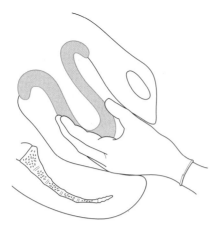

Figure 37.1   Manual replacement of uterine inversion

Uterine rupture is uncommon. It can occur when Syntocinon is used in multiparae or in women with a scar from a previous Caesarean section. Scar dehiscence or rupture tends to cause less bleeding, as it is generally lower segment. Rupture of an unscarred uterus is usually upper segment. Often the degree of shock is inconsistent with the revealed bleeding, as much will be into the abdominal cavity. In very rare cases, uterine rupture is as a result of a rotational vaginal delivery.

Uterine inversion is very rare. At presentation, the fundus cannot be palpated abdominally and a mass that is the uterine fundus can be felt within the vagina or at the introitus (Figure 37.1). Because of the vagal effect of traction on the infundibulopelvic ligaments, the pulse rate can be low, despite heavy bleeding.

Very occasionally, clotting disorders may present with PPH. Von Willebrand's disease (VWD) is the most commonly recognized inherited bleeding abnormality, with a prevalence of 0.8–1.3 per cent. VWD arises as a result of inherited deficiency of von Willebrand factor and is divided into several types and subtypes. In all types, women are at risk of severe bleeding during delivery if the defect remains uncorrected. Some women will not be aware they have this problem until they present with severe PPH.

Diagnosis and Clinical Assessment

Blood loss at delivery is notoriously difficult to quantify. Blood loss significant enough to produce a

fall in blood pressure is usually in excess of 1500 mL. Sometimes the true degree of loss only becomes apparent when a postnatal haemoglobin check is performed.

Whilst resuscitation is taking place, a diagnosis of the cause must be made and treatment rapidly instituted.

> **Key questions**
>
> Is the placenta delivered?
> Does the uterus feel well contracted?
> Is there obvious bleeding from perineal lacerations or episiotomy?
> Were there any predisposing factors that may be important?

Management

> **Priorities**
>
> Rub up a contraction
> Summon help
> Resuscitation
> Identify and treat the underlying cause
> Replace blood loss

When excessive blood loss is recognized, the patient must be resuscitated and the cause dealt with as quickly as possible.

Resuscitation

Resuscitation follows similar lines to that outlined in Chapter 25. A team consisting of the obstetrician, anaesthetist and senior midwife is needed.

> **Basic tenets of resuscitation**
>
> Site two i.v. cannulae of at least 16 gauge
> Take blood for full blood count, clotting and cross-match
> Give 1 L of crystalloid initially, followed by blood, if available, or colloid if not
> Site a Foley catheter to monitor urine output
> Measure pulse and blood pressure every 5 minutes

Ensure that the Uterus is Contracted

Uterine atony is the commonest cause of PPH. The management is therefore to produce rapid and long-acting contraction. The uterus can be contracted by rubbing up a contraction abdominally or by bimanual compression, with one hand on the fundus

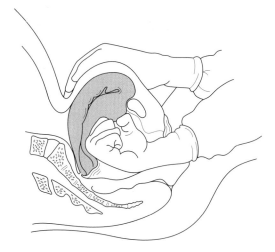

Figure 37.2 Bimanual compression of the uterus

and one in the vagina (see Figure 37.2). This can produce a holding situation whilst oxytocics are administered; 10 IU Syntocinon i.v. will produce a rapid contraction. Syntometrine (which contains 5 IU Syntocinon and 500 μg ergometrine) can also be given. This should be followed by a Syntocinon infusion of 40 IU in 500 mL 5 per cent dextrose over 4 hours.

If this fails to produce adequate contraction, synthetic prostaglandins can help. Carboprost (prostaglandin F2α) is administered intramuscularly. It takes approximately 15 minutes to achieve an effect, but usually produces long-lasting contraction. It causes bronchospasm in a small number of women and asthmatics are especially at risk.

Examination under Anaesthetic

If conservative management is failing, a further cause must be sought. Examination of the genital tract and uterus under general anaesthetic should be performed. Clotting defects should be corrected.

Trauma to the genital tract can involve the perineum, vagina and cervix. If bleeding is not subsiding despite good uterine contraction, this is the most likely cause. A careful examination with good lighting is vital. Tears to the cervix may be especially difficult to see, as they are high and can bleed torrentially. An examination of the uterine cavity may sometimes suggest a uterine rupture. Laparotomy must then be undertaken without delay.

Retained Placenta

Examination of the uterine cavity is undertaken when the placenta is fully or partially retained. This is done under anaesthetic, as it is particularly uncomfortable. If an epidural is *in situ* and the maternal condition is stable, this can be topped up.

The operator passes a hand behind the placenta to find a plane of cleavage, and the placenta is removed. Syntocinon and antibiotics should be given. If no plane of cleavage is found, a placenta accreta is suspected. Further attempts to remove the placenta piecemeal will cause torrential bleeding.

Hysterectomy is the safest form of management. If preservation of fertility is of paramount importance, conservative options have been tried, with some limited success. These include:

- curettage with Syntocinon;
- leaving the entire placenta in place (if it has not been partially removed and bleeding is not heavy);
- resection of part of the uterus with the adherent placenta.

These are dangerous options as heavy bleeding may occur at any time. If they are tried, early recourse to hysterectomy is vital if heavy bleeding occurs.

Hysterectomy

When bleeding from the uterus is uncontrollable by conservative means, hysterectomy is always the safest option.

Other surgical options

Ligation of the internal iliac arteries
Ligation of the uterine arteries
The B-lynch (belt and braces) suture

Arterial ligation reduces uterine perfusion. Successful pregnancies have been reported following this. The B-lynch suture compresses the uterus in three places, reducing blood supply to the placental bed, and has met with some success (Figure 37.3).

Postoperative Management

The patient should be managed in a high-dependency unit for at least 4 hours, to ensure that her condition is stable. Most labour wards have facilities for high-dependency care.

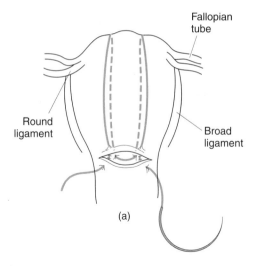

Fallopian tube

Round ligament

Broad ligament

(a)

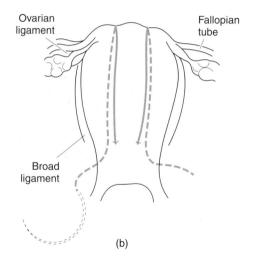

Ovarian ligament

Fallopian tube

Broad ligament

(b)

Figure 37.3 The B-lynch brace suture to control bleeding from the atonic uterus after Caesarean section. (a) Anterior view. (b) Posterior view

Observations to continue

Blood pressure
Pulse rate
Urine output
Blood loss

Only when the patient's condition has been stable for at least 4 hours should transfer to a lower dependency area be considered. If the measured haemoglobin is <8 g/dL, a top-up transfusion should be considered, as making up the deficit will take approximately 3–4 weeks.

Learning Points

- **PPH is a life-threatening situation**
- **Uterine atony is the commonest cause**
- **Bleeding from the genital tract can be persistent and lead to excessive loss**
- **Resuscitation and treatment must be instituted together**

See Also

Antepartum haemorrhage (Chapter 25)
Maternal collapse (Chapter 32)

Preterm labour

Definition

Preterm labour is the onset of labour before 37 weeks' gestation and after fetal viability. This usually means 24 weeks, when dates are certain.

Importance

Preterm labour occurs in approximately 4 per cent of pregnancies. Gestations of 34–36 weeks are generally not problematic to the neonate. Babies born before this gestation can have significant problems. The perinatal mortality rate is directly proportional to both gestation and birthweight. At 24 weeks, mean survival is less than 15 per cent. At 34 weeks, more than 99 per cent will survive.

In addition to death, there is significant morbidity attached to preterm delivery, including cerebral palsy, blindness/deafness, learning difficulties and lung disease.

Causes

Risk factors associated with preterm labour

Previous preterm delivery

Infection

Bleeding and abruption

Uterine distension (multiple pregnancy, hydramnios)

Growth restriction

Fetal abnormality

Cervical incompetence

Women who have had a preterm labour previously have a 15 per cent risk of subsequent preterm labour.

After two previous preterm deliveries, this increases to 40 per cent.

The commonest cause of spontaneous preterm labour is infection. Labour is usually preceded by rupture of membranes. The earlier the gestation, the more likely infection is to be implicated.

Abruption is covered in Chapter 25. It is common for significant abruption to trigger uterine activity and labour. There may be marked fetal compromise associated with this condition. Recurrent bleeding precedes 18 per cent of all preterm labours.

Multiple pregnancy is a common cause of preterm delivery. It is particularly a risk in multiple pregnancies complicated by other pathological conditions such as twin to twin transfusion syndrome, intra-uterine growth restriction or fetal abnormality. Polyhydramnios (see Chapter 13) is associated with spontaneous preterm delivery, as a result of uterine overdistension. There may also be underlying fetal abnormality, which is also contributory.

Babies born after spontaneous preterm labour tend to be smaller than those fetuses that remain *in utero*. The exact mechanism by which labour is triggered is not understood.

Cervical incompetence is a rare cause of recurrent preterm labour. Labour presents at a late stage with little evidence of uterine activity. Commonly delivery occurs between 16 and 24 weeks. Transvaginal ultrasound can show funnelling of the cervix, which is more apparent if fundal pressure is applied.

Smoking is associated with preterm labour in a dose-dependent way. As a single risk factor, however, its effect on gestation at delivery is only marginal. Other socioeconomic factors are likely also to have some impact and interact with smoking. Cocaine abuse is a potent trigger to both abruption and preterm labour. Additionally, drug withdrawal can also precipitate uterine activity.

Diagnosis and Clinical Assessment

History

Ask about:

Gestation

Contraction frequency and duration

Bleeding or show

Loss of fluid

A full history must also include previous obstetric history, events in the current pregnancy and enquiry about the above risk factors.

Because of the rapidly changing prognosis with gestation, dates must be accurately established. If an early scan (before 20 weeks) has been performed, this must be used to confirm dates.

Examination

Key findings

Maternal or fetal tachycardia

Pyrexia

Uterine tenderness

Cervical dilatation

Premature rupture of membranes

Abruption is associated with maternal tachycardia and, if severe, hypotension. The presence of a fever suggests possible chorioamnionitis or urinary tract infection.

Carry out an abdominal examination for tenderness, which may suggest infection or abruption, measure fundal height to assess fetal growth, and estimate liquor volume. Auscultation of the fetal heart should be performed.

Vaginal examination is important. If there is any suggestion of premature rupture of the membranes without contractions, only a sterile speculum examination should be performed. If there is uterine activity, a digital examination to assess cervical changes is important.

Investigations

Perform:

✓High vaginal swab

✓Full blood count

✓Ultrasound assessment of:

- Fetal presentation
- Fetal size
- Liquor volume

✓Cardiotocograph

Ultrasound can be a useful test to acquire extra information, but is irrelevant if the woman is admitted in established labour, except if the presentation is undefined. Swabs for bacteriology (including *Chlamydia*) must be taken. If the gestation is 26 weeks or more, cardiotocography should be performed.

Management

The aim of treatment of suspected preterm labour is to delay delivery for long enough for fetal lung maturity to be enhanced with corticosteroid therapy or so transfer can be arranged to a unit with neonatal facilities.

Steroid Therapy

Steroid therapy has a proven role in improving outcome at gestations of 26–34 weeks. The effect is maximal from 24–48 hours and lasts for 7 days.

Steroid therapy reduces:

Respiratory distress syndrome

Necrotizing enterocolitis

Oxygen dependence

There is increasing evidence that recurrent courses of corticosteroids may lead to childhood or adolescent hypertension and so, whilst having an undoubted benefit in the preterm infant, steroids must be used with care.

Tocolysis

There are a number of drugs that have been shown to have activity against uterine activity (tocolytics). Tocolytic therapy can successfully, albeit temporarily, inhibit preterm labour. Its main role is to delay labour until 24 hours after completion of corticosteroid therapy. In obstetric units with no neonatal facilities, tocolytics may be used to delay labour to allow intrauterine transfer to a unit with better facilities. All efforts should be made to assess the likely benefit or harm to the mother and the fetus if delivery is delayed.

Contraindications to tocolyis

Gestation more than 34 weeks

Advanced labour (contractions and cervical dilatation of
   3–4 cm)

Clinical signs of chorioamnionitis

Placental abruption

Evidence of fetal compromise or intrauterine fetal death

Evidence of maternal compromise

Tocolytics should not be used when fetal well-being is in jeopardy, as in suspected fetal acidosis, placental abruption or chorioamnionitis, or where maternal well-being is compromised, e.g. severe antepartum haemorrhage. Cardiac disease and diabetes are relative contraindications. After 34 weeks, there is no benefit in preventing labour.

The classes of tocolytic drugs available include:

- beta-sympathomimetics (ritodrine, salbutamol, terbutaline)
- calcium antagonists (nifedipine)
- magnesium sulphate
- nitric oxide donors (glyceryl trinitrate, isosorbide mono/dinitrate)
- prostaglandin synthetase inhibitors (indomethacin)
- oxytocin antagonists

Beta-sympathomimetics are widely used to inhibit uterine contractions. Ritodrine is the most commonly used drug in the UK and is effective in delaying labour for an average of 48 hours. It is usually given intravenously and has a number of significant side-effects.

Side-effects of ritodrine

Maternal and fetal tachycardia

Palpitations and shortness of breath

Hypotension

Tremor

Nausea and vomiting

Nervousness and restlessness

Hyperglycaemia and hypokalaemia

Careful monitoring of fluid balance is essential, as pulmonary oedema and maternal death have been reported, especially when beta-sympathomimetics are administered in conjunction with corticosteroids. Close monitoring of mother and fetus is important and must include:

- maternal pulse rate every 15 minutes, which should not rise above 140 beats/min;
- at least 4-hourly auscultation of maternal lung bases to check for developing pulmonary oedema;
- continuous fetal heart rate monitoring.

Hyperglycaemia and hypokalaemia are due to the influx of potassium to the intracellular compartment. Neonatal hypoglycaemia, as a result of maternal hyperglycaemia, can occur and careful neonatal glucose monitoring is needed if delivery occurs soon after stopping treatment.

Calcium channel blockers act by inhibiting the entry of calcium through the cell membrane, inhibiting the contractions of smooth muscles. Nifedipine in tablet form is an effective oral tocolytic agent. It is considered more effective than oral ritodrine with fewer side-effects. Its administration may be associated with headache, flushing, tachycardia and palpitations. It can be used where ritodrine is contraindicated or not tolerated.

Magnesium sulphate is used as a uterine muscle relaxant of choice in the USA. It is as effective as beta-sympathomimetics in delaying preterm labour. During administration, regular monitoring of blood pressure, urine output, respiratory rate and patellar reflexes is important and measurement of plasma magnesium concentration is recommended, as overdosage can cause respiratory depression, weakness, slurred speech, double vision, drowsiness, cardiac arrest and even death. Recently some concerns regarding fetal effects have been raised. It is rarely used in the UK.

Nitric oxide donors such as glyceryl trinitrate have the advantage of easy application (patches) and are widely used in some units. They appear to be effective, although there is little research into their effectiveness.

Labour is associated with an increase in type 2 cyclo-oxygenase in the fetal membranes. Therefore, cyclo-oxygenase inhibitors have been found to be effective in the suppression of uterine activity in this context. Indomethacin is the most widely used prostaglandin synthetase inhibitor used in the UK. It is associated with a number of deleterious effects, including premature closure of the ductus arteriosus and decreased fetal renal perfusion. It is not widely used except in the presence of idiopathic poly-hydramnios.

Recently an oxytocin antagonist (Atosiban) has been developed to overcome the side-effects encountered by alternative medications. The results of clinical trials assessing its effectiveness are still awaited, but animal work suggests a clinically useful effect.

Antibiotics

Infection is the most common cause of preterm delivery. Despite this, there is not yet convincing evidence that antibiotics are useful in disrupting the pathological process. They must certainly be used, however, in cases of confirmed vaginal infection, and in mothers who threaten preterm labour and have a history of group B streptococcal infection.

Cervical Cerclage

Emergency cervical cerclage has been attempted in cases that appear to be due to cervical incompetence. Some benefit has been shown in a small number of women.

Intrauterine Transfer

One of the most important reasons for attempting to defer delivery of the very preterm infant is to allow transfer of the patient to a unit with full neonatal facilities. Neonatal outcome has been shown to be improved by this strategy. It is vital that the conditions of the mother and fetus are fully assessed, as in 50 per cent of cases, transportation of the patient will be hazardous and neonatal transfer will be safer.

Management if Labour Continues

The fetal gestation at which preterm birth presents influences management and fetal outcome. The earlier the gestational age at presentation, the higher the possibility of an infective cause, which is usually followed by rapid progress in labour and delivery, regardless of treatment.

The mode of delivery will be determined by a number of factors. The preterm infant is at risk of hypoxia, which can cause damage to the immature fetal brain. The threshold for expediting delivery in cases of abnormal fetal heart rate patterns is lower. Continuous fetal heart rate monitoring should be instituted after 26 weeks.

Because of the higher risk of fetal head entrapment by an incompletely dilated cervix, the preterm breech is usually delivered by Caesarean section. There is, however, little concrete evidence to support this management.

When delivery is anticipated, it is vital for the parents to receive some counselling with regard to the likely outcome and degree of resuscitation the infant may need. This is especially important at the margins of viability, when full resuscitation may not be appropriate. Parental wishes in these cases must be ascertained before delivery if possible.

After delivery, every effort should be made to allow the parents easy and quick access to their infant. One of the advantages of *in utero* transfer is that splitting of mother and child should not occur. This is particularly important if the baby is delivered by Caesarean section, as the mother may not be able to travel for 24 hours after delivery.

Learning Points

- **Accurate estimate of gestational age is a vital starting place in the assessment of preterm labour**
- **Infection is the commonest cause of preterm delivery**
- **Steroid therapy is the mainstay of management and tocolysis should only be given with this in mind**
- **The preterm fetus is sensitive to hypoxia and acidosis and early recourse to delivery in cases of suspected fetal compromise is important**

See Also

Rupture of membranes while not in labour (Chapter 39)
Antepartum haemorrhage (Chapter 25)

Rupture of membranes while not in labour

Importance

Rupture of membranes (ROM) without labour occurs in 10 per cent of women. Most of these women will be at term (37 weeks), but 2 per cent of all pregnancies will be complicated by preterm premature rupture of membranes (PPROM). The major risk to both mother and fetus is of infection. Some cases of rupture of membranes are associated with small abruptions and will increase the risks of fetal compromise. Prolonged ROM can lead to significant oligohydramnios. This carries extra risks to the fetus, with poor lung development and limb contractures.

The treatment plans will change as the risks of prematurity become outweighed by the risks of infection, as gestation advances. Thus, the management can be broadly divided into dealing with the mature and dealing with the premature fetus. When a fetus becomes mature in this setting is open to debate. For the purposes of this chapter, we will define mature as being 34 weeks or more. At this gestation, neonatal survival will match that at term.

Diagnosis and Clinical Assessment

History

The important aspects of the history will focus on the relevant facts. The patient should be carefully questioned about events leading up to the suspected rupture of membranes. These may include passing urine or having a bath. Both of these can lead to a loss of fluid after the event that may not be liquor. A his-

tory of a gush of fluid followed by a continuous loss is very suspicious of ROM. Women who have laboured prematurely in previous pregnancies are more likely to do so in subsequent pregnancies, and ROM precedes labour in many cases.

A history of heavy vaginal discharge may point to vaginal infection, which, particularly in the case of bacterial vaginosis, may be enough to mimic ROM, but equally can predispose to ROM.

Establishment of the correct gestational age is vital, and any problems encountered in the pregnancy should be sought. Bleeding after 20 weeks is an important factor that should be identified, as it carries extra risks to the fetus.

Examination

Check for:

Pyrexia
Maternal or fetal tachycardia
Fundal height
Presentation
Uterine tenderness
Liquor seen on speculum examination

A general examination is very important. This should include temperature, pulse rate and blood pressure. The finding of a pyrexia is a particularly important feature.

An abdominal examination should next be performed. The salient features are:

- The fundal height – a smaller fundal height than expected may be found if liquor has leaked away.

In addition, growth restriction is a cause of premature labour, and ROM may precede this.

- The presentation – this is pertinent because delivery will be likely if ROM is confirmed and prelabour rupture of membranes is associated with abnormal presentations.
- Uterine tenderness or uterine contractions – both can indicate early infection.

At gestations of 26 weeks or more, monitoring of the fetus is vital. Fetal tachycardia is the earliest sign of impending chorioamnionitis, the major complication of ROM.

The diagnosis of ROM will usually rely on the finding of liquor draining. A speculum examination should be performed. The follow features are helpful in diagnosis:

- Pooling of liquor in the posterior blade of the speculum. This is pathognomonic for ROM.
- Liquor is alkaline in comparison to vaginal secretions. A positive nitrazine stick test indicates an alkaline pH. This can be false positive in the presence of semen, blood or bacterial vaginosis.

Liquor shows a characteristic pattern when a film is placed on a microscope slide, termed 'ferning'. This is a simple and easy test to perform, but it is rarely done.

At this point a digital examination of the cervix should not be performed, unless contractions are occurring and labour is thought to be likely.

Investigations

Relevant investigations

Vaginal and endocervical swabs
Full blood count
C-reactive protein
Ultrasound

Swabs must be taken from the vagina and cervix for bacteriological assessment, including an endocervical swab for *Chlamydia*. Full blood count and C-reactive protein can also be helpful in diagnosing impending chorioamnionitis. Remember that maternal white cell count will be elevated for 24–48 hours following steroid injections. Erythrocyte sedimentation rate is not useful in pregnancy, as this naturally rises.

Ultrasound scanning can be helpful if a decreased liquor volume is noted. Whilst this may not necessarily indicate ROM (placental dysfunction being another major cause), it may heighten the need for induction of labour or increased fetal surveillance. Ultrasound may also help confirm presentation.

At all stages of pregnancy, confirmation of fetal well-being must be undertaken. This is especially the case if a conservative management plan is to be implemented.

Tests to confirm fetal well-being

Cardiotocograph (CTG) assessment
Ultrasound for growth
Measurement of remaining liquor volume
Assessment of fetal breathing movements

Fetal breathing movements disappear in the presence of intrauterine infection, and therefore if seen can be reassuring.

Management

Priorities

Carefully reassess the gestation
Establish whether there is leakage of liquor
Evaluate fetal well-being
Carefully assess for infection
Decide whether to deliver or manage conservatively

In general, regardless of gestation, 70 per cent of women will go on to labour within 48 hours of ROM. The earlier the gestation at ROM, the higher the likelihood of infection.

Deciding Whether to Deliver

Signs of infection

Maternal pyrexia
Maternal tachycardia
Fetal tachycardia
Uterine tenderness

If there are signs of obvious infection, delivery should be considered. Antibiotics will not treat acute chorioamnionitis without delivery and delay may threaten the life of the mother if a severe infection develops. Additionally, it is recognized that the incidence of cerebral palsy is much higher in infants who suffered prolonged intrauterine infection, particularly if hypoxia supervenes.

If there are no signs of infection, the management will be influenced by the gestation of the pregnancy.

Gestation > 36 Weeks

At this point, there is no benefit to the fetus from prolonging the pregnancy. The risk of infection increases as the duration of ROM becomes longer. The intervention will, in part, be influenced by the prevailing incidence of vaginal infection. In most areas, where the risk of chorioamnionitis is reasonably low, allowing a delay of 24 hours is acceptable, as most women will labour in this time.

When labour does not occur, augmentation of labour is the most common management, although if no signs of infection are present, mothers who wish to defer this may be allowed to do so, with appropriate monitoring.

Methods of augmentation are the same as for induction of labour (see Chapter 30). Induction with prostaglandins or oxytocin infusion is equally effective regardless of the status of the cervix. There is little to choose in either case, as 10 per cent of women will require Caesarean section for failed augmentation, whichever method is chosen.

When the history is suspicious of ROM but no liquor has been seen, a repeat speculum examination after a period of rest in bed (e.g. overnight) can be helpful to demonstrate pooling of liquor. If this repeat examination is still negative, an assessment of liquor volume by ultrasound may be undertaken. If the liquor volume is normal, no further action needs to be taken. If a further loss occurs, this should be reported and re-investigated.

Gestation 34–36 Weeks

At gestations of 34–36 weeks, many choose the above strategy, as there is little to be gained in terms of fetal maturity. However, if the cervix is very unfavourable, the chances for a vaginal delivery may improve with waiting. It is important to ensure that there are no signs of infection and to confirm fetal well-being.

Gestation < 34 Weeks

Below 34 weeks the risks of prematurity must be balanced at all times against the risks to the mother and/or fetus of continuing the pregnancy. Fetal lung maturity can be compromised if delivery occurs.

Steroid injections (see Chapter 38) and antibiotic treatment with erythromycin should be given, and a delay of at least 24 hours gained, if possible. A delay of several weeks for the very immature fetus may be accomplished. The steroid dose may be repeated if delivery does not occur.

Nothing should delay delivery if infection supervenes, and thus if a conservative policy is introduced, fetal and maternal monitoring must occur.

Extreme Prematurity

Two main problems are likely with PPROM from very early gestations:

- pulmonary hypoplasia
- limb contractures.

At gestations of <24 weeks, fetal lung development can be compromised by a lack of liquor, and despite good overall fetal growth an infant can be born with significant lung hypoplasia, which prevents adequate oxygen delivery and may result in neonatal death. When rupture of membranes occurs at very early gestations (especially <20 weeks), termination of the pregnancy may be considered. The outlook is generally poorer if ROM occurs spontaneously rather than after a procedure such as amniocentesis. This is almost certainly because the forewaters are usually ruptured when spontaneous ROM occurs, leading to complete loss of liquor and a higher incidence of infection, whereas in procedure-related ROM there is a hindwater rupture which limits liquor loss and the opportunity for ascending infection.

Conservative Management

Fetal Monitoring

- Fetal heart rate (CTG) – a rise in the baseline and loss of variability are features of developing chorioamnionitis.
- Biophysical profile including fetal breathing movements.

Maternal Monitoring

The mainstay of maternal surveillance is temperature measurement. Even a small (0.5 °C) rise needs to be taken seriously, with a full search for infection. C-reactive protein can occasionally be helpful if a rise is seen over time. Full blood count performed weekly can show a rising white count before obvious infection is demonstrated.

The degree of monitoring needed usually requires prolonged hospitalization. This can be extremely difficult, especially if there are other children at home. After a period of monitoring of a few days, outpatient monitoring may be considered in some circumstances, with the risks carefully outlined and appropriate strategies for maternal and fetal monitoring put in place. Most women can be taught to monitor their own temperature and report any rises.

Antibiotics

A positive vaginal swab should be treated. The results of the ORACLE study have shown that the use of prophylactic erythromycin in preterm ruptured membranes is associated with a reduction in neonatal morbidity and increased gestational age at delivery.

Management During Labour

Labour usually ensues within 72 hours after ROM. If delivery does not occur in this time, the chances of a significant delay in delivery improve.

Labour remains a constant risk. If the fetal presentation is not cephalic, Caesarean section may be considered if labour occurs. The relative risks to the mother and fetus must be balanced on an individual basis. During labour, continuous fetal monitoring must be undertaken and signs of fetal compromise managed by expeditious delivery. Under no circumstances can a potentially infected preterm fetus be allowed to become hypoxic.

High doses of antibiotics must be started immediately if infection occurs. These must be in doses to allow rapid placental transfer and include adequate cover against group B *Streptococcus* and Gram-negative rods. The following combination is acceptable in most cases:

- ampicillin 2 g i.v. followed by 1 g 8-hourly until delivered;
- metronidazole 500 mg i.v. 8-hourly.

After delivery, antibiotics should be continued for at least 24 hours, and in significant infections for 5 days.

If swabs are found to be positive after delivery, a full maternal reassessment should take place and appropriate antibiotics considered if true infection is thought to be present or likely. Not all cases of positive swabs will require treatment. Positive blood cultures usually represent significant maternal infection and will only have been taken in the presence of pyrexia, necessitating treatment. A check of bacterial sensitivities should be undertaken to ensure appropriate antibiotics were used, and changes made as necessary.

The paediatricians should be made aware of any positive bacteriology, even if maternal treatment is not required.

Learning Points

- **ROM is a clinical diagnosis made on the basis of history and confirmation of leakage of liquor**
- **Infection, both maternal and fetal, is the major risk**
- **At term, augmentation of labour is usually considered**
- **Preterm management is generally conservative if no signs of infection are present**
- **If conservative management is adopted, careful fetal and maternal surveillance must be undertaken**
- **Steroids are indicated to enhance lung maturity in the preterm fetus**
- **Antibiotic treatment with erythromycin should be given**
- **Delivery must be expedited if infection occurs, and antibiotics should be promptly administered**
- **The combination of intrauterine infection, hypoxia and prematurity massively increases the risk of cerebral palsy**

See Also

Preterm labour (Chapter 38)
Infections in pregnancy (Chapter 12)

Shoulder dystocia

Definition

A 'practical' definition of shoulder dystocia is difficulty in extracting the shoulders after delivery of the head. A more specific definition is a situation in which manoeuvres are required to deliver the shoulders in addition to gentle downward traction and episiotomy.

Importance

Shoulder dystocia is an obstetric emergency. The incidence of shoulder dystocia is 0.15 to 1.7 per cent of all vaginal deliveries, which varies depending on its definition. Transient or permanent injury to the baby may occur. Rarely, the baby will not survive.

Causes

Mechanics of Shoulder Impaction

In order to understand how to deliver the baby whose shoulders are impacted it is important to understand how the situation arises:

- After delivery of the head, spontaneous external rotation returns the head to its perpendicular relationship to the shoulders, which are usually in an oblique axis under the pubic rami, and expulsive efforts by the mother drive the anterior shoulder under the pubis.
- If the shoulder fails to rotate into the oblique axis and remains in the anteroposterior position, the expulsive efforts drive the anterior shoulder against the symphysis.

- Strong maternal expulsive efforts then drive the anterior shoulder forward and upward, above the symphysis.
- If gentle downward traction to assist the delivery of the anterior shoulder is applied, the brachial plexus may be significantly stretched, leading to injury to the brachial plexus.
- As the fetus becomes hypoxic, after delivery of the head, the fetus loses muscle tone, which initially protects against undue stretching, and brachial plexus injury becomes easier to inflict.

Predisposing Factors

Factors associated with macrosomia

Diabetes
Prolonged pregnancy
Maternal obesity
Previous delivery of large infant

Certain conditions which predispose to fetal macrosomia carry a higher incidence of shoulder dystocia. The problem is that these do not always cause shoulder dystocia, and many babies that experience this complication are not macrosomic.

The incidence of shoulder dystocia increases to 31 per cent in diabetics whose infants weigh more than 4000 g. The incidence of shoulder dystocia in non-diabetic mothers is 22.6 per cent when their infants weigh more than 4500 g. However, almost half (47.6 per cent) of all shoulder dystocias occur in infants weighing less than 4000 g.

Even mothers who have previously had an infant with shoulder dystocia do not usually experience this again. Even if the infant is larger, only about 10 per cent will have similar problems.

Risks

The major maternal risks are of extended perineal trauma, and bony injury if symphysiotomy is needed as one of the manoeuvres.

The classic fetal injury is trauma to the brachial plexus. Duchenne made the connection to traumatic delivery in 1872 and Erb, in 1874, noted that the trauma most commonly affected the fifth and sixth cervical nerves. The lower trunk lesion (C8 and T1), described by Klumpke, generally affects the forearm and wrist. Horner's syndrome may be present on the affected side due to the involvement of the sympathetic fibres that traverse T1.

Rarely, a severe injury will involve the entire plexus and cause complete paralysis of the arm. Most infants that do have an observable palsy at birth have only transitory symptoms and recover with no permanent injury. Complete recovery may take up to a year, and between 4 and 15 per cent demonstrate some permanent sequelae.

Clinical Assessment

Recognizing which fetuses are large is not easy. There are three methods of establishing fetal size:

- abdominal palpation with fundal height measurement;
- ultrasound assessment, utilizing the abdominal circumference;
- ask the mother (if she has had babies before).

These are all valid methods. In some circumstances, they may be equally reliable. Ultrasound carries a margin of error of at least 15 per cent. This is greatest in the large fetus.

The only labour abnormality that has been shown to increase the incidence of shoulder dystocia is prolonged second stage. The head may be seen to deliver up to the nose and then retract back into the vagina, the 'turtle sign'.

With each additional risk factor, the risk of shoulder dystocia becomes higher, but the only factor that carries even a reasonable predictive value is the macrosomic fetus of a diabetic mother.

Management

Priorities

Suspect the problem in advance
Call for help when the problem becomes apparent
Go through the manoeuvres in turn
Accurately document the procedure
Carefully explain to the parents after the event

Difficulty with delivery of the shoulders should be anticipated in the presence of risk factors for macrosomia, previous shoulder dystocia and poor progress in the second stage of labour. In a minority of cases, delivery by elective Caesarean section may be recommended. This will usually be the case where there has been a history of significant shoulder dystocia in a previous delivery of a similar or smaller sized infant, or where there is evidence of significant macrosomia in a pregnancy complicated by diabetes. Where vaginal delivery is planned, an experienced obstetrician should be present at delivery and careful assessment made of any failure to progress in labour or the need for instrumental delivery.

Everyone who delivers babies must be able to go through the shoulder dystocia drill, as even with the best predictive indices only half of infants who experience this problem will have been suspected. With good management, the risk of injury to the baby can be minimized.

Shoulder dystocia drill

Anticipate a shoulder dystocia
Call for help and do not panic
Stop traction on the head
Make a large episiotomy
Move the mother into McRobert's position (Figure 40.1). This
    means flexing and abducting the thighs up onto the
    maternal abdomen, which flattens the sacral curve and
    gives more room for the shoulders
Apply suprapubic pressure to the anterior shoulder in the
    same direction as the fetal face and apply gentle
    downward traction
Avoid excessive traction on the neck

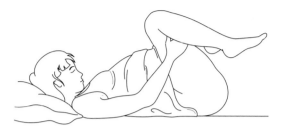

Figure 40.1 The McRobert's position for shoulder dystocia

With these manoeuvres, the majority of babies will be delivered. The next stage moves on to trying to rotate the shoulders to disimpact them:

- Perform a rotation manoeuvre, by pressure on the anterior shoulder in the direction of the fetal face (the wood screw manoeuvre).
- Extract the posterior arm.

If these are not possible or unsuccessful, there are three options:

- Partially divide the symphysis pubis (symphysiotomy);
- Replace the head and perform a Caesarean delivery (Zavanelli manoeuvre);
- Break the clavicle of the baby.

Symphysiotomy is the most tried and tested of the above. Cephalic replacement appears to be a difficult procedure in practice. Breaking the clavicle of the baby runs the risk of damage to the lung, vessels and nerves, and in these hearty, well-grown babies is very difficult.

Permanent neurological sequelae secondary to hypoxia become increasingly likely if delivery is not accomplished after 15 minutes.

All the manoeuvres attempted, and the time taken, must be carefully documented.

Counselling the Parents

Significant shoulder dystocia is very frightening for parents. Full counselling with both an experienced obstetrician and a paediatrician is important. Careful paediatric follow-up must be undertaken if there has been any injury. Most clinicians would advise that, if there has been significant injury to the baby, the next delivery should be by Caesarean section, even though it is realized that most women would not experience this again.

Learning Points

- **Shoulder dystocia is generally unpredictable**
- **Everyone delivering babies must know the drill**
- **Long-term neonatal sequelae are uncommon**

See Also

Large for gestational age (Chapter 13)
Diabetes (Chapter 8)
Failure to progress in the second stage (Chapter 28)

Section 4

On the maternity wards

41. Difficulty with breast-feeding 169
42. The confused or withdrawn mother 172
43. The febrile patient 175
44. Venous thrombosis 178

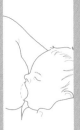

Difficulty with breast-feeding

Importance

Breast milk is the ideal food for the newborn baby. Breast-feeding provides nutrition, immunological and antimicrobial protection, aids digestion and facilitates mother–infant bonding. In addition, there is no risk of contamination, as may occur in the preparation of artificial feeds. The resulting protection against infection provides a distinct survival advantage (especially in the developing world). There is also a suggestion that breast-feeding may protect against later diseases (cancer, ischaemic heart disease, malabsorption syndromes), sudden infant death syndrome and child abuse, and may lead to higher cognitive performances.

Normal Physiology

After delivery, reduced oestrogen levels allow prolactin to initiate lactation. Suckling induces prolactin secretion and thus more breast milk. In response to suckling, oxytocin is released and causes milk ejection. During pregnancy and for the first 2–3 days after childbirth, colostrum (rich in protein and immunoglobulins) is secreted. Thereafter, breast secretion changes and milk volume increases.

Causes

Difficulties in breast-feeding may result from psychological, physiological or anatomical causes. They may be due to the mother, the baby or the health care professional, or a combination of these.

Causes of difficulty with breast-feeding

Mother
- Insufficient secretion
- Breast engorgement
- Sore or cracked nipples
- Flat or inverted nipples
- Breast infection

Baby
- Inability to suck
- Lethargy
- Breast refusal

Insufficient secretion is usually a temporary condition where the mother is tired, tense or overly anxious. The mother may have a poor knowledge of breast-feeding. Breast engorgement typically occurs on the third or fourth day after delivery. This early engorgement is due to lymphatic and venous stasis. The engorgement then interferes with milk flow along the lactiferous ducts. The condition can also occur at a later time during lactation whenever there is inadequate removal of milk from the breasts.

When the baby starts breast-feeding, the nipples are most likely to become sore or cracked if the baby is incorrectly fixed to the breast. The baby may cause an abrasion which can develop into a painful fissure or crack (the sensitivity of the nipples increases after delivery). Cracked nipples can be exacerbated by irritants such as soaps or perfumes.

Flat or inverted nipples increase the chance of the baby incorrectly fixing on the breast. However, babies should not feed from the nipple but should feed from the breast (with much of the areola in its mouth); thus breast-feeding is often successful despite flat or inverted nipples.

Breast infection or mastitis usually follows breast engorgement and cracked nipples. The infective organism is *Staphylococcus aureus*. If the mastitis is not treated adequately, an abscess may form.

A variety of conditions may prevent the baby from sucking properly, including prematurity, congenital anomalies such as cleft lip and palate, neurological disease or acute systemic infections. Lethargy may be temporary or may result from intrapartum sedatives. If persistent, possible causes include congenital heart or neuromuscular disease, and dysmorphic syndromes such as Down's syndrome. Refusal of a baby to take to the breast is usually temporary and the result of poor technique.

There are also a few contraindications to breast-feeding. These include severe maternal debilitating conditions or infections such as tuberculosis, human immunodeficiency virus (HIV) or recently acquired syphilis. Drugs that are contraindicated during breast-feeding include cytotoxic agents, radioactive compounds, lithium and chloramphenicol. Babies with rare metabolic disorders such as galactosaemia, lactose intolerance and phenylketonuria will not be able to take breast or cow's milk.

Diagnosis and Clinical Assessment

A careful history and examination of the mother, baby and the feeding process will allow an accurate diagnosis to be made.

History

Ask about:

Timing of the problem
Symptoms of pain and soreness
Previous/antenatal education and experience
Mother's attitude to breast-feeding

As detailed above, the timing of any breast-feeding difficulty may indicate the cause of the problem. Difficulties due to breast engorgement typically present on days 3–4, diminished secretion may be related to increased fatigue, and an ill baby may suddenly stop feeding. Painful breasts suggest engorgement or mastitis, whilst painful nipples may be due to nipple soreness or cracking. If a mother has previously breast-fed and is experiencing difficulties, there is an increased likelihood of the baby being the source of any problem. The mother's mental attitude plays an important role in the success of breast-feeding. Fear of failure, a poor self-image, misinformation and a lack of education may all contribute to breast-feeding problems.

Examination

Both the mother and baby should be examined, before and during breast-feeding. The mother's breasts and nipples should be examined carefully. The breasts may be engorged or there may be evidence of mastitis, with hard, reddened and tender breast(s) (there may also be axillary lymphadenopathy and pyrexia). The nipples may be flat, inverted, sore or cracked.

The baby should be examined thoroughly for any evidence of systemic illness or disease. Anatomical problems such as a cleft lip or palate should be excluded. Signs of dehydration (increased skin turgor, lethargy, oliguria) indicate an inadequate supply of breast milk.

The technique of breast-feeding should be observed to check the attachment and position of the baby on the breast. The baby should be held securely, should be brought to the breast rather than vice versa, and should attach adequately by taking much of the areola into the mouth (Figure 41.1).

Management

Prevention: Antenatal Preparation and Postnatal Support

Many breast-feeding difficulties can be prevented by mothers receiving antenatal education and encouragement regarding breast-feeding. Following delivery, the baby should be put to the breast as soon as possible, in a calm and supportive setting. Mothers should be helped to breast-feed and shown how to position the baby optimally.

Treatment of the Underlying Cause

Any underlying cause should be treated. Breast engorgement can be prevented or treated by allowing the baby unrestricted suckling; expression of milk between feeds may also be necessary. Sore or cracked

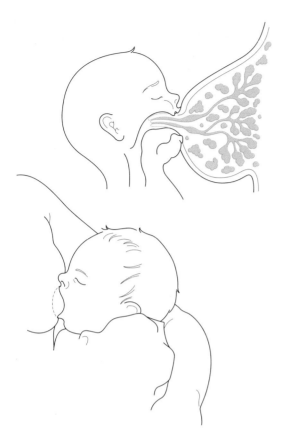

Figure 41.1 The correct position for breast-feeding

or manual expression) and the appropriate antibiotics (determined by culture of the milk) prescribed. Inadequate treatment may lead to an abscess which needs incising and draining. If there is a reason why the baby is unable to suck (such as prematurity), milk can be expressed and the baby fed via an intragastric tube until the ability to suck develops.

Artificial Feeding

Mothers may choose not to breast-feed or may abandon their attempts. Artificial formula feeds meet the nutritional requirements of the baby; unmodified cow's milk does not, and should not be used.

A baby that is thriving will have a lusty, vigorous cry, take feeds eagerly, sleep well and appear contented. There will be no apparent discomfort after feeds, no vomiting, and normal stools. Body weight will gradually increase.

Learning Points

- Breast milk provides nutrition and immunological and antimicrobial protection, aids digestion and facilitates bonding
- Difficulties in breast-feeding may result from the mother's attitude, problems with the breast/nipple, anatomical or systemic disorders affecting the baby, or poor breast-feeding technique

Further Reading

Sweet BR. The breast and breast-feeding. In: *Mayes' Midwifery*. Baillière Tindall, London, 1984, pp. 454–64.

nipples can be prevented by correct technique. If identified, the nipples should be checked for candidal infection (the baby's mouth should also be examined). Care must be taken to avoid infection. If mastitis does develop, the breast should be emptied (by suckling

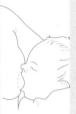

The confused or withdrawn mother

Importance

Childbirth is a major life event and is associated with significant psychological adaptation. Pregnancy and childbirth can cause or exacerbate mental illness, and psychiatric disorders are particularly common in the puerperium. Psychiatric disorders range from a mild depression ('maternity blues') to frank psychosis with schizophrenic, manic or depressive features. Suicide accounts for 4 per cent of maternal deaths.

Causes

Common causes of altered mood or behaviour in the puerperium

Maternity blues
Puerperal psychosis
Postnatal depression
Exacerbation of pre-existing psychiatric condition
Medical disorders presenting as acute confusional states

More than half of women experience 'maternity blues' or 'baby blues', characterized by transient episodes of tearfulness, emotional vulnerability and mild depression 2–5 days after childbirth. The condition is so common that biological rather than psychological causes have been proposed; factors such as hospitalization, medication, sleep deprivation, physical pain and adaptation to the needs of the baby may all be involved in the development of the blues.

Puerperal psychosis affects 1 in 500–1000 mothers and usually presents within 2 weeks of delivery, often with catastrophic impact on the mother, her baby and her family. The basic disorder is not understood; the predilection for the puerperium suggests that the associated endocrine, metabolic or psychological changes may be superimposed on a genetic predisposition.

Postnatal depression occurs in 10–15 per cent of women between 6 and 12 weeks after delivery and the clinical picture is typical of depression in other situations. Any pre-existing psychiatric condition may be exacerbated following childbirth. These include depressive and anxiety neuroses, phobic disorders, drug dependence, severe personality disorder and certain types of psychotic illness.

Occasionally, medical disorders can present as acute confusional states in the puerperium. Relevant conditions include 'all the failures', i.e. cardiac, respiratory, renal and liver failure; severe infections including meningitis, pneumonia and malaria; drug overdose, e.g. alcohol, amytriptyline or cannabis; small cerebrovascular accidents; hypoglycaemia or hyperglycaemia; and endocrine conditions such as thyroid problems.

Diagnosis and Clinical Assessment

History

A careful and detailed psychiatric history is crucial to establishing the diagnosis. A history from relatives and care-givers may provide important information.

As detailed above, maternity blues usually present on days 2–4, at the initiation of lactation, and persist for 24–48 hours. Puerperal psychosis presents within a month of delivery and most women become ill within a fortnight of delivery. The early days after delivery are often unremarkable and many observers have commented on the presence of a 'lucid' interval. In contrast, the peak incidence of postnatal depression is between 6 and 12 weeks after childbirth.

A history of weepiness, emotional lability, irritability and anxiety typifies women with maternity blues. These women may also suffer mild impairments of attention, concentration and memory. These clinical features also characterize women in the early stages of puerperal psychosis. However, of more sinister significance, there may also be signs of suspiciousness, irrational ideas and unusual reactions to the baby. The full clinical picture of puerperal psychosis usually takes the form of an affective disorder, manic or depressive in type, or schizophrenic features may predominate. In addition, there may be clouding of consciousness, perplexity and confusion, but not actual disorientation. Although there is some overlap between the clinical features of puerperal psychosis and postnatal depression, women with postnatal depression do not lose touch with reality. They present with several of the features of depression: lowered mood and self-esteem, tearfulness, hopelessness, guilt and self-reproach, fatigue, loss of appetite and libido, insomnia, irritability, inability to cope, isolation and social withdrawal.

A previous history of a psychiatric disorder should alert care-givers to the possibility of an exacerbation of that disorder, and also increases the risk of both puerperal psychosis and postnatal depression. A previous history of postnatal depression conveys a two-fold to four-fold increased risk in subsequent pregnancies, whereas a previous history of puerperal psychosis increases the risk 100-fold (to about 1 in 5–10). A positive family history of a psychiatric disorder also increase the risks of puerperal psychosis or postnatal depression developing.

In addition to a previous or family history, other risk factors for psychiatric disorders after childbirth include maternal age (over 30 years), subfertility, marital conflict or doubts about continuing with the pregnancy, poor parental relationships and major obstetric complications.

Examination and Investigations

The findings on clinical examination and the results of investigations rarely contribute to the diagnosis. Occasionally, however, clinical signs will indicate a possible medical disorder contributing to the confusional state, and further investigation is warranted. For example, a high fever may be noted (Chapter 43) or a tremor and a tachycardia may suggest thyroid disease.

Management

The appropriate management is dependent on the diagnosis. However, in severe disease, a multidisciplinary team approach is essential; there should be good communication and close collaboration between obstetricians, midwives, psychiatrists and general practitioners.

Maternity Blues

This is usually self-limiting, although occasionally the condition will progress to either puerperal psychosis or postnatal depression. Women should receive empathy and understanding and be encouraged to express their emotions.

Puerperal Psychosis

The management of puerperal psychosis should involve psychiatrists. Early recognition is preferable. An adequate psychiatric history should be taken from all pregnant women and those at high risk should be monitored carefully after delivery. Ideally, women at particularly high risk will have been in contact with psychiatric services before delivery. Early warning signs should prompt immediate evaluation. If psychosis is present, hospitalization is usually necessary. 'Mother and baby' units provide a therapeutic setting for the mother to care for her baby with the appropriate supervision and help. (In cases where there is concern about infanticidal impulses, some temporary separation may be necessary.) Therapeutic options include psychotherapy and a range of antipsychotic medication. Phenothiazines are appropriate where manic or schizophrenic features predominate. In depressed women, tricyclic antidepressants are commonly used. Tricyclic antidepressants can be prescribed in the knowledge that they do not enter breast milk in sufficient quantities to affect the infant (unlike phenothiazines). Lithium carbonate is of particular value as maintenance therapy. The immediate prognosis is fair and the majority of mothers are able to leave hospital within 2–3 months, but careful outpatient follow-up is essential.

Postnatal Depression

Early diagnosis is also crucial to the management of postnatal depression. Indeed, women with risk factors should receive prophylactic antenatal counselling. After delivery it is important to ensure that a network of family and friends is available to provide help and support; this network should complement the health care team. In mild cases, medication is usually avoided. However, in severe cases, or if there is a slow or inadequate response to supportive measures, antidepressant drugs (such as tricyclic agents) are often necessary. Hospitalization may occasionally be needed. Again, the use of specialist 'mother and baby' units is preferable.

Learning Points

- Psychiatric complications after childbirth include maternity blues, puerperal psychosis, and postnatal depression
- A detailed psychiatric history, including the timing and precise nature of signs and symptoms, any previous or family history of psychiatric disorders, and the presence of any risk factors, is crucial to establishing the diagnosis
- In the management of severe disease, a multidisciplinary team approach is essential

See Also

The febrile patient (Chapter 43)

Further Reading

Kumar R. Pregnancy, childbirth and mental illness. In: Studd J, ed. *Progress in Obstetrics and Gynaecology*, vol. 5. Churchill Livingstone, Edinburgh, 1985, pp. 134–45.

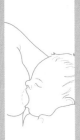

The febrile patient

Importance

Because of the nature of the labour process, both the genital and urinary tracts are particularly prone to infection. Following an operative procedure (such as a Caesarean section) additional avenues of infection are opened. Puerperal pyrexia is commonly defined as a temperature elevation to 38 °C on two occasions after the first 24 hours postpartum.

Causes

Differential diagnosis of a postpartum fever

Endomyometritis
Haematomas/abscesses
Wound infection
Urinary tract infection
Chest infection
Deep venous thrombosis
Septic pelvic/ovarian vein thrombophlebitis
Mastitis/breast abscess

A uterine infection or endomyometritis is a common and serious infection of the puerperium. The incidence is approximately 2–3 per cent following vaginal delivery and 15–20 per cent after Caesarean section (in the absence of prophylactic antibiotics). Following delivery there is a loss of the epithelial covering at the placental site which predisposes to infection by organisms that are commensals in the bowel or lower genital tract (*Escherichia coli*, anaerobic streptococci and *Bacteroides*). Any retained placental tissue will act as a nidus for infection.

As discussed in Chapter 18, pregnancy predisposes to urinary tract infections and asymptomatic bacteriuria may be present. Stasis of urine may be exacerbated during the labour and urinary retention may follow regional anaesthesia or result from reflex inhibition from the pain or abdominal or perineal wounds. Catheterization may lead to colonization by organisms of the lower urethra. These factors contribute to the development of cystitis and pyelonephritis.

Haematomas/abscesses may be in the lower vagina or vulva (vulval haematomas may extend into the ischiorectal space). Haematomas above the pelvic diaphragm may arise from high vaginal lacerations, cervical lacerations or vessels of the broad ligament.

The incidence of wound infections after Caesarean section ranges from 3 to 20 per cent (in the absence of prophylactic antibiotics) and is much higher after emergency than after elective procedures. Infection is caused by a mixture of anaerobic and aerobic bacteria similar to those found in endomyometritis (*Escherichia coli*, *Proteus mirabilis*, *Bacteroides*, β-haemolytic streptococci). *Staphylococcus aureus* is isolated in 25 per cent of cases and originates from the skin rather than the endometrium. Infection at the site of an episiotomy or perineal tear is relatively uncommon (about 3 per cent) and usually takes the form of a stitch abscess or infected haematoma.

Virchow's triad of thrombosis – abnormal coagulation, venous stasis and abnormal vessel walls – is present in pregnancy. Infection also accelerates vascular damage and promotes thrombosis. Septic thrombophlebitis of the pelvic or ovarian veins is a rare puerperal complication, but is more likely after Caesarean section.

Breast infections and deep venous thrombosis are discussed in Chapters 41 and 44. A drug-induced fever or a viral syndrome may also be considered.

Diagnosis and Clinical Assessment

An accurate diagnosis can usually be made after a careful history and examination.

History

Ask about:

Associated symptoms
Associated risk factors

Lower abdominal pain is suggestive of a urinary tract infection or endomyometritis. Symptoms of urinary frequency, urgency, incontinence or loin pain may be elicited in cases of urinary tract infections, depending on the severity of the ascending infection. Endomyometritis is often characterized by a heavy, offensive vaginal loss. Unilateral leg swelling and pain suggest a deep venous thrombosis, whereas breast pain indicates mastitis or a breast abscess. Vulval haematomas are painful.

A history of a Caesarean section (particularly an emergency procedure) suggests a possible wound infection and increases the likelihood of a urinary tract or chest infection or endomyometritis. Other risk factors for endomyometritis include prolonged rupture of membranes, multiple vaginal examinations and manual removal of a retained placenta.

Examination

Check for:

Tachycardia and hypotension for evidence of septic/
   haemodynamic shock
Lymphadenopathy
Unilateral leg tenderness and swelling
Breast tenderness
Tenderness, erythema or discharge from any wound
Crepitations on chest auscultation
Uterine tenderness
Offensive vaginal discharge
Vulval or vaginal haematomas

If hypotension is found, septic shock should be suspected; haematomas above the pelvic diaphragm may produce rapid haemorrhage and result in a haemodynamically unstable patient. A systematic examination should be performed in order to identify any of the localizing signs listed above.

Investigations

Cultures that may be indicated

An uncontaminated midsteam urine/catheterization sample
Blood
Swabs from any wound
High vaginal and endocervical swabs
Breast milk (if breast abscess/mastitis suspected)
Sputum (if chest infection suspected)

In addition, ultrasonography, computerized tomography or magnetic resonance studies may be necessary to diagnose a pelvic haematoma/abscess. The investigation of a suspected deep venous thrombosis is discussed in Chapter 44.

Management

General principles in the management of febrile patients

Antibiotic therapy
Intravenous fluids
Analgesia
Drainage of abscesses

Antibiotics

The dose and route of antibiotic therapy will depend on the severity of the infection. Broad-spectrum antibiotics should be given until the results of culture and sensitivity studies are available. Intravenous fluids should be given if the infection is severe, or if the woman is nauseous or vomiting. Pain should be relieved by analgesic drugs. Additional measures including central venous pressure monitoring may be necessary in cases of septic shock. If an abscess has developed, surgical drainage is usually required.

Other Measures

The appropriate management also depends on the cause of the pyrexia. Additional treatment with heparin resolves fever caused by septic pelvic/ovarian vein thrombophlebitis. Infected Caesarean section wounds should be drained and any necrotic tissue debrided; the wound may then be reapproximated once granulation tissue appears, or allowed to close by secondary intention. Salt baths and infrared treatment have been advocated in the management of infected episiotomy wounds. Physiotherapy will aid resolution of a chest infection. The management of breast infections and deep venous thrombosis is discussed in Chapters 41 and 44.

Learning Points

- **The differential diagnosis of a postpartum febrile patient includes endomyometritis, haematomas/abscesses, wound infection, urinary tract infection, chest infection, deep venous thrombosis, septic pelvic/ovarian vein thrombophlebitis and mastitis/breast abscess**

See Also

Infections in pregnancy (Chapter 12)
Proteinuria (Chapter 18)
Difficulty with breast-feeding (Chapter 41)
Venous thrombosis (Chapter 44)

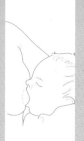

Venous thrombosis

Importance

Accurate diagnosis and management of deep vein thrombosis (DVT) are vitally important in preventing the development of a pulmonary embolism. Thromboembolic disease (DVT and pulmonary embolism) is a major cause of maternal mortality (1 in 50 000–100 000 in the developed world) and is the leading cause of maternal mortality in the UK. Although thromboembolic disease can present at any stage of pregnancy, the puerperium is the most hypercoagulable time and is the time of greatest risk.

Causes

Risk factors for thromboembolic disease

A previous thromboembolic event
An identified thrombophilia (this may be indicated by a family history of thromboembolic disease)
An operative delivery (especially a Caesarean section)
Prolonged bed rest
Obesity
Increased maternal age (>35 years)
High parity (>4)
White ethnic group
Sickle cell disease
Blood group other than O
Dehydration

Less commonly identified risk factors include malignant disease, congestive cardiac failure and oestrogen therapy (rarely prescribed in the puerperium; bromocryptine is now used if suppression of lactation is required).

Diagnosis and Clinical Assessment

A high index of suspicion is crucial to establishing a diagnosis. Any suggestive symptom or sign must be carefully investigated.

History

Ask about:

Current symptoms
Previous DVT or pulmonary embolism
Any family history of thrombosis
Other risk factors

A DVT may not lead to any symptoms, although women often complain that one or other leg feels heavy or painful. DVT is more common in the left leg than the right, as blood flow is slower on the left side.

The features of a pulmonary embolism depend on the size of the embolus. A small embolus may be asymptomatic, whereas a larger embolus may lead to symptoms of chest tightness or pain, wheezing and a frothy or blood-stained cough.

A previous history or a family history is suggestive of a thrombophilia, an abnormality in the blood which predisposes to thromboembolism. Thrombophilic defects include antiphospholipid antibodies (lupus anticoagulant and anticardiolipin antibodies) that are directed against the phospholipid components of cell membranes which control cell fusion. In recent years, there has been an increased focus on genetically determined defects, including deficiencies of antithrombin III, factor XII, protein C and its co-factor protein S. Identified mutations of the prothrombin gene and the factor V gene are also thrombophilias. (A single point mutation in the factor V gene, factor V Leiden, causes a resistance to activated protein C.) The thrombophilias also predispose to recurrent miscarriage (Chapter 59), intrauterine growth restriction (Chapter 21) and pre-eclampsia (Chapter 11).

Examination

Deep Vein Thrombosis

An otherwise unexplained tachycardia or pyrexia may be present. The calf and thigh of the affected leg may be tender and turgid. Tender, hard veins may be palpable in deep tissues. When the foot is dorsiflexed, there may be pain in the calf (Homan's sign). However, the clinical diagnosis is notoriously inaccurate; many cases of DVT are not clinically evident, and when 'classical' features are present, the diagnosis is only confirmed in approximately 30 per cent of cases.

Pulmonary Embolism

As with symptoms, there may be minimal signs, or alternatively tachypnoea and cyanosis may be found.

Investigation

It is essential to have an objective form of diagnosis. Any unusual leg symptoms, unexplained tachycardia or fever must be investigated.

Techniques used to establish a diagnosis
DVT
Ultrasonography
Venography
Pulmonary embolism
Chest X-ray
Electrocardiogram (ECG)
Blood gas analysis
Isotope lung scanning
Pulmonary angiography

Ultrasonography has replaced venography for the diagnosis of DVT in many centres. The technique accurately identifies the site and extent of the thrombus; Doppler assessment of blood flow may also be helpful. Ultrasonography cannot be used to diagnose DVT accurately above the inguinal ligament or in the calf; however, calf DVTs rarely embolize.

Venography is an alternative to ultrasonography, particularly for the diagnosis of calf DVT. However, pelvic shielding is required if the woman is pregnant, and the technique is time-consuming, expensive and invasive.

In the diagnosis of a pulmonary embolism, chest X-ray, ECG and blood gas analysis all have a place. However, none can be relied upon if the clinical presentation is anything but obvious. A ventilation and perfusion lung scan should be performed; underperfusion of one or more parts of the lung which are radiologically normal establishes the diagnosis. Pulmonary angiography is a more precise but more traumatic investigation.

Investigation or confirmation of a thrombophilic tendency is best performed outside pregnancy and the puerperium, as the levels of certain parameters (particularly protein S) are altered in pregnancy.

Management

Prevention

Simple prophylactic measures (should be utilized for all patients)
Early mobilization
Rapid restoration of blood volume after haemorrhage
Early correction of dehydration
Avoid unnecessary pressure on veins (e.g. when legs are held in stirrups)

Additional measures (considered when there is a history of thromboembolism or after a Caesarean section)
Anticoagulant prophylaxis
Elastic stockings (which should be properly fitted)
Calf muscle stimulators during Caesarean section

Previous History of Thromboembolism

Because of the side-effects of anticoagulants (see above), prophylaxis throughout pregnancy is not recommended for all women with a previous thromboembolic event. Women are subdivided on the basis of their risk:

- low risk (single previous episode, few additional risk factors) – heparin in labour and heparin/warfarin for 6 weeks post-delivery;
- high risk (multiple episodes or additional risk factors such as family history or thrombophilia) – heparin throughout pregnancy (from booking) and in labour; heparin/warfarin for 6 weeks post-delivery.

Operative Delivery

Delivery by Caesarean section increases the risk of thromboembolism two-fold to ten-fold. The appropriate prophylactic therapy again depends on whether women are deemed to be at low or high risk:

- low-risk women – should have calf stimulation during the Caesarean section or wear elastic stockings; some centres prescribe prophylactic doses of heparin until women retain mobility postoperatively;
- high-risk women with risk factors (detailed above) – should receive heparin/warfarin for up to 6 weeks post-delivery.

Established DVT or Pulmonary Embolus

Without treatment, about 10 per cent of DVTs lead to a pulmonary embolus. It has been estimated that untreated pulmonary embolus has a mortality of 13 per cent. Thus if there is doubt regarding the diagnosis, anticoagulant treatment should be instigated prior to the definitive results of investigations. Therapy can be stopped if negative results are obtained.

Heparin

An initial dose of 40 000 IU heparin/24 hours is given by intravenous infusion. Conventional monitoring is by the partial thromboplastin time; the target is to double the control level.

After about 1 week, the risk of further thromboembolism is reduced and it is reasonable to aim for lower levels of anticoagulation. The standard prophylactic dose of heparin is 10 000 IU b.d. (monitored using the thrombin time or heparin assay). Increasingly, low-molecular-weight forms of heparin are used; these may have fewer side-effects than heparin and only need to be given once a day.

> Side-effects of long-term heparin
>
> Haemorrhage
> Thrombocytopenia
> Osteoporosis

If haemorrhagic complications occur, the effects of heparin can be rapidly reversed with 1 per cent protamine sulphate.

Warfarin

After the initial period of heparin administration, warfarin is an alternative to prophylactic heparin therapy. However, the effects of warfarin are more difficult to adjust and reverse (reversal requires vitamin K administration). Unlike heparin, warfarin crosses the placenta and is contraindicated in early pregnancy.

> Side-effects of warfarin
>
> Maternal:
> - Haemorrhage
> Fetal:
> - Haemorrhage
> - Optic atrophy
> - Chondrodystrophy

Anticoagulation therapy is not a contraindication to breast-feeding.

If there has been a major pulmonary embolism, pulmonary embolectomy or thrombolytic therapy with streptokinase or tissue plasminogen activator should be considered in this life-threatening situation.

Learning Points

- **Thromboembolic disease is the leading cause of maternal mortality in the UK**
- **The puerperium is the time of greatest risk**
- **The clinical features of thromboembolic disease are very variable and it is essential to establish the diagnosis by positive evidence from relevant investigations**
- **Side-effects of long-term heparin include haemorrhage, thrombocytopenia and osteoporosis**
- **Additional prophylactic measures should be planned when there is a history of thromboembolism or after a Caesarean section**

See Also

The febrile patient (Chapter 43)

Further Reading

Royal College of Obstetricians and Gynaecologists (RCOG). *Report of the RCOG Working Party on Prophylaxis Against Thromboembolism in Gynaecology and Obstetrics.* RCOG, London, 1995.

Section 5

In the gynaecology clinic

45. The abnormal cervical smear test 183

46. Amenorrhoea and oligomenorrhoea 188

47. Chronic pelvic pain 194

48. Contraception 199

49. Heavy periods 205

50. Hirsutism and virilization 211

51. Infertility 214

52. Intermenstrual bleeding 219

53. Menopausal symptoms 222

54. Painful intercourse 227

55. The pelvic mass 230

56. Postmenopausal bleeding 234

57. Premenstrual syndrome 238

58. Prolapse 242

59. Recurrent miscarriage 246

60. Sterilization 248

61. Termination of pregnancy 250

62. Urinary frequency 253

63. Urinary incontinence 255

64. Vaginal discharge 259

65. The swollen or painful vulva 261

66. Vulval pruritus 265

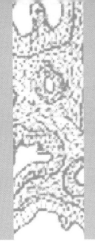

Chapter 45

The abnormal cervical smear test

Importance

Cervical cancer is the second commonest cause of female cancer deaths worldwide. Up to 30 per cent of new cases occur in women under the age of 45. The pre-invasive stage of the disease (cervical intraepithelial neoplasia, CIN) can be detected by microscopic examination of cells (cytology) sampled from the ectocervix using a spatula. Treatment of pre-invasive disease is effective in preventing the development of cervical cancer. In the UK all women between the age of 20 and 65 are offered 3-yearly cervical smears. Ten per cent of cervical smears will be reported as abnormal or technically unsatisfactory and about half of these will be referred for further investigation. The incidence of cervical carcinoma has fallen by 40 per cent in the UK since the introduction of regular cervical screening.

Causes

Cervical smear results

Normal
Inflammatory
Inadequate
Borderline nuclear atypicalities
Dyskaryosis
- Mild
- Moderate
- Severe
Malignant
Atypical glandular cells

Under the influence of oestrogen, the columnar epithelium of the endocervical canal extends onto the ectocervix. This epithelium has a darker red appearance than the adjacent squamous epithelium and when visible on the ectocervix is sometimes described as an ectropion or erosion. When exposed to the low pH of the vagina, it gradually changes back to squamous epithelium by a process of squamous metaplasia. The junction between the columnar epithelium of the endocervical canal and the squamous epithelium of the ectocervix is called the squamocolumnar junction (SCJ). This tends to move back towards the external cervical os as the columnar epithelium reverts to squamous. Neoplastic change occurs in the region known as the transformation zone, which corresponds to the area on the ectocervix between the current and previous SCJ. There is a strong association with infection by certain serotypes (16, 18 and 33) of the human papilloma virus (HPV) and cervical neoplasia.

Cytological abnormalities are graded as borderline, mild to severe dyskaryosis, malignant cells and abnormal glandular cells. Smears will be reported as unsuitable for analysis if the cervical cells are obscured by inflammatory or red blood cells. Screening at 3-yearly intervals identifies 98 per cent of abnormalities that would be detected by annual testing. False-negative rates are typically between 10 and 20 per cent (but may be up to 40 per cent) and the specificity of the method is approximately 94 per cent.

An inadequate smear may be due to insufficient squamous epithelial cells being present for analysis. This may occur if the sample consists mainly of columnar epithelial cells sampled from a large ectropion or in conditions where oestrogen levels are low (e.g. after the menopause). Persistently inadequate smears require colposcopic examination to exclude any coincidental abnormality.

In inflammatory smears, squamous epithelial cells are obscured by inflammatory cells or microorganisms.

Atypical glandular cells may represent premalignant disease of the endocervix or endometrium. Premalignant disease of the endocervix cannot be excluded by colposcopy and will require cone biopsy for diagnosis. Endometrial disease should be excluded by hysteroscopy.

CIN is a histological diagnosis usually made from colposcopically directed biopsy. CIN is graded as mild (CIN 1), moderate (CIN 2) or severe (CIN 3). The correlation between the degree of abnormality assessed by cytology and biopsy is poor. Twenty-five per cent of cases of CIN 1 will progress to higher-grade lesions over 2 years; 30–40 per cent of CIN 3 will progress to carcinoma over 20 years; 40 per cent of low-grade lesions (CIN 1) will regress to normal within 6 months without treatment.

Cervical intraglandular neoplasia (CIGN) is the equivalent change occurring in the columnar epithelium and is associated with the development of adenocarcinoma of the cervix. Two-thirds of cases coexist with CIN. Cervical cytology cannot be used to reliably detect adenocarcinoma of the cervix or CIGN and screening has had no impact on its incidence.

Diagnosis and Clinical Assessment

History

> Ask about:
>
> Results and dates of previous smears
> Previous treatment for abnormal smears
> Abnormal vaginal bleeding
> Last menstrual period and contraception
> Smoking

CIN is asymptomatic. Abnormal (intermenstrual or postmenopausal) bleeding may be a sign of invasive disease. Ask about previously abnormal smears (and treatment). Cervical neoplasia is rare in women over the age of 45 who have had previously normal smears. Pregnancy affects the appearance of the cervix and increases the risk of bleeding following cervical biopsy and treatment (see below). Smoking may act as a co-factor in the development of CIN.

Examination

This is usually carried out either at the time the smear is taken or at colposcopy.

Colposcopy

When to Refer for Colposcopy

Women with moderate or severe dyskaryosis, abnormal glandular cells or in whom the appearance of the cervix or the smear suggests malignancy should be referred for colposcopy within 4 weeks. Smears showing borderline changes or mild dyskaryosis are repeated after 6 months and referral is made if these abnormalities persist or worsen. Inadequate or unsatisfactory smears should be repeated after 3 months and referred for colposcopy if two further unsatisfactory smears are obtained. Patients with a previous history of CIN and those who have had an abnormal smear should have three normal smears at annual intervals before returning to the normal programme.

Colposcopic Examination

> Key features at colposcopy
>
> Squamocolumnar junction
> Abnormal vessels
> Changes with acetoacetic acid
> - Acetowhite epithelium
> - Punctation
> - Mosaicism

Colposcopy is inspection of the cervix using a binocular microscope with a light source (colposcope). It is usually an outpatient procedure performed using a speculum to expose the cervix. Squamous neoplasia most often occurs in the areas adjacent to the junction of the columnar (velvety red) and squamous (smooth pink) epithelium or SCJ. If this cannot be seen in its entirety, CIN cannot be excluded by colposcopic examination and a cone biopsy will be required. CIN appears as a white area with a well-defined edge following application of 5 per cent acetic acid solution. Small blood vessels beneath the epithelium may be seen as dots (punctation) or a crazy-paving pattern (mosaicism). CIN can also be identified by the use of

Schiller's iodine solution, which stains normal cervical epithelium dark brown. The diagnosis is confirmed by biopsies taken from the most abnormal looking areas. Early invasive disease (cancer of the cervix) is characterized by a raised or ulcerated area with abnormal vessels, friable tissue and coarse punctation with marked mosaicism. It feels hard on palpation and often bleeds on contact. In more advanced disease, the cervix becomes fixed or replaced by a friable, warty looking mass.

Women with evidence of dyskaryosis on cervical cytology in pregnancy should be referred for colposcopy to differentiate premalignant from invasive disease. If an area of atypical epithelium is identified, this should be biopsied if clinically suspicious of high-grade CIN or invasive disease. There is some increased risk of bleeding following biopsy during pregnancy but the risk of miscarriage is low. Colposcopic assessment without biopsy may be acceptable if there is no suggestion of invasive disease on cytology and colposcopy, and the assessment is carried out by an experienced colposcopist.

Management

Explanation

Many woman associate abnormal cytology with a diagnosis of cancer, and the knowledge that their cervical smear is abnormal causes considerable anxiety. In most cases they can be reassured with an explanation that an abnormal smear does not indicate cancer, although it may indicate an increased risk of developing cancer later.

Persistently Inadequate Smears

Once coexisting neoplastic disease has been excluded by colposcopy, atrophic changes can be reversed by topical oestrogen or hormone replacement therapy and infections treated with systemic or topical antibiotics before repeating the smear.

Cervical Intraepithelial Neoplasia

CIN 1 can be managed by cytological and colposcopic surveillance at 6-monthly intervals, as progress to invasive disease does not occur within 6 months, or it can be treated as for higher-grade lesions (see below).

Conservative treatment of CIN 1

Not suitable if:
- Patient is likely to be lost to follow-up
- Patient would prefer immediate treatment

Advantages
- 40 per cent of cases will resolve
- Avoids complications of treatment

Disadvantages
- Possible delay in treatment if higher-grade lesion missed at biopsy
- More hospital visits
- More expensive
- Increased anxiety

Higher-grade lesions (CIN 2 and 3 and dyskaryotic glandular cells) are an indication for immediate treatment by either excision or destruction of the affected area (usually the whole of the transformation zone).

Destructive therapies include laser ablation and coagulation diathermy. Excision can be carried out using scalpel, laser or a diathermy loop wire (large loop excision of the transformation zone, LLETZ) (Figure 45.1). Laser and LLETZ can be carried out under local anaesthetic. Ectocervical lesions can be adequately treated by removing tissue to a depth of 1 cm, but where the SCJ cannot be seen or a lesion of the glandular epithelium is suspected, a deeper 'cone' biopsy is required to ensure that all of the endocervix is sampled (Figure 45.2). Patients are advised to abstain from intercourse and not to use tampons for 4 weeks after treatment, to reduce the risk of

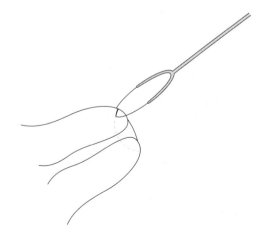

Figure 45.1 Large loop excision of the transformation zone

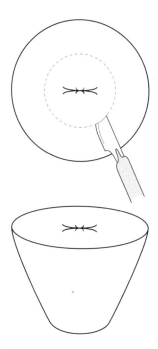

Figure 45.2 Knife cone biopsy

infection and secondary haemorrhage. Cervical stenosis or incompetence is rare and is usually associated with cone biopsy rather than LLETZ.

Complications of treatment for CIN

Bleeding
Discharge
Cervical stenosis
Cervical incompetence

Hysterectomy is rarely indicated for treatment of CIN but may be used if indicated for another reason such as heavy periods.

Treatment for CIN in pregnancy is usually deferred until 3 months after delivery, with colposcopic surveillance during pregnancy to exclude the development of invasive disease.

Follow-up

Approximately 5 per cent of women will have persistent or recurrent disease following treatment. Cervical cytology and/or colposcopy are used to carry out follow-up. Two examinations are carried out in the first 12 months after treatment, followed by annual smears for 4 years before returning to the normal 3-yearly screening programme.

Carcinoma of the Cervix

The majority of carcinomas (60 per cent) are squamous, although both the relative proportion and overall number of adenocarcinomas have increased over the last 10 years. The commonest presenting symptoms are intermenstrual or postmenopausal bleeding and vaginal discharge. Pain is uncommon and occurs late in the disease. The diagnosis may be made from colposcopic or cone biopsy, but where there is a strong clinical suspicion from examination, histological confirmation should be made from a larger biopsy as part of a formal staging examination. Spread is by local invasion and lymphatic metastases to the iliac, presacral and obturator nodes.

Treatment is determined by the clinical stage (Table 45.1) of the disease, usually established by an examination under anaesthetic including (knife) biopsy, cystoscopy, rectal examination and intravenous urography.

Microinvasive lesions can be managed by cone biopsy if the patient wishes to preserve her fertility. Extended hysterectomy or radiotherapy can be used to treat stage Ia–Ib. The cure rate is similar for both surgery and radiotherapy but the former is generally associated with less long-term morbidity from vaginal stenosis. Stage II–IV disease is usually treated with intracavity and external beam radiotherapy.

Surgery

Extended or Wertheim's hysterectomy involves removal of the uterus, paracervical tissues and pelvic lymph nodes. The ovaries can be conserved. The more extensive dissection required to remove the tissues surrounding the cervix and the pelvic lymph nodes increases the risk of complications, such as urinary tract injury and bleeding, compared with standard hysterectomy. The vagina is shortened by 2–3 cm but this does not generally affect sexual function. Patients with lymph node involvement are treated with adjuvant radiotherapy.

Radiotherapy

This is given by a combination of external beam irradiation of the whole of the pelvis and internal sources placed in the vagina or canal of the cervix. The external beam therapy is given in a series of outpatient treatments over a 5-week period. Some bowel and bladder symptoms occur in most patients and a radiation-induced menopause is likely in premenopausal patients. The use of dilators and early

Table 45.1 FIGO staging of cervical cancer

Stage	Description
I	Cervical carcinoma confined to the uterus
Ia	Microscopic lesion less than 5 mm deep or 7 mm in area (microinvasive)
Ib	Any clinically visible lesion or microscopic lesion > 5 mm deep or 7 mm in area
II	Tumour invades beyond the uterus into the upper third of the vagina or into the parametrium
III	Tumour extends to the lower third of the vagina or the pelvic side wall
IV	Tumour invades bladder or rectal mucosa or distant metastases (liver or lung)

reintroduction of intercourse help to reduce the risk of vaginal stenosis and dyspareunia. Radiotherapy and chemotherapy may be used as palliative treatment in advanced disease to reduce vaginal bleeding.

Complications of treatment

Surgery
- Bleeding
- Voiding difficulties
- Damage to bladder, bowel, ureter
- Venous thromboembolism
- Fistulae (2–5 per cent)
- Lymphoedema

Radiotherapy
- Diarrhoea, obstruction, rectal bleeding
- Haematuria, cystitis
- Vaginal stenosis, dyspareunia
- Fistula

Follow-up

Following treatment, patients are seen at 3-monthly intervals for 3 years, 6-monthly for 2 years and then annually. Recurrence tends to occur locally at the vault or in the lymph nodes and is treated by radiotherapy or exenteration.

The prognosis depends on stage (5-year survival rates are 90 per cent for stage I, 84 per cent for stage II, 20–45 per cent for stage III, 5 per cent for stage IV) and is approximately halved where there is node involvement. Recurrence is unlikely after 5 years.

Learning Points

- Regular cervical screening reduces the risk of developing cancer of the cervix by 75 per cent
- 40 per cent of cervical malignancies in the UK are adenocarcinomas
- Low-grade lesions may regress spontaneously to normal

See Also

History-taking and examination in gynaecology (Chapter 3)
Intermenstrual bleeding (Chapter 52)
Postmenopausal bleeding (Chapter 56)

Further Reading

Anderson MC, Coulter CAE, Mason WP, Soutter WP, Tidy J. Malignant disease of the cervix. In: Shaw RW, Soutter WP, Stanton SL, eds. *Gynaecology*. Churchill Livingstone, Edinburgh, 1992, ch. 36.

Soutter WP. Premalignant disease of the lower genital tract. In: Shaw RW, Soutter WP, Stanton SL, eds. *Gynaecology*. Churchill Livingstone, Edinburgh, 1992, ch. 34.

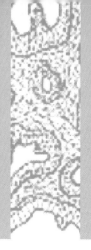

Chapter 46

Amenorrhoea and oligomenorrhoea

Definition

Amenorrhoea is the absence of menstruation. Secondary amenorrhoea is the cessation of periods for more than 6 months in a normal woman of child-bearing age in whom menstruation has previously occurred. Primary amenorrhoea is defined as the failure to start menstruation by the age of 16 in a girl with normal secondary sex characteristics (or 14 where there is a failure to develop secondary sex characteristics). Oligomenorrhoea is menstrual bleeding that occurs between 6 weeks and 6 months apart.

Importance

At any time, approximately 1–2 per cent of non-pregnant women will have absent or infrequent periods. In many cases this will be self-limiting, but there may still be concerns about fertility and contraception. Rarely, it may be a presenting symptom of an underlying endocrine or neoplastic disorder which itself requires diagnosis and treatment. Even where this is not the case and fertility is not an issue, there may be long-term health implications due to reduced or unopposed oestrogen production.

Normal Menstrual Cycle

Normal menstruation requires the pulsatile release of gonadotrophin-releasing hormone (GnRH) from the hypothalamus to stimulate the release of the gonadotrophins, follicle-stimulating hormone (FSH)

and luteinizing hormone (LH), from a functioning anterior pituitary. The ovaries must be able to respond to these signals and produce oestrogen and progesterone. Finally the endometrial cavity must be intact and the lower genital tract must be patent to allow shedding of the endometrium if conception does not occur.

Hypothalamus and Pituitary

Gonadotrophin-releasing hormone is a decapeptide released by the median eminence of the hypothalamus. It stimulates the anterior pituitary to release FSH and LH. The negative feedback of oestrogen and progesterone on FSH and LH is less in the first half of the cycle so there is a gradual increase in FSH levels. Around 35–42 hours prior to ovulation there is a surge in LH (and to a lesser extent FSH) levels. FSH and LH levels tend to fall during the second half of the cycle, whilst prolactin levels increase.

Ovary

Approximately 30 follicles begin development each month, only one of which normally releases an ovum (the dominant follicle). As the follicles develop, the granulosa cells surrounding the ovum divide into an inner and outer layer separated by a fluid-filled space (the antrum). The ovarian stromal cells around the outer layer differentiate into the theca interna and externa. Up to the formation of the antrum, follicular development is independent of FSH and LH release. Prior to ovulation LH stimulates production of androgens from cholesterol in the thecal cells. These are then converted into oestrogen in the granulosa cells by a process of aromatization under the influence of FSH.

FSH also stimulates granulosa cell proliferation and increased levels of LH receptors. The surge in LH levels on day 12 triggers a resumption of meiosis in the ovum and rupture of the dominant follicle. After ovulation, LH and prolactin stimulate the remaining granulosa and theca interna cells to undergo a process known as luteinization to form the corpus luteum. This produces progesterone, with maximal levels reached 7 days after ovulation. In the absence of human chorionic gonadotrophin (pregnancy) the corpus luteum begins to regress and progesterone levels fall.

Endometrium

The endometrium responds to changes in oestrogen and progesterone levels. It consists of three layers. The basal zone (zona basalis), in contact with the myometrium, contains compact stromal cells. The endometrial glands and supporting stroma in the zona spongiosa and zona compacta comprise the functional layers of the endometrium. Four distinct phases can be identified in the endometrial cycle. During the menstrual phase (days 1–5) shedding of the functional layers (upper 75 per cent) of the endometrium occurs. Menstruation ceases as a result of vasoconstriction. Endometrial repair (days 5–7) then occurs with glandular and stromal regeneration. In the proliferative or follicular phase (days 7–14), rising levels of oestrogen cause elongation of the endometrial glands and expansion of the adjacent stroma. The endometrium increases in thickness from less than 0.5 to 5 mm. After ovulation in the luteal or secretory phase (days 14–28), the glands become more convoluted under the influence of progesterone. There is vacuolation in the glandular epithelium and secretory activity. Towards the end of the secretory phase, the stroma becomes oedematous and decidualized. Unless pregnancy occurs, falling oestrogen and progesterone levels lead to vasoconstriction of the spiral arterioles and shedding of the endometrium.

Causes

Commonest causes of absent or infrequent periods

Physiological
- Pregnancy
- Breast-feeding
- Menopause

Pathological
- Polycystic ovarian disease (PCOS)
- Hypothalamic dysfunction (weight loss/stress)
- Hyperprolactinaemia
- Premature menopause

Rarer causes of secondary oligomenorrhoea

Anatomical – cervical stenosis, Asherman's syndrome
Endocrine – thyroid disease, Cushing's, ovarian or adrenal tumours
Hypothalamic–pituitary – tumours, radiotherapy or surgery, renal failure
Ovarian – autoimmue, radiotherapy/chemotherapy

In *primary amenorrhoea*, also consider:

- hypothalamic failure – Kallmann's syndrome, cranial tumours
- ovarian – Turner's syndrome, gonadal dysgenesis
- anatomical – imperforate hymen, absent uterus or vagina
- androgen insensitivity (testicular feminization).

Remember that pregnancy and breast-feeding are the commonest causes of secondary amenorrhoea in women of reproductive age. Late menarche is usually constitutional.

Polycystic Ovarian Syndrome

Polycystic ovarian syndrome (PCOS) accounts for 90 per cent of cases of oligomenorrhoea. The classical picture of subfertility, weight gain and infrequent periods and hirsutism (Stein–Leventhal syndrome) is present in only a minority of cases. The aetiology is probably related to insulin resistance, with a failure of normal follicular development and ovulation.

Hypothalamic and Pituitary Causes

Hypothalamic dysfunction is the single commonest pathological cause of secondary amenorrhoea (33 per cent of cases) and is most often seen as a result of stress, excessive weight loss or exercise, and eating disorders. Hypothalamic failure accounts for 30 per cent of cases of amenorrhoea and 5 per cent of cases of oligomenorrhoea. It may be congenital (Kallmann's syndrome) or due to tumour, infarction, thrombosis or inflammation. Pituitary failure may be congenital or acquired as a result of trauma, treatment of pituitary tumours or infarction after massive blood loss (Sheehan's syndrome). It may be associated with other endocrine abnormalities including hypothyroidism.

Hyperprolactinaemia accounts for a further 20 per cent of cases of amenorrhoea. Prolactin inhibits GnRH release from the hypothalamus. Up to 40 per cent of cases of hyperprolactinaemia are idiopathic and a further 40–50 per cent are associated with pituitary adenomas. Prolactin release is inhibited by dopamine, which can be blocked by tumours or antidopaminergic drugs.

Drugs that may cause hyperprolactinaemia

Phenothiazines

Antihistamines

Butyrophenones

Maxolon

Cimetidine

Methyldopa

The incidence of amenorrhoea after stopping the combined oral contraceptive pill is not increased, although the pill may conceal an underlying cause of oligomenorrhoea, which only becomes evident when it is stopped.

Ovarian

Premature ovarian failure occurs in approximately 1 per cent of women before the age of 40. Ovarian failure may occur after chemotherapy or radiotherapy and following surgery for conditions such as endometriosis. Ovarian failure may also occur as a result of autoimmue disease and following viral infection. Certain karyotypic abnormalities such as Turner's syndrome (XO) are associated with abnormal ovarian development (streak gonads). In testicular feminization syndrome, patients have a male karyotype but female appearance and external genitalia as a result of congenital insensitivity to endogenous testosterone. In addition to the implications for fertility and menstruation, there is an increased risk of malignancy developing in these gonads.

Endocrine Disorders

Androgen-secreting tumours of the ovaries or adrenal glands and endocrine disorders such as Cushing's disease, Addison's disease and acromegaly interfere with the normal functioning of the hypothamlic–pituitary–ovarian axis and may present with amenorrhoea. High levels of thyroxine will inhibit both FSH and thyroid-stimulating hormone (TSH) release from the anterior pituitary. It is important to remember that pituitary failure may affect FSH release as well as causing hypothyroidism.

Anatomical

Anatomical causes for secondary amenorrhoea are usually due to previous surgery. In practice, the commonest example of this would be hysterectomy or endometrial ablation (see Chapter 49). Damage to the endometrium with adhesion formation within the uterine cavity may occur after curettage for retained products of conception (Asherman's syndrome) and the cervix may become stenosed after cone biopsy. Congenital absence of the uterus may occur on its own or as part of testicular feminization syndrome. An imperforate hymen prevents the escape of blood from the lower genital tract and presents with primary amenorrhoea and cyclical abdominal pain.

Diagnosis and Clinical Assessment

History

Ask about:

Age of menarche

Previous menstrual history

Previous pregnancies

Contraception

Weight change

Associated symptoms

Previous gynaecological surgery

Chronic illness

Lifestyle

Drugs

The possibility of pregnancy should always be considered by asking about sexual activity and contraception. If pregnancy has ever occurred, most causes of primary amenorrhoea, including congenital anatomical problems and karyotypic abnormalities, can be excluded (although menstruation can occur in some patients with Turner's syndrome).

Amenorrhoea may be due to recent pregnancy or lactation. In Asherman's syndrome there will usually be a history of endometrial curettage for retained products of conception. Severe postpartum bleeding with hypotension can lead to pituitary infarction

(Sheehan's syndrome). If the periods have always been infrequent, the most likely diagnosis will be of PCOS. For girls with primary amenorrhoea a history of cyclical abdominal pain and bloating suggests cryptomenorrhoea due to an imperforate hymen. Congenital hypothalamic failure (Kallmann's syndrome) is associated with lack of sense of smell (anosmia) and infantile sexual development. PCOS is associated with weight gain, whilst weight loss is a common cause of hypothalamic dysfunction.

Other associated symptoms that may be significant include headache and visual disturbance (cranial tumours including pituitary adenomas), male pattern hair growth (usually associated with PCOS but also with androgen-secreting tumours) and galactorrhoea (hyperprolactinaemia). Thirty per cent of women will be amenorrhoeic whilst using injectable progestogens for contraception, as will 20 per cent of women using the levonorgestrel intrauterine device. Previous gynaecological surgery may have resulted in cervical stenosis or endometrial ablation, or early ovarian failure. Untreated thyroid disease, treatment for malignancy and renal failure may all be associated with amenorrhoea. Major life events that are stressful are a common cause of hypothalamic dysfunction.

Examination

Check:

Body mass index
Blood pressure
Secondary sex characteristics
Abdominal masses, ascites
Imperforate hymen, cervical stenosis
Pelvic masses

A body mass index (BMI) of less than in 19 kg/m^2 is likely to be associated with a weight loss-related cause. Blood pressure is elevated in Cushing's disease and PCOS. The features of Turner's syndrome are short stature and poorly developed secondary sex characteristics. Hirsutism, when associated with infrequent periods, is most often due to PCOS, whilst the presence of adult virilization suggests an androgen-producing tumour of the ovary or adrenal glands (see Chapter 52).

Haematometra due to an imperforate hymen or cervical stenosis may be palpable as an abdominal mass. Ovarian tumours may cause ascites. Look for the scars of previous gynaecological surgery.

A careful inspection of the external genitalia is essential in any girl with primary amenorrhoea, to look for imperforate hymen as a bluish membrane covering the introitus. Ovarian tumours may be palpable as a pelvic mass.

Investigations

Initial investigations

Pregnancy test
FSH, LH
Prolactin
Thyroid function tests
Progestogen challenge test (PCT)

Once pregnancy has been excluded, the common causes of secondary oligomenorrhoea can be differentiated by the above tests. The PCT involves taking an oral progestogen for 5 days and seeing if this provokes a withdrawal bleed when stopped. A positive result indicates that the endometrium has been oestrogenized and excludes most anatomical defects.

A persistently raised FSH level indicates that the pituitary is trying to stimulate an unresponsive ovary. Oestrogen levels are low so the PCT will be negative (hypergonadotrophic hypogonadism). In secondary amenorrhoea, this is usually as a result of ovarian failure due to premature menopause, although an autoantibody screen should be taken to exclude autoimmune disease. For cases of primary amenor-rhoea, check the karyotype and arrange ultrasound or laparoscopy to look for ovarian tissue or streak gonads.

Disorders of hypothalamic and pituitary function are characterized by normal or low FSH levels and a negative PCT (hypogonadotrophic hypogonadism). If prolactin levels are elevated, arrange computerized tomography (CT) or magnetic resonance imaging (MRI) of the pituitary fossa to look for pituitary tumours and a formal assessment of visual fields. Remember that prolactin levels are also elevated in 15 per cent of women with PCOS, during lactation and pregnancy and even after breast examination. If the prolactin levels are normal, the most likely diagnosis will be hypothalamic dysfunction related to weight loss or stress. However, thyroid function should be checked as pituitary failure may also lead to hypothyroidism, and thyrotoxicosis may cause suppression of pituitary function.

PCOS is characterized by normal FSH levels with increased levels of LH, typically to more than three times that of the FSH. Patients are not usually oestrogen deficient and therefore will have a positive PCT. An ultrasound examination of the ovary shows a thickened capsule with multiple subcapsular follicles and stromal hypertrophy. Not all these findings are present in all cases. The diagnosis is also supported by increased levels or testosterone, a raised free androgen index and a reduced level of sex hormone binding globulin, although these are rarely needed to confirm the diagnosis. Endometrial sampling should be considered to exclude endometrial hyperplasia.

Anatomical causes and other endocrine or medical conditions associated with amenorrhoea will usually be suggested by the history or examination. An ultrasound assessment should be arranged wherever there is a pelvic mass or primary amenorrhoea to exclude ovarian tumours and haematometra. Congenital malformations of the reproductive tract are associated with an increased incidence of renal tract malformations. If the uterus is absent, check for testicular feminization by taking blood for karyotyping (XY).

Management

Absent or infrequent menstruation is a symptom and does not require treatment *per se* (although in some cases this may be requested). The need for treatment depends partly on the underlying cause (including any associated long-term health risks), on whether the woman is currently trying to conceive and, if not, on her need for contraception. In many cases, the condition will be self-limiting and all that will be required will be an explanation of the cause and reassurance. In some cases, it may be that other associated symptoms, such as hirsutism, are the primary concern (see Chapter 50).

Key considerations of management

Is there any underlying cause for the infrequent periods that demands treatment?
Is the patient wishing to get pregnant?
If she does not wish to get pregnant, does she need contraception?
Does she wish to have regular 'periods'?

Underlying Cause

Cranial tumours, including macroadenomas of the pituitary, should be referred to a neurosurgeon.

Androgen-producing tumours of the ovary and adrenals should be removed. The gonads in patients with testicular feminization, gonadal dysgenesis and Turner's syndrome should be removed because of the risk of malignancy. These patients will then require hormone replacement therapy. Cryptomenorrhoea due to imperforate hymen or cervical stenosis is treated by surgical incision or dilatation of the cervix. Thyroid disease and other associated endocrine disorders or chronic renal failure should be treated as appropriate. Eating disorders are associated with significant morbidity and mortality and specialist psychiatric help may be required for their treatment.

Any condition resulting in a prolonged hypo-oestrogenic state will be associated with an increased risk of osteoporosis, cardiovascular and cerebrovascular disease. Oestrogen replacement (with progestogen if the uterus is present) can be given either as hormone replacement therapy (HRT) or using the combined oral contraceptive pill (COCP, see Chapter 53).

Women with amenorrhoea due to PCOS are at increased risk of endometrial hyperplasia and malignancy. The endometrium can be protected by using either the COCP or cyclical progestogens to induce regular withdrawal bleeds. Patients with PCOS should be aware of the risks associated with insulin resistance and hyperinsulinaemia, including the increased long-term risks of cardiovascular disease (smoking, diet).

Fertility

The prognosis for those women with confirmed ovarian failure is poor. If ovarian biopsy shows evidence of remaining follicles, a proportion of women will respond to treatment with high-dose gonadotrophin therapy, but in most cases assisted conception with donor oocytes will be required for pregnancy.

Endometrial ablation due to Asherman's syndrome may respond to hysteroscopic division of adhesions followed by insertion of an intrauterine contraceptive device (IUCD), but subsequent fertility rates are low and there is an increased risk of miscarriage and abnormal placentation.

In contrast, the prognosis for patients with PCOS and hypothalamic failure is excellent with appropriate treatment. Ovulation may resume if some weight loss can be achieved in patients with PCOS; if not, the first line of treatment is to use the anti-oestrogen clomiphene (see Chapter 51). Second-line therapy may involve the use of gonadotrophins or laparoscopic drilling of the ovaries. Treatment with oral hypoglycaemic agents such as metformin may be effective in some PCOS patients with anovulation. Patients with PCOS will be at increased risk of miscarriage and should be screened for gestational diabetes during pregnancy.

Hyperprolactinaemia will usually respond to stopping any dopamine-inhibiting drugs or to treatment with dopamine agonists such as bromocriptine or carbergoline.

In patients with hypothalamic dysfunction due to stress or weight loss, the emphasis should be on maintenance of normal weight and changes in lifestyle. In other cases of hypothalamic or pituitary dysfunction, ovulation can be induced by the use of exogenous gonadotrophins (see Chapter 51) or pulsatile GnRH therapy.

All women undergoing treatment with clomiphene or gonadotrophins for ovulation induction should be warned about the risk of multiple pregnancy and ovarian hyperstimulation (see Chapter 51). Ovulation induction therapy should be carried out under the supervision of a specialist fertility clinic and monitored by ultrasound.

Contraception

Most women with confirmed ovarian failure (whether this is congenital, iatrogenic or due to premature menopause) will not require contraception. Women having the menopause below the age of 50 should be advised to continue using contraception for 2 years from their last period. However, spontaneous ovulation may resume in women with autoimmue ovarian disease. Ovulation may occur intermittently in women with hypothalamic dysfunction or PCOS, so these women should be advised of the need for contraception. Oral contraceptives are the method of choice if there is a need for endometrial protection or oestrogen replacement, although preparations containing androgenic progestogens should be avoided in PCOS. IUCDs should be avoided in nulliparous and hypo-oestrogenic patients. Pregnancy may occur after endometrial ablation.

Regular Bleeding

This can be most conveniently engineered for those women who prefer to have a regular withdrawal bleed by the use of a combined oral contraceptive or hormone replacement therapy. If oestrogen levels are adequate (such as in PCOS), a cyclical regime of oral progestogens can be used instead.

Treatment options for oligomenorrhoea

Medical treatment options
- Combined pill
- HRT
- Clomiphene
- Dopamine agonists for hyperprolactinaemia
- FSH/LH
- GnRH

Surgical treatment
- Removal of streak gonads
- Incision of imperforate hymen
- Laparoscopic ovarian drilling for PCOS

Learning Points

- **Always exclude pregnancy and consider the need for contraception**
- **There may be long-term health implications associated with conditions causing amenorrhoea**
- **The prognosis for fertility is good with appropriate treatment in most women**

See Also

Menopausal symptoms (Chapter 53)
Infertility (Chapter 51)
Hirsutism and virilization (Chapter 50)

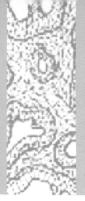

Chronic pelvic pain

Importance

Fifty per cent of women experience some degree of pain with menstruation, and in 10 per cent this is sufficiently severe to interfere with daily activity. Pelvic pain accounts for 5 per cent of new referrals to gynaecological outpatient clinics.

Causes

Common diagnoses

Primary dysmenorrhoea
Endometriosis/adenomyosis
Chronic pelvic inflammatory disease
Irritable bowel syndrome
No apparent organic cause

Primary dysmenorrhoea is the occurrence of painful menstruation in the absence of pelvic pathology. It may be associated with an underlying defect in prostaglandin action within the uterus or congestion of the pelvic venous circulation. The pain may begin prior to the onset of bleeding but always in the second half of the cycle and usually resolves by the time bleeding ceases. It may occur for the first time in later life but is commonly present from menarche. It is often associated with heavy menstrual bleeding and tends to be familial. It usually improves after pregnancy.

Adenomyosis is the presence of endometrial glands within the myometrium and is usually diagnosed by histological examination of the uterus after hysterectomy, although the diagnosis may be suspected from the history and examination. Endometriosis is the presence of ectopic deposits of endometrium outside the uterus and can be diagnosed at laparoscopy. The aetiology is unknown but possible mechanisms include:

- implantation of endometrial glands and tissue after retrograde menstruation;
- de-differentiation of the epithelium lining the peritoneal cavity;
- implantation following surgical procedures;
- blood spread.

It is more common in nulliparous women and those with congenital abnormalities of the lower genital tract. The sites most commonly affected are the ovaries, uterosacral ligaments and pouch of Douglas. The amount of disease may vary from one or two isolated deposits 1–2 mm in size resembling matchstick heads up to large endometriotic cysts containing altered blood (chocolate cysts). Extensive disease is often associated with adhesion formation. The pain may occur throughout the month but tends to worsen during menstruation and with intercourse. Symptoms are often not proportional to the amount of disease present.

Isolated adhesions alone rarely cause pain unless involving other organs such as bowel. Chronic pelvic inflammatory disease (PID) can cause pain through acute infective exacerbations but more often as a result of a chronic inflammatory response to previous infections. This is characterized by multiple adhesions and hydrosalpinges. The pain is less cyclical than endometriosis and usually associated with discomfort during intercourse.

Although a variety of musculoskeletal, urinary and bowel problems can present as chronic pain, irritable bowel syndrome (IBS) is the commonest non-gynaecological cause of lower abdominal pain in young women. It is characterized by intermittent colicky pain associated with abdominal bloating and changes in bowel habit.

Pelvic pain may also be a presenting symptom of sexual dysfunction, depression or anxiety about cancer or infection.

Diagnosis and Clinical Assessment

History

Ask about:

Duration and onset of symptoms
Is the pain cyclical (i.e. related to the menstrual cycle)?
Pain with intercourse
Associated gastrointestinal symptoms
Previous investigations and treatments
Effect of pain on quality of life
Plans for further pregnancies

An accurate history is essential in making a diagnosis and assessing how disabling pain is in order to plan appropriate therapy.

Recent-onset menstrual pain is more likely to be associated with pathology. Cyclical pain is more likely to be associated with endometriosis and adenomyosis, whereas pain occurring throughout the month is less likely to be gynaecological. Pelvic pathology is less likely in the absence of deep dyspareunia. Bloating, constipation and diarrhoea suggest a diagnosis of irritable bowel syndrome. Valuable diagnostic information may be available if the patient has already had a laparoscopy.

Examination

Check for:

Abdominal scars
Site of any tenderness
Any pelvic mass
A bulky tender uterus
An immobile retroverted uterus

In the absence of any abnormal features, you are unlikely to find significant pathology by further investigations. A pelvic mass on abdominal or pelvic examination may be associated with PID or endometriosis but demands exclusion of malignancy by further investigation or surgery. A bulky tender

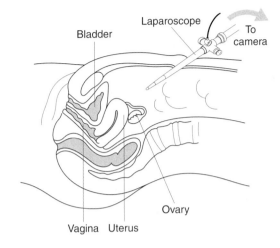

Figure 47.1 Laparoscopic examination of the pelvic organs

uterus may be the only finding in adenomyosis. An immobile retroverted uterus suggests pathology in the pouch of Douglas, such as endometriosis or PID. Thickening or nodularity of the uterosacral ligaments is characteristic of endometriosis.

Investigations

Investigations are primarily indicated to confirm diagnoses suggested by findings at examination but may be of value in providing reassurance to patients with no pelvic pathology.

Endocervical swabs may be useful in excluding early or acute infective exacerbations of PID. Ultrasound is indicated if examination has revealed a pelvic mass. Laparoscopy is the definitive investigation for endometriosis and PID but it has an operative morbidity (see Chapter 67) (Figure 47.1).

Management

Management is determined by:

Diagnosis
Degree of disability
Side-effects of treatment
Need to preserve fertility and effect of treatment on fertility
Response to treatment

A clear explanation of the diagnosis and proposed treatment is essential. In some cases, reassurance (if necessary directed towards specific fears about the cause of the pain) is all that is required. Even where pathologies such as minimal endometriosis or an isolated omental adhesion are identified, it should be remembered that such findings are common in asymptomatic women and may be coincidental. Chronic pelvic pain is rarely due to conditions such as malignancy, which demand treatment irrespective of symptoms. More often the morbidity of therapy must be balanced against that of the pain. Some treatment options will not be available to patients who are actively trying to conceive, although on occasions it may be necessary to postpone this while the cause of the pain is treated.

Primary Dysmenorrhoea

Treatment is with:

- non-steroidal anti-inflammatory drugs (NSAIDs)
- combined oral contraceptive pill
- progestogens
- hysterectomy.

Non-steroidal anti-inflammatory agents inhibit the synthesis of prostaglandins thought to play an important role in mediating the pain. They also reduce the amount of blood loss during menstruation, which may help to reduce the amount of cramping pain felt as the uterus contracts to expel blood clots.

The oral contraceptive pill taken cyclically reduces pain significantly for some women but this effect is variable. It has the additional advantage of reducing blood loss, providing contraception and having relatively few side-effects. Taken continuously it should suppress all menstruation and dysmenorrhoea. This may be a useful short-term measure to gain relief from symptoms or act as a diagnostic tool to distinguish true dysmenorrhoea from other causes of chronic pain.

Progestogens have no proven benefit but may be of value to some women with the characteristic features of pelvic venous congestion when given in the second half of the cycle. More potent drugs such as danazol can be used as for endometriosis for short-term relief or as a diagnostic tool but are unsuitable for long-term therapy.

Where a woman has completed her family, hysterectomy with ovarian conservation should provide a definitive cure. Unless this is indicated for other reasons, such as menorrhagia, it is advisable to suppress menstruation medically first and show that this abolishes the symptoms. Laparoscopic ablation of the nerve fibres in the uterosacral ligaments by diathermy or laser has been used in some centres, but response rates vary considerably.

Endometriosis/Adenomyosis

Medical Treatment

Treat with:

NSAIDs
Progestogens
Suppress ovulation using:
- Combined oral contraceptive
- Danazol
- Gonadotrophin-releasing hormone analogues (GnRHa)

NSAIDs have the advantages of being compatible with trying for pregnancy, of needing only be taken at the time of symptoms and of reducing any associated menorrhagia. They will not alter the underlying disease and may cause gastrointestinal irritation.

The oral contraceptive pill inhibits ovulation by negative feedback, suppressing the release of luteinizing hormone (LH) and follicle-stimulating hormone (FSH) from the pituitary. The normal proliferative and secretory changes in the endometrium cease and ectopic endometrium atrophies. To be effective in this context, the pill must be taken on a continuous basis (i.e. without the 7-day break for a withdrawal bleed). Patients should be warned that they will not have a bleed. Treatment should be continued for 6 months. This treatment has the advantage of being relatively free from unpleasant side-effects and the incidental benefit of providing contraception. However, it is not suitable for women over 35 who smoke or those at increased risk of deep vein thrombosis (DVT). Symptoms recur in up to 40 per cent of women.

Synthetic progestogens (medroxyprogesterone, dydrogesterone) produce decidual changes in ectopic endometrium when given continuously. Side-effects are breakthrough bleeding, weight gain and fluid retention.

Danazol acts at a number of sites and causes a hypogonadotrophic state, which again leads to atrophy of the ectopic endometrium. Treatment is normally given for up to 6 months at a dose sufficient to induce amenorrhoea. Side-effects are common. These are both hypo-oestrogenic (hot flushes, vaginal dryness, loss of libido) and androgenic (acne, weight gain, mood changes, voice changes). Additional contraceptive measures must be taken. Up to 50 per cent of women are unable to tolerate this drug and counselling patients as to the potential side-effects is essential. Symptoms may recur after treatment is completed.

GnRHa competes with GnRH for binding sites on the pituitary and inhibit the production of LH and FSH, again effectively inducing a menopausal-like state and causing atrophy of the endometrium. They tend to be associated with more marked hypo-oestrogenic but fewer androgenic symptoms than danazol. In particular, they are associated with a loss of bone mass which limits their use to 6 months. They are given as monthly injections or as a nasal spray.

Surgical Treatment

Conservative surgical treatment includes diathermy or laser ablation of individual deposits of endometriosis, usually laparoscopically. This may improve symptoms and avoid the side-effects of medical therapy but requires appropriate equipment and operator expertise. Larger endometriotic deposits such as ovarian cysts can be removed by cystectomy or oophorectomy as either an open or laparoscopic procedure, often in combination with medical therapy.

Where the woman no longer wishes to preserve her fertility, the definitive treatment for adenomyosis is simple hysterectomy, but for endometriosis this must be accompanied by bilateral salpingo-oophorectomy to prevent recurrence of the disease. Hormone replacement therapy can and should be given to women under the age of 50 following such treatment.

Chronic Pelvic Inflammatory Disease

Antibiotic therapy
Simple analgesics
Adhesiolysis
Salpingectomy
Hysterectomy and bilateral salpingectomy

Isolated adhesions alone rarely cause pain unless involving other organs such as bowel. It may be possible to divide them surgically (adhesiolysis), laparoscopically or by means of open laparotomy.

Patients should be aware that not only may this be unhelpful but it may actually cause further adhesion formation. Patients with isolated non-vascular adhesions which do not involve other structures may be better managed as for the group with no apparent pathology.

Treatment with antibiotics may improve symptoms in acute exacerbations of pelvic inflammatory disease but will not improve chronic symptoms.

The only definitive cure is likely to be removal of the pelvic organs by total abdominal hysterectomy and bilateral salpingo-oophorectomy. However, it may be possible to preserve fertility by more limited surgery, such as removal of one tube, or by the use of assisted conception techniques after bilateral salpingectomy.

Irritable Bowel Syndrome

Irritable bowel syndrome is a diagnosis of exclusion, although it characteristically affects young women who may be going through a period of anxiety or stress. It is often associated with periods of loose stools followed by constipation, with faecal urgency. The pain can be continuous or intermittent and occasionally excruciating. Abdominal bloatedness is often reported. It can be difficult to differentiate from chronic PID, except on laparoscopy, which is normal in irritable bowel syndrome.

Initial management should include a clear explanation of the nature of the problem and the importance of an adequate fibre intake. There are a number of treatments and it is usually a case of experimentation to find which suits the particular individual. These include:

- dietary modification, eliminating triggers and adding fibre supplements;
- drug therapies, such as antispasmodics, e.g. mebeverine, peppermint oil capsules, antidiarrhoeals and occasionally low-dose antidepressants.

Prevention of irritable bowel syndrome
Eating a healthy diet, with plenty of fibre, fruit and vegetables
Excluding any trigger foods
Taking regular exercise
Avoiding unnecessary stress
Relaxation techniques

No Apparent Pathology

Whilst most patients with pain will be reassured by being told there is no abnormality, it will leave some feeling frustrated that there is no clear explanation for their symptoms. It may be necessary to reconsider the use of investigations such as laparoscopy, if not already done, to provide adequate reassurance to such patients.

Carefully review and possibly revisit your history for any evidence of depression, psychosexual disorders (see Chapter 54) and anxiety about underlying illness. There is often insufficient time to explore these issues in the general outpatient clinic, so consider arranging referral to an appropriate counsellor.

In the majority of cases, the pain will resolve spontaneously within 6 months. If this does not occur, review the original diagnosis and consider further investigation or a therapeutic trial of treatment for IBS or endometriosis. Refer to a pain clinic.

Learning Points

- Pelvic pain is a common presenting symptom for non-organic problems
- Significant pelvic pathology is unlikely in the absence of abnormal findings on clinical examination
- Most cases of pelvic pain with a normal laparoscopy resolve within 6 months

See Also

Infertility (Chapter 51)
Painful intercourse (Chapter 54)
The pelvic mass (Chapter 55)
Acute abdominal pain (Chapter 67)

Further Reading

Lewis TLT, Chamberlain GVP (eds). *Gynaecology by Ten Teachers.* Arnold, London, 1990, ch. 9 (Pelvic pain)

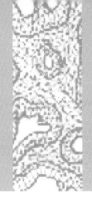

Contraception

Definitions

Pregnancy rates are expressed as the number of pregnancies per 100 women-years of use of a contraceptive (Pearl index). Failure rates may be the lowest expected for the method or a typical failure rate depending on compliance (Table 48.1).

Importance

Twenty-one per cent of unwanted pregnancies result from unprotected intercourse. Worldwide there are approximately 500 000 pregnancy-related deaths a year, including 500 per day from abortion. Historically breast-feeding has been the major factor in spacing pregnancies.

Clinical Assessment

History

Ask about:

Age
Menstrual history
Previous contraception
Sexually transmitted infections
Thromboembolism
Breast-feeding
Contraceptive needs
Smoking

Current pregnancy should be excluded. An intrauterine contraceptive device (IUCD) is usually not the first method of choice in nulliparous women

Table 48.1 Failure rates of different methods of contraception

	Failure rates/ 100 women-years	
	Method	Typical user
Combined oral contraceptive pill	0.1	2–8
Progestogen-only pill	3	10
Depo-provera	0.4	0.4
Mirena	0.2	0.2
Barrier	4–28	4–28

or those at greater risk of sexually transmitted disease. Conversely, barrier contraception will offer some protection against infection in at-risk groups. Compliance with oral contraceptives may be more difficult for the very young. Fertility rates fall after the age of 40. The combined oral contraceptive pill (COCP) is contraindicated in women who are currently breast-feeding, although progestogen-only preparations may still be used. Women with a family history of thromboembolism should be investigated for evidence of hereditary thrombophilia before being prescribed the combined pill. Menstrual blood loss may be increased by using an IUCD (except for the levonorgestrel intrauterine system) but is reduced in women using hormonal contraception.

Drugs may reduce the effectiveness of hormonal contraception by increasing the metabolism of oestrogen or by affecting gut flora and altering absorption. The COCP may interfere with the action of other drugs such as anticoagulants.

Drugs that alter effectiveness of the oral contraceptive pill (OCP)

Anticonvulsants
- Carbamazepine, phenytoin, primidone

Antibiotics
- Rifampicin, griseofulvin

Phenylbutazone

Barbiturates

Examination

Before prescribing contraception, check:

Blood pressure

Body mass index (BMI)

Up-to-date cervical smear if over 20 years old

Pelvic examination

Obesity and raised blood pressure are associated with an increased risk of thrombosis. Combined oral contraceptives are contraindicated in women over the age of 40 who smoke.

If the uterus is enlarged and pregnancy has been excluded, this is most likely to be due to uterine fibroids. These may enlarge in patients on the OCP or distort the uterine cavity making the IUCD less effective. Any pelvic mass should be investigated and, if indicated, swabs should be taken and infection treated before an IUCD is inserted.

Investigations

Routine investigation is not usually required. A full blood count should be taken if there is history of heavy menstrual bleeding and, if necessary, a pregnancy test performed to exclude current pregnancy. An ultrasound scan should be requested for any pelvic mass. Women with a strong family history of venous thrombosis should be investigated for hereditary thrombophilia.

Choosing an Appropriate Method

Methods of contraception

Hormonal

Barrier methods

Intrauterine devices

Non-medical methods

Sterilization (see Chapter 60)

Each method has advantages and disadvantages that need to be discussed with each woman in the light of her own circumstances. Even where there are other contraindications, these may be relative and have to be balanced against the need to prevent unplanned pregnancy (see Table 48.1).

Hormonal

- Combined oral contraceptive pill
- Progestogen-only pill
- Injectables
- Implants

Oral Contraceptive Pill

There are two types: the combined pill that contains both oestrogen and a progestogen (a synthetic progesterone) and the progestogen-only pill.

Progestogen content of contraceptive pills

Combined
- Norethisterone (Norimin, Ovysmin)
- Norgesterol (Eugynon)
- Levonorgestrel (Eugynon 30, Microgynon)
- Desogestrel (Mercilon)
- Gestodene (Femodene)

Progestogen only
- Norethisterone (Norriday)
- Levonorgestrel (Neogest)

The combined pill contains 20–50 μg of ethinyl-oestradiol and 150 μg–4 mg of progestogen. It works by inhibiting ovulation and by altering cervical mucus. It is taken for 21 days followed by a 7-day pill-free interval during which there is a withdrawal bleed. Everyday (ED) preparations include seven placebo pills that are taken instead of a pill-free week. If a pill is missed for more than 12 hours (or absorption is uncertain because of vomiting or antibiotics), alternative methods of contraception should be used for the next 7 days. If this would include the pill-free week, the woman should be advised to start the next pill packet without the normal break. The concentration of the hormones may be the same throughout the 21 days (monophasic preparations) or vary across the cycle (biphasic and triphasic preparations) in order to reduce breakthrough bleeding. Pills containing lower doses of oestradiol are more likely to be associated with irregular bleeding. The risks of arterial and venous thrombosis are higher with higher doses of oestrogen. Norethisterone and levonorgestrel adversely affect the ratio of high-density to low-density lipoproteins in the blood. Pills containing gestodene and desogestrel are associated with a twofold greater risk of venous thrombosis than other progestogens.

The progestogen-only pill is taken every day. Its main method of action is through its effect on the cervical mucus and the endometrium. It must be taken at the same time every day and additional contraceptive methods should be used if there is a delay of more than 3 hours.

Contraindications to the combined contraceptive pill

Absolute
- Known or suspected pregnancy
- Undiagnosed vaginal bleeding, endometrial pathology
- Oestrogen-dependent tumours (including trophoblastic disease)
- Circulatory disease (venous thrombosis, ischaemic heart disease, hyperlipidaema, thrombophilia, cerebrovascular accident (CVA), valvular), hypertension
- Acute or severe liver disease (cholestasis, porphyria, gallstones, jaundice)
- Focal migraine

Relative
- Family history of ischaemic heart disease, hyperlipidaemia or thrombosis
- Smoker (> 35 years old or > 40 cigarettes/day)
- Diabetes
- Generalized migraine
- Sickle cell disease

Advantages

The combined pill has a failure rate of less than 1 per 100 women-years. Menstrual blood loss is reduced by 40 per cent and there is a reduction in fibroids and benign ovarian tumours. The risk of ovarian and endometrial cancer is reduced in women taking the pill by up to 50 per cent, although there may be some increase in the risk of breast cancer. The effect on cervical mucus provides some protection against ascending infection.

The progestogen-only pill is associated with fewer serious side-effects and is compatible with breast-feeding.

Disadvantages

Both methods are dependent on compliance. The risk of venous thrombosis is increased from 5 per 100 000 to 15 per 100 000 and further increased in smokers and women with a previous history of the condition. There is an increase in arterial disease with a 1.5-fold to two-fold increase in CVA and a three-fold to five-fold increase in myocardial infarction (although there is no significant increase in women under 25 or in non-smokers). However, both these conditions are rare in women under 35, so the overall risk remains low.

There is an increase in gallstone formation and cholecystitis and an increase in glucose intolerance.

The progestogen-only pill has a higher failure rate and is more likely to be associated with irregular bleeding. If it fails, there is a higher risk of ectopic pregnancy.

Emergency contraception using the pill (after unprotected intercourse, missed COCP or burst condom)

A single 750 mg levonorgestrel tablet is taken within 72 hours of intercourse followed by a second dose exactly 12 hours later. The levonorgestrel-only method has fewer side-effects than the previously used combined method and is available as Levonelle to women over 16 from pharmacists. Side-effects include nausea, vomiting (an additional pill should be taken if vomiting occurs within 2–3 hours of the first dose) and bleeding. The woman should be advised that:

- her next period might be early or late;
- she needs to use barrier contraception until then and should continue taking the oral contraceptive pill;
- she needs to return if she has any abdominal pain or if the next period is absent or abnormal.

If the next period is more than 5 days overdue, pregnancy should be excluded. Emergency contraception prevents 85 per cent of expected pregnancies. Efficacy decreases with time from intercourse.

Follow-up

This should be at 4 weeks after starting the pill to check blood pressure, side-effects and compliance, and then yearly.

Injectables

There are currently two main types of injectables. Depo-provera contains 150 mg of medroxyprogesterone acetate and is given as a 3-monthly intramuscular injection. Norplant silastic rods containing levonorgestrel are implanted subdermally and last for

5 years. These injectables work by making the cervical mucus hostile and the endometrium hypotrophic.

Contraindications

Pregnancy
Undiagnosed vaginal bleeding
Neoplasia
Acute liver disease

Advantages
They are long-acting but easily reversible, effective, avoid first-pass effect liver metabolism, require minimal compliance and avoid side-effects associated with oestrogens.

Disadvantages
They may cause irregular bleeding or amenorrhoea, which can be a source of anxiety because of the possibility of pregnancy. Removal of the implants may be difficult. Some women will experience systemic progestogenic effects such as mood changes and weight gain or symptoms of oestrogenic deficiency.

Failure rates are low, at 0.2 per 100 women-years in the first year, rising to 3.9 per 100 women-years over 5 years. Failures mostly relate to women already pregnant at the time of implantation, so it is essential that depot injections are given at the time of termination or within the first 5 days of menstruation.

Intrauterine Contraceptive Device

- Silastic non-medicated (Lippes loop)
- First-generation copper devices (Cu 7, Cu T)
- Second-generation copper-coated devices (Multiload 250, Nova T)
- Third-generation copper devices (Multiload 375, Cu T 380)
- Progestogen-releasing devices (levonorgestrel).

Non-medicated devices are no longer available although some women may still have them *in situ*. IUCDs work by causing a foreign body reaction in the endometrium which inhibits implantation and sperm transport. The levonorgestrel-releasing intrauterine system, or IUS (Mirena®), also causes atrophy of the endometrium and affects cervical mucus. It is normally effective for 5 years but in women over the age of 40 will usually be effective until the menopause.

Counselling for IUCD insertion

Failure rate
Risk of miscarriage and ectopic pregnancy in the event of
    failure
Possible increase in menstrual blood loss and pain (copper
    devices)
Increased risks of sexually transmitted infection
Risk of perforation at insertion and migration of device
Need for follow-up

Patient selection and counselling are essential. Any contraindication, especially the possibility of pregnancy, should be excluded and any vaginal infection treated. Insertion is best carried out at the time of, or shortly after, menstruation. A vaginal examination is performed to determine the size and position of the uterus. The cervix is cleaned with antiseptic solution and the length of the uterine cavity measured using a uterine sound before inserting the device under aseptic conditions whilst holding the anterior lip of the cervix with a tenaculum (Figure 48.1).

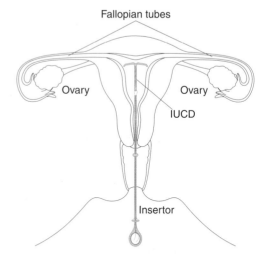

Figure 48.1   Insertion of an intrauterine contraceptive device

Absolute contraindications to the IUCD

Pregnancy (known or suspected)
Undiagnosed bleeding
Current pelvic inflammatory disease (PID; except *Candida*) or
    within the last 12 months
Lack of informed consent
Uterine malformation

Advantages

Low failure rates and high compliance.

Disadvantages

Perforation at the time of insertion occurs in 2/1000 cases but can be reduced by having an experienced operator, adequate examination before insertion and good technique. It should be suspected if there is excessive pain at the time of insertion or if the threads of the device can no longer be seen at follow-up. If suspected, arrange an ultrasound scan and plain abdominal X-ray and remove laparoscopically (laparotomy required in 10 per cent of cases).

There is a twofold increased risk of PID, mostly within the first 3 months after insertion. Menorrhagia and dysmenorrhoea occur in 40 per cent of women after insertion of copper-containing devices and are the commonest reasons for requesting removal, although they may respond to treatment with non-steroidal anti-inflammatory drugs (NSAID). Menstrual loss is reduced by up to 90 per cent at 6 months after insertion of the levonorgestrel IUCD, although irregular bleeding affects 40–60 per cent of women in the first 3 months after insertion.

Expulsion of the device occurs in 1–10 per 100 cases, usually in the first 3 months, and is increased if the device is inserted less than 3 weeks after delivery. If the threads are lost, arrange an ultrasound scan to locate the device. If this shows it is correctly positioned in the uterus, it can be left if removal is not required for other reasons. The threads can usually be brought down by coil retriever. Although the overall risk of ectopic pregnancy is reduced (1.2/1000 woman-years), 3–4 per cent of pregnancies that occur with an IUCD *in situ* will be ectopic. If intrauterine pregnancy occurs with an IUCD present, the risk of miscarriage, and later of preterm rupture of membranes, is increased fivefold. The device should be removed if the threads are visible. The long-term risk of infertility is not increased by IUCD use unless PID occurs.

Barrier Contraception

- Condoms
- Diaphragm
- Cervical cap
- Vaginal sponges or rings.

These act by preventing the entry of sperm into the cervical canal and are most effective when used in conjunction with a spermicide. The size of diaphragm or cervical cap needs to be determined by examination by a doctor or nurse. The woman is then shown how to insert it herself before intercourse and instructed to leave it in for 8 hours afterwards.

Advantages

There are no systemic side-effects, they offer protection against sexually transmitted infection and condoms are widely available.

Disadvantages

They require premedication and may reduce sensation during intercourse. They have relatively high failure rates and occasionally cause vaginal irritation as a result of allergic reaction.

Follow-up

After 6 weeks, and then yearly to ensure correct fitting of the diaphragm (this will also need to be refitted after a pregnancy).

Non-medical Contraception

- Withdrawal (coitus interruptus)
- Abstinence during fertile periods (rhythm method)
- Breast-feeding.

The fertile period extends across the 4–5 days before and after ovulation. In a regular 28-day cycle this occurs on the 14th day after the start of the last period. It is associated with changes in cervical mucus that a woman can learn to recognize by self-examination and hormone changes that can be measured by home urine testing kits. Avoidance of the fertile period can be an extremely effective method in well-motivated couples.

Advantages
There are no side-effects.

Disadvantages
The rhythm method depends on having a regular cycle and a high degree of motivation by the couple.

Learning Points

- **Always exclude the possibility of pregnancy before prescribing hormonal contraception or fitting a contraceptive device**
- **Provide advice about what to do in the event of method failure**
- **Relative contraindications may have to be balanced against the need for an effective method to prevent unwanted pregnancy**

See Also

Sterilization (Chapter 60)
Termination of pregnancy (Chapter 61)

Further Reading

Anonymous. Practical guidance on the supply of emergency hormonal contraception as a pharmacy medicine. *The Pharmaceutical Journal* 2000; 265: 890–92.

Chapter 49

Heavy periods

Definitions

The normal menstrual cycle is between 21 and 35 days with bleeding lasting 2–5 days. Menorrhagia is defined as the occurrence of heavy or prolonged (>7 days) regular menstrual bleeding. Polymenorrhoea is the occurrence of regular periods at intervals of less than 21 days. In (meno)metrorrhagia there is (heavy/prolonged) irregular and frequent uterine bleeding. Intermenstrual bleeding is bleeding or spotting between normal periods (see Chapter 54).

Importance

Ten per cent of women in the UK have hysterectomies by the age of 60 where the main indication is heavy periods. Each year 5 per cent of women aged 30–49 see their GP because of menorrhagia. Menstrual disorders are the commonest single cause for referral to gynaecology outpatient clinics.

Causes

Causes of heavy periods

Dysfunctional uterine bleeding
Structural lesions of the uterus
- Fibroids
- Adenomyosis
- Polyps

Malignancy
Chronic infection
Bleeding disorders
Hypothyroidism
Iatrogenic

The median blood loss per month in menstruation is 40 mL. Blood loss of more than 80 mL/month is considered abnormal. The physiology of the normal menstrual cycle is described in Chapter 46.

Dysfunctional bleeding is the term used to describe abnormally heavy or prolonged menstrual bleeding where there is no uterine or systemic cause. It accounts for more than 80 per cent of cases of menorrhagia and can be either ovulatory or anovulatory. Anovulatory bleeding tends to occur at the extremes of reproductive life and is associated with a shortening of the luteal phase of the cycle (Figure 49.1).

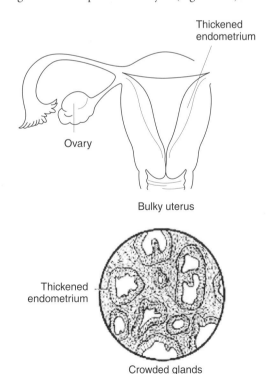

Figure 49.1 Metropathia haemorrhagica – caused by 'unopposed' oestrogen in anovulatory cycles

Fibroids are the commonest structural lesion to cause heavy regular bleeding (see Chapter 55). Endometrial carcinoma is rare under the age of 40 and is more likely to cause irregular bleeding. Adenomyosis (implantation of endometrial glands in the myometrium) is associated with a uniformly enlarged, tender uterus and is normally diagnosed following hysterectomy.

Diagnosis and Clinical Assessment

History

Ask about:

Age
Duration of symptoms
Length and duration of bleeding
Heaviness of loss
Effect on work/social/sex life
Any intermenstrual bleeding
Associated pain
Contraception
Previous treatment
Last cervical smear

An accurate history is essential to establish the pattern of bleeding and the duration of symptoms. Pregnancy should always be excluded before considering other causes of abnormal uterine bleeding in any woman of reproductive age. Assessment of the heaviness of periods is necessarily subjective. Less than 50 per cent of patients complaining of heavy periods have a measured blood loss of more than 80 mL/month. The presence of clots in the menstrual loss, the need to change sanitary protection at night and 'flooding' (the soiling of bedclothes or underwear during menstruation) are more likely to indicate significant bleeding. A recent change in the pattern of menstruation and associated pain are more likely to be associated with the development of pelvic pathology. Pain is associated with adenomyosis and chronic pelvic inflammatory disease. Structural lesions of the uterus and cervix are more likely in the presence of intermenstrual bleeding. The commonest iatrogenic cause of heavy bleeding is the presence of an intrauterine contraceptive device (IUCD).

Examination

Check for evidence of:

Anaemia
Hypothyroidism
Pelvic mass
Structural lesions of the lower genital tract

All women with abnormal bleeding should have a pelvic examination, including a cervical smear if indicated.

A pelvic mass is most likely to be due to uterine leiomyomata (fibroids) but may indicate a uterine malignancy or ovarian tumour.

Investigation

A full blood count is the only investigation needed before starting treatment, provided that examination is normal. Patients should be referred for further investigation if:

- there is a history of irregular or intermenstrual bleeding or of risk factors for endometrial carcinoma (see Chapter 56);
- their cervical smear is abnormal (see Chapter 45);
- pelvic examination is abnormal;
- they do not respond to first-line treatment after 6 months.

Risk factors for endometrial carcinoma include diabetes, hypertension, polycystic ovarian syndrome (PCOS), obesity and a family history. However, malignancy is extremely rare under the age of 40.

Further investigations

Endometrial biopsy
Pelvic ultrasound
Hysteroscopy
Thyroid function tests
Clotting studies

Endometrial biopsy can be performed as an outpatient procedure either alone or in conjunction with hysteroscopy.

Hysteroscopy is visualization of the uterine cavity using an endoscope introduced through the cervix. It can be performed under general anaesthetic or as an outpatient investigation. It has a higher sensitivity for endometrial pathology than dilatation of the cervix and endometrial curettage alone (see Chapter 56).

Pelvic ultrasound may be of value in distinguishing fibroids from other causes of pelvic mass such as ovarian tumours but is unlikely to help in the assessment of the endometrium itself (see Chapter 56).

Investigations for systemic causes of abnormal menstruation are only indicated if there are other features to suggest these on examination or in the history.

Management

Medical treatment of menorrhagia

Treat anaemia with ferrous sulphate 200 mg b.d.

Mefenamic acid 500 mg t.d.s.

Tranexamic acid 1 g t.d.s.

Combined oral contraceptive pill (COCP) (see Chapter 48)

Levonorgestrel intrauterine system (IUS)

Progestogens

Danazol

The treatment chosen will depend on whether contraception is required, whether irregularity of the cycle is a problem and the possible contraindications to certain treatments (Figure 49.2). Where a conventional IUCD is in place, mefenamic or tranexamic acid can be used or the device replaced by a levonorgestrel IUS (Figure 49.3).

Non-steroidal Anti-inflammatory Drugs

Mefenamic acid is a non-steroidal anti-inflammatory which blocks prostaglandin synthase. It reduces blood loss by 30–40 per cent and its analgesic properties may be an advantage if there is associated dysmenorrhoea. Its principal side-effects are gastrointestinal irritation and possible exacerbation of asthma (ask about any history of peptic ulceration).

Antifibrinolytics

Tranexamic acid is an antifibrinolytic agent which reduces blood loss by 50 per cent. It increases the risk of thrombosis and so is contraindicated in patients with a previous history of thromboembolic disease.

Mefenamic acid and tranexamic acid have the advantage of only needing to be taken during menstruation.

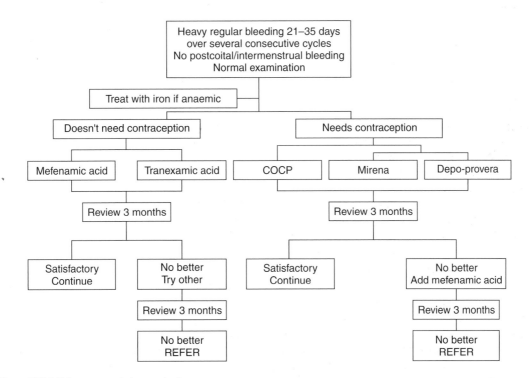

Figure 49.2 Initial management of menorrhagia

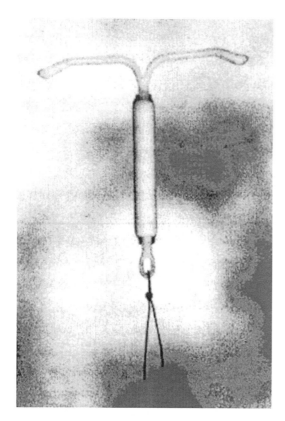

Figure 49.3 Levonorgestrel intrauterine device

Hormonal Treatments

Use of the COCP and the levonorgestrel IUS (Mirena®) is associated with a 30 and a 90 per cent reduction in average monthly blood loss, respectively. Hormone replacement therapy (HRT) may be useful in perimenopausal women to control ovulatory dysfunctional uterine bleeding (DUB).

Progestogens such as norethisterone and medoxyprogesterone actetate given in the second half of the cycle have not been shown to reduce blood loss, although they may have a role in establishing a more predictable cycle in patients with irregular bleeding. They are sometimes used in an acute situation to control heavy menstrual bleeding (oral medoxyprogesterone acetate 10 mg daily for 10 days).

Danazol is a synthetic androgen derivative that acts on the hypothalamic–pituitary axis and endometrium. Given at high doses it will normally cause amenorrhoea but is associated with significant side-effects in 50 per cent of patients and is normally limited to 6 months' use. However, at a lower dose (200 mg) given continuously it reduces menstrual loss by up to 60 per cent and is better tolerated. It is normally used as a second-line treatment in women where other medical treatment has failed.

Surgical treatment

Surgical treatment of menorrhagia

Myomectomy
Endometrial ablation or resection
Hysterectomy

Surgical treatment is normally used when first-line measures fail to control symptoms or where indicated by an underlying cause such as pelvic malignancy. Dilatation and curettage (D & C) is a diagnostic procedure and has no long-term effect on menstrual loss.

Myomectomy

Myomectomy is the removal of benign leioymomata from the uterine wall. It can be performed endoscopically for some pedunculated fibroids but requires a laparotomy for largely intramural lesions. It is indicated for women with symptomatic fibroids who wish to preserve their fertility. The fibroids may recur. There is a risk of bleeding and a possible need for hysterectomy.

Endometrial Resection and Ablation

Endometrial resection is the removal of the endometrium down to the myometrium using an operating hysteroscope and an electrocautery loop under general anaesthetic. Endometrial ablation can be carried out by vaporization using a fibreoptic laser, diathermy or thermal balloon.

There is a 1 per cent risk of hysterectomy at the time of operation. In addition to the risk of bleeding, the major complications are perforation of the uterus (with possible damage to bowel or bladder) and excessive absorption of the fluid used to irrigate and distend the uterus.

The major advantages of the procedure over hysterectomy are the shorter recovery period and lower morbidity. Approximately 25 per cent of patients will have no improvement in their symptoms and 6 per cent will eventually undergo hysterectomy. Success rates are lower when:

- uterus >10 cm in size
- patient < 35 years old
- moderate/severe dysmenorrhoea present.

Table 49.1 Comparison of endometrial resection and hysterectomy

	Hysterectomy	Resection
Effect on periods	100 per cent amenorrhoea	13–64 per cent amenorrhoea 62–77 per cent improved
Effect on pain	Abolished	13 per cent increased
Patient satisfaction	Higher long term	Higher at 1 month
Recovery	8–12 weeks	2–3 weeks
Postoperative complications	Up to 45 per cent	0–15 per cent
Mortality	0.4–2/1000	1/1000
Long-term risks	Inclusive bowel/urinary	Unknown/pregnancy

Pretreatment with danazol or gonadotrophin-releasing hormone (GnRH) antagonists is usually given to thin the endometrium 6 weeks prior to surgery. Endometrial histology should be obtained to exclude malignancy or hyperplasia prior to surgery.

Neither operation is compatible with preservation or fertility, although pregnancy may occur rarely after endometrial resection (Table 49.1).

Hysterectomy

The most definitive but also the most invasive treatment, this can be performed through a vaginal or abdominal approach. The cervix is normally removed with the uterine corpus but may be conserved at the patient's request or if technically difficult to remove (subtotal hysterectomy). The ovaries are more normally left *in situ* in vaginal surgery and in women under the age of 45. Unless indicated for known ovarian disease, women over 45 undergoing abdominal hysterectomy should be counselled about the benefits and disadvantages of oophorectomy.

Removal of normal ovaries at the time of hysterectomy

Advantages – removes risk of benign and malignant ovarian tumours

Disadvantages – causes premature menopause or the need for HRT to be taken

Vaginal hysterectomy is the route of choice because of the lower incidence of postoperative complications (15 per cent compared with 25–30 per cent for abdominal surgery), quicker return to normal activity and better cosmetic effect.

Complications of hysterectomy

Intraoperative
- Anaesthetic
- Bleeding
- Damage to the bladder/bowel/ureter

Immediate postoperative
- Bleeding – wound, vault, pelvic haematoma, pedicle
- Infection – wound, urinary, pelvic, chest
- Thromboembolism
- Fistula

Long term
- Prolapse
- Early ovarian failure

The overall mortality for hysterectomy is 0.2–2 per 1000 operations. Major bleeding occurring within 24 hours is more likely to be from a slipped pedicle; later bleeding is due to secondary haemorrhage associated with infection.

Ovarian failure occurs 12–18 months earlier following hysterectomy with ovarian conservation.

Learning Points

- **All women complaining of heavy periods should have a pelvic examination and a full blood count**
- **The commonest cause of regular heavy bleeding is dysfunctional uterine bleeding**
- **Progestogens are of no value in reducing menstrual blood loss**

See Also

Intermenstrual bleeding (Chapter 52)
The pelvic mass (Chapter 55)
Postmenopausal bleeding (Chapter 56)

Further Reading

Royal College of Obstetricians and Gynaecologists. The initial management of menorrhagia. *Evidence Based Clinical Guidelines No. 1*. RCOG, London, 1998.

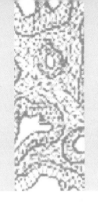

Chapter 50

Hirsutism and virilization

Definition

Hirsutism is excessive hair growth in an abnormal position that worries the patient. Virilization includes changes in voice, male pattern baldness, clitoral hypertrophy and breast atrophy.

Importance

Ten per cent of women are hirsute. Virilization may be a presenting symptom of an androgen-secreting tumour or adult-onset adrenal hyperplasia.

Causes

Causes of abnormal hair growth

Familial/racial
Polycystic ovarian syndrome
Ovarian tumours
Adrenal
- Cushing's disease
- Adrenal tumours
- Congenital adrenal hyperplasia
Acromegaly
Iatrogenic
Postmenopausal

Most women presenting will in fact have normal variations of hair growth related to familial or racial differences. Polycystic ovarian syndrome (PCOS) is associated with weight gain, subfertility and infrequent periods (see Chapter 46) and is the commonest cause of true hirsutism in premeno-pausal women.

Falling levels of oestrogen after the menopause are associated with a reduction in sex hormone binding globulin (SHBG) levels and an increase in free testosterone levels.

Androgen secretion is more likely to occur in sex-cord stromal ovarian tumours than the commoner epithelial types. Androgen-secreting tumours of the adrenals or ovaries may be accompanied by other signs of virilization (deepening of the voice, breast atrophy and enlargement of the clitoris).

As well as testosterone implants given for hormone replacement therapy, other drugs with androgenic effects include danazol, some progestogens, anabolic steroids and corticosteroids.

Diagnosis and Clinical Assessment

History

Ask about:

Age
Duration/onset of symptoms
Menstruation
Weight gain
Medical history
Drugs (including contraception)
Family history

Hirsutism of rapid onset is more likely to be associated with androgen-producing tumours. Weight gain and gradual onset of symptoms starting in the late teens are more typical of PCOS. Symptoms of hirsutism or virilization before puberty are likely to be due to congenital adrenal hyperplasia or tumours. Patients may not volunteer information about the use of non-prescription anabolic steroids unless asked directly or be aware of the potential for androgenic side-effects of other medication. Drugs used to treat epilepsy (such as phenytoin) are associated with a generalized increase in hair growth. A diagnosis of endocrine disorders may have already been made.

Examination

Significant findings

Male pattern hair distribution
Hypertension
Abdominal distension/striae
Clitoral hypertrophy
Pelvic masses

Assessment of hair distribution involves examination of the face, chest, abdomen, back and legs. Male pattern hair distribution typically includes extension of pigmented hair over the face, chest, nipples and lower abdomen (Figure 50.1). Temporal hair loss, deepening of the voice and clitoral hypertrophy indicate virilization, usually due to adrenal tumours or hyperplasia or ovarian tumours. Hypertension is associated with both PCOS and non-gynaecological endocrine causes of hirsutism such as Cushing's syndrome, which is also suggested by the presence of fresh striae on the abdomen.

Investigations

Relevant investigations

Testosterone
SHBG
Luteinizing hormone (LH):follicle-stimulating hormone (FSH)
Androstenedione
17-OHP
DHAS
Cortisol
Ultrasound, computerized tomography, laparoscopy

Testosterone levels may be elevated in PCOS but a markedly raised level (>5 mmol/L) suggests an ovarian or adrenal tumour. Adrenal tumours will also be associated with increased levels of androstenedione and dehydroepiandrosterone

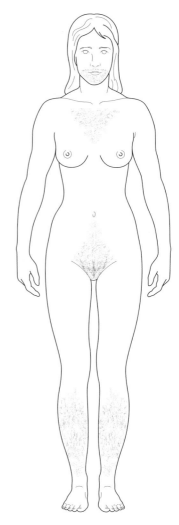

Figure 50.1 Male pattern hair growth

sulphate (DHAS). 17-hydroxyprogesterone (17-OHP) levels are raised in adrenal hyperplasia. SHBG levels are reduced in PCOS and after the menopause. FSH will be increased in postmenopausal women but within the normal range in PCOS. The LH:FSH ratio is increased in PCOS. Cortisol levels are increased in Cushing's disease.

Ultrasound imaging is used to confirm the diagnosis of PCOS and to identify ovarian tumours. Magnetic resonance imaging is indicated if biochemical investigation suggests the possibility of an adrenal tumour.

Management

Priorities

Identify cases due to hormonally active tumours or endocrine
    disorders
Discuss cosmetic treatment
Assess the need for additional drug therapy
Arrange suitable monitoring for patients on drug therapy

Ovarian tumours are treated by surgical removal (see
Chapter 55). Non-gynaecolgical endocrine disorders
should be referred to an appropriate medical
endocrine clinic for further management. If possible,
androgenic drugs should be stopped or a less androgenic alternative used. For further details on the
treatment of PCOS, see Chapter 46.

Treatment for abnormal hair growth

Cosmetic measures
Combined oral contraceptive pill
Cyproterone acetate
Corticosteroids

Hirsutism due to other causes may not require
treatment if mild. Weight loss may help improve
ovarian function in PCOS. Cosmetic measures such
as electrolysis, shaving and waxing may be as effective
as drug therapy in mild or moderate cases. Some
improvement in symptoms can be achieved in 30 per
cent of women using the combined oral contraceptive pill (COCP), which has the advantage of being
suitable for long-term maintenance therapy. More
severe cases can be treated with cyproterone acetate
(CPA) (an anti-androgenic progestogen). This can be
given in the form of the COCP Dianette or at higher
doses with additional ethinyloestradiol tablets from
day 5 to 21. Using this regime, up to 75 per cent

of women will report an improvement in their
symptoms by 12 months. Patients taking CPA should
have their liver function checked after 1 month and
then 6-monthly because of the potential risk of
hepatotoxicity. The diuretic spironolactone has some
anti-androgenic effects. Corticosteroids are effective
in about 50 per cent of women but tend to cause
weight gain. Long-term use is associated with a risk
of osteoporosis and adrenal suppression.

Learning Points

- **Most women seeking help for hirsutism have
  normal familial or racial variants of hair growth**
- **Polycystic ovarian disease is the commonest
  cause of true hirsutism**
- **Virilization or very elevated levels of testosterone
  require further investigation for possible
  hormonally active adrenal or ovarian tumours**
- **Cosmetic treatments may be more appropriate
  than drug therapy in some cases**
- **Drug therapy tends to inhibit new hair growth
  rather than reverse hirsutism and takes several
  months to show any effect**

See Also

Amenorrhoea and oligomenorrhoea (Chapter 46)

Further Reading

Jacobs HS. Hirsutism. *Current Obstetrics and Gynaecology* 1991; 1:
17–20.

Eden JA. Hirsutism. In: Studd J, ed. *Progress in Obstetrics and
Gynaecology*. Churchill Livingstone, Edinburgh, 1991, pp. 319–34.

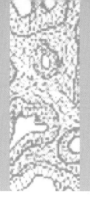

Chapter 51

Infertility

Definition

Infertility is defined as failure to conceive after 12 months of regular unprotected intercourse. It is primary if there have been no previous pregnancies, and secondary if the woman has previously been pregnant.

Importance

Affects 1 in 7 couples in the UK.

Normal Conception

Migration of sperm into the cervical mucus occurs rapidly after intercourse. The cervical mucus is most receptive in mid-cycle. During the passage through the Fallopian tubes, the sperm undergo a process known as 'capacitation', enabling them to penetrate the zona pellucida of the oocyte. A small number of spermatozoa reach the oocyte in the ampullary region of the tube. The adherence of sperm to the oocyte induces the loss of the plasma membrane over the head of the sperm, allowing the release of lytic enzymes which facilitate penetration of the oocyte membrane (the acrosome reaction). The sperm head decondenses inside the oocyte to form the male pronucleus which becomes apposed to the female pronucleus in the fertilized egg (zygote). The chromosomes of the pronuclei fuse (syngamy) and this is followed by the first cleavage division.

The fertilized egg is transported through the tube by the peristaltic action of its ciliated epithelium and undergoes further cleavage divisions to form a morula (16-cell stage) and then a blastocyst. Six days after fertilization the blastocyst implants by its embryonic pole, usually near the mid-portion of the uterine fundus. Endometrial cells are destroyed by the cytotrophoblast and the cells are incorporated into the trophoblast. Endometrial stromal cells become large and pale (decidual reaction).

The chance of conception per cycle in a normal young couple is approximately 20 per cent; 60 per cent of couples will conceive within 6 months, and 85 per cent within 12 months.

Causes of Infertility

Principle causes

Ovulation failure
Tubal disease
Male factor
Coital failure
Cervical hostility
Endometriosis

Ovulation failure may be congenital (Turner's syndrome) or acquired as a result of impaired follicle-stimulating hormone (FSH)/luteinizing hormone (LH) release (e.g. polycystic ovarian syndrome [PCOS] or hyperprolactinaemia) or ovarian failure (see Chapter 46).

Tubal damage may occur as a result of previous sexually acquired infection, peritonitis from other causes (such as appendicitis) and as a result of previous surgery.

Endometriosis may also impair fertility by causing tubal damage or impairing oocyte transport from the ovary to the tube by adhesion formation. Endometriosis is associated with subfertility even in the absence of obvious tubo-ovarian disease.

Male factor infertility occurs in 5 per cent of men, is the major cause of infertility in 30 per cent of couples and is a contributory factor in a further 20 per cent. The major causes are testicular hypospermatogenesis (due to chromosome disorders in 2 per cent of infertile men), cryptorchidism (failure of the testes to descend by 2 years) or toxins. Orchitis affects up to 30 per cent of adults contracting mumps and is bilateral in 17 per cent of cases. Obstruction of the vas deferens may be due to congenital agenesis of the Wolffian duct, cystic fibrosis or infection. Varicoceles arising from the internal spermatic vein/renal vein may increase the temperature around the testes and impair spermatogenesis but are not always associated with infertility.

Toxins affecting spermatogenesis

Radiation
Cytotoxic drugs
Sulphasalazine
Steroids
Anticonvulsants
Alcohol
Cannabis

Coital disorders include erectile dysfunction and ejaculatory failure as a result of drugs, depression, spinal cord injury, bladder neck surgery, diabetes, alcohol or chronic illness.

Diagnosis and Clinical Assessment

History

Both partners should be involved in both the assessment and treatment of infertility. Ask about the frequency of, and any problems with, intercourse.

Ask female partner about:

Age
Previous pregnancies
Menstrual cycle
Previous abdominal/pelvic surgery
Previous pelvic inflammatory disease (PID)/sexually transmitted disease (STD)
Drug history
Cervical smear

Ask male partner about:

Previous children
Previous urogenital surgery or trauma
Genital pathology
Previous STD
Systemic disease
Occupation
Drug history

Female fertility declines with age, particularly after the age of 37. Previous pregnancy excludes most congenital causes of infertility, whilst complications of previous pregnancies such as Asherman's syndrome may themselves be a cause of secondary infertility. A history of regular menstruation is likely to indicate ovulation. Tubal damage is more likely to be present if there is a history of infection with Chlamydia and gonorrhoea or of previous tubal surgery. The risk of ascending infection is greater if infections occur when an intrauterine device is being used.

Excessive drinking can affect reproductive function in men and cause fetal abnormalities. Other drugs of addiction including smoking can affect both male fertility and the developing fetus. Environmental factors (e.g. excessive heat) can affect fertility in men.

Chronic illness such as renal disease is associated with anovulation and reduced sperm quality.

Previous genital pathology of relevance in men includes torsion, cryptorchidism, orchitis (mumps) and varicocele.

Examination

Check:

Body index index BMI
Secondary sex characteristics
Lower genital tract
Pelvic masses

A body mass index (BMI) of less than $19\,\text{kg/m}^2$ is likely to be associated with anovulation as a result of hypothalamic dysfunction (see Chapter 46). PCOS is associated with weight gain. Female genital tract examination should include taking swabs if there is any abnormal discharge, and a cervical smear if due. Ovarian tumours, fibroids and inflammatory masses of the tubes may be palpable as a pelvic mass.

Genital examination in the male partner consists of inspection for evidence of hypospadias or varicocele and palpation of the testicles and epididymis. Small testes may be associated with primary testicular failure.

Investigations

Investigations should be carried out according to local protocols, with each stage fully explained to the couple. They need to be interpreted in the context of the couple's age and the duration of infertility.

Initial investigation of infertile couple

Day 21 progesterone level
Tubal patency
Rubella status
Semen analysis

Ovulation should be confirmed by a mid-luteal (i.e. day 21) serum progesterone level of greater than 60 pm/L. There is no need to measure thyroid function or prolactin levels in women with regular periods unless they have symptoms of galactorrhoea or thyroid disease.

Diagnostic laparoscopy with dye insufflation is the procedure of choice for evaluation of the pelvis and tubal patency. Where there is no history of pelvic surgery or infection, tubal patency can be assessed by instillation of radio-opaque contrast media through the cervix and X-ray imaging (hysterosalpingography). This is normally carried out in the first 10 days of the menstrual cycle to avoid inadvertent X-ray exposure in early pregnancy. Ultrasound may be useful in evaluation of the uterine cavity and of the ovaries for conditions such as PCOS.

In addition, all women presenting with infertility should have their immunity to rubella checked and, if seronegative, be offered vaccination before undertaking further treatment for their infertility.

A minimum of two semen analyses should be performed. These samples should be obtained by masturbation into a suitable container (not a condom) after a period of abstinence of 3 days.

Normal semen analysis (WHO reference values)

Volume 2–5 mL
Count > 20 million/mL
Motility > 50 per cent progressive motility at 1 hour (25 per cent linear)
Morphology > 30 per cent normal
Liquefaction time: within 30 minutes
White cells in sample < 10^6/mL

If the sperm count is low, an elevated FSH level suggests testicular damage and a low-level hypogonadotrophism, whilst obstructive causes are associated with normal levels. A chromosome analysis should be carried out where the FSH is elevated. Testicular biopsy is indicated for suspected obstruction.

Management

Treatment options

Ovulation induction
Surgery (open or laparoscopic)
Intrauterine insemination ± ovarian stimulation
Assisted conception techniques
Donor gametes

No treatment is required for women under the age of 35 where there are no abnormal features in the history or after examination or investigation in both partners if the duration of infertility is less than 18 months. Where treatment is required, the couple should be referred to a specialist infertility clinic.

Couples should be advised to have intercourse throughout the month. Although ovulation can be detected in some cases by detecting a rise in basal body temperature or by LH detection kits, there is no evidence that using these to time intercourse improves fertility rates.

All women undergoing investigation or treatment for infertility should be advised to take 0.4 mg folic acid whilst trying to conceive and for the first 12 weeks of pregnancy, to reduce the risk of neural tube defects. Both partners should be advised to stop smoking and limit their intake of alcohol. Women with a BMI of more than 30 should be encouraged to join a supervised programme of weight loss.

All techniques involving gamete manipulation are regulated in the UK by the Human Fertilisation and Embryology Authority (HFEA).

Ovulation Induction

Ovulation induction should be carried out under specialist supervision with a full explanation of the potential complications. Treatment should be monitored with serial ultrasound scans.

The simplest method is clomiphene citrate, given orally at a dose of 50–100 mg daily for 5 days each month for up to 12 cycles. Other methods of ovulation induction involve injections of gonadotrophins (FSH and LH) with daily monitoring of ovarian response by ultrasound and serum oestrogen levels. Ovulation is triggered by an additional injection of human chorionic gonadotrophin (hCG) at day 13. In some cases, treatment with gonadotrophin-releasing hormone (GnRH) antagonists may be given beforehand to suppress any endogenous pituitary activity. Administration of GnRH is possible in cases of hypothalamic failure using pulsatile administration by subcutaneous infusion. Where anovulation is associated with high prolactin levels, treatment with a suitable dopamine agonist such as bromocriptine is effective in up to 80 per cent of cases.

Complications of ovulation induction

Multiple pregnancy
Increased risk of miscarriage
Ectopic pregnancy
Ovarian hyperstimulation

Ovarian hyperstimulation affects 1–5 per cent of patients undergoing ovulation induction treatment. It typically presents 3–6 days after hCG administration and is characterized by bilateral ovarian enlargement, tenderness, and nausea and vomiting. There is a marked loss of fluid and protein into the peritoneal cavity, resulting in hypoalbuminaemia, haemoconcentration and ascites. The condition tends to be worse when pregnancy occurs.

Tubal Surgery

Surgical correction (other than reversal of sterilization) of tubal damage has a relatively low success rate and is only suitable in cases of mild distal or proximal obstruction. This can be performed as an open or endoscopic procedure using microsurgical techniques. In more severe disease or where pregnancy does not occur within 12 months of surgery, the treatment of choice is in vitro fertilization (IVF). There is an increased risk of ectopic pregnancy following surgical correction of infertility.

Intrauterine Insemination

Intrauterine insemination (IUI) with the partner's sperm and ovulation induction with hCG and gonadotrophins are indicated for unexplained infertility or where there are problems with the interaction between the sperm and cervical mucus. The pregnancy rate per treatment cycle is approximately 10 per cent.

Assisted Conception Techniques

In vitro Fertilization and Embryo Transfer (IVF-ET)

In vitro fertilization involves fertilization of the ovum outside the body with the partner's sperm. Follicular development is stimulated using gonadotrophin (FSH/LH) injections until follicles reach 18–20 mm in diameter (12–14 days). Ovulation is triggered with an injection of hCG and oocyte collection carried out 34–36 hours later by transvaginal aspiration of the follicle under ultrasound guidance. Pretreatment with GnRH analogues prevents any spontaneous LH release, allowing better control over the timing of egg collection. The oocytes are mixed with prepared sperm 4–6 hours after collection and fertilization is confirmed 16–18 hours later by the presence of two polar bodies. Two embryos are then transferred to the uterus after 2–3 days and any remaining embryos cryopreserved for future use. Low-dose hCG or progesterone is given to provide luteal phase support and a pregnancy test is performed 14 days after embryo transfer.

The procedure has a pregnancy rate of approximately 30 per cent, although this is significantly lower in women over 40. IVF is indicated for tubal disease, some male factor causes of infertility and unexplained fertility. Donor gametes (sperm or oocytes) can be used in cases of primary ovarian failure or azoospermia.

Intracytoplasmic Sperm Injection (ICSI)

This involves the direct injection of immobilized sperm into the cytoplasm of the oocyte. Pregnancy rates are similar to those for IVF-ET. This technique allows treatment of couples with severe oligospermia or, using sperm aspirated from the testes or epididymis, some causes of azoospermia.

Gamete Intra-Fallopian Tube Transfer (GIFT)

The ooctyes are collected laparoscopically and mixed with sperm before being replaced into the Fallopian tubes so that fertilization occurs in vivo. This is an effective alternative in couples with unexplained infertility.

Male Factor

Men should be advised to stop smoking and avoid excessive alcohol consumption. Obstructive causes of oligospermia may be correctable by surgery.

Treatment of varicocele in oligospermic men improves pregnancy rates. Any infection should be treated. Gonadotrophin drugs are effective in men with hypogonadotrophic hypogonadism and bromocriptine in men with hyperprolactinaemia. IUI with a partner's sperm is effective in cases of poor sperm quality or sexual dysfunction, but IVF techniques such as ICSI are the treatments of choice for severe oligospermia.

Learning Points

- Both partners should be involved in the management of infertility
- Male factors are involved in 50 per cent of cases
- Treatment can be deferred for up to 3 years in couples with unexplained fertility under 35

- Couples requiring ovulation induction or assisted conception techniques should be referred to a specialist clinic

See Also

Amenorrhoea and oligomenorrhoea (Chapter 46)

Further Reading

Royal College of Obstetricians and Gynaecologists. The initial investigation of the infertile couple. *RCOG Evidence-based Clinical Guidelines No. 2*. RCOG, London, 1998.

Royal College of Obstetricians and Gynaecologists. The management of infertility in secondary cares. *RCOG Evidence-based Clinical Guidelines No. 3*. RCOG, London, 1998.

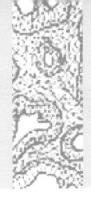

Chapter 52

Intermenstrual bleeding

Definition

This is bleeding from the genital tract occurring between periods. It may be unprovoked or occur only after intercourse (postcoital bleeding).

Importance

Intermenstrual bleeding (IMB) may be the presenting symptom of cervical or endometrial cancer. In women who are taking the combined oral contraceptive pill (COCP), persistent breakthrough bleeding may indicate an increased risk of pregnancy.

Causes

Common causes of IMB
- Structural lesions of the reproductive tract
  - Malignancy of the cervix or uterus
  - Cervical or endometrial polyps
  - Cervical ectropion
- Infections
- Iatrogenic
  - Intrauterine contraceptive device (IUCD)
  - Oral contraceptive pill (OCP) or hormone replacement therapy (HRT)

A cervical ectropion (sometimes wrongly called a cervical erosion) is an outgrowth of columnar epithelium onto the ectocervix. This gives the area around the external cervical os a dark red, velvety appearance. Cervical ectropion is a normal physiological variant, although a large ectropion may bleed when touched. Cervical polyps are commonly benign

overgrowths of the cervical epithelium. Cervical intraepithelial neoplasia (CIN) is normally asymptomatic; bleeding tends to be associated with the presence of cervical carcinomas. Bleeding may occur from either the cervix (cervicitis) or the endometrium in the presence of infection.

Bleeding that occurs between normal withdrawal bleeds on the contraceptive pill (breakthrough bleeding) and HRT will occur if a pill is missed or something interferes with absorption (broad-spectrum antibiotics, vomiting) or increases hepatic metabolism (anticonvulsants). Persistent breakthrough bleeding in a compliant user may indicate a pill of too low a strength to prevent ovulation.

Irregular bleeding commonly occurs in women using the levonorgestrel intrauterine system during the first 3 months after insertion but will usually settle after this.

Diagnosis

History

Ask about:

Age
Last menstrual period LMP.
Bleeding
- Onset
- Precipitating factors
Associated symptoms
Contraception
Compliance/other medication
Last cervical smear

Irregular bleeding and even continued cyclical bleeding may occur in early pregnancy and this possibility should always be excluded by history and, if necessary, a pregnancy test. Pelvic inflammatory disease (PID) is associated with pelvic pain and dyspareunia. Malignancy is more likely in the older age group, although up to a third of cases of cervical cancer occur in women under the age of 40. Broad-spectrum antibiotics interfere with oral oestrogen uptake by altering the normal gut flora, whilst antituberculous therapy induces liver enzymes that increase first-pass liver metabolism.

Drugs that may interfere with OCP/HRT

Antibiotics
- Broad spectrum
- Antituberculous

Anticonvulsants

Examination

Key findings

Abdominal or pelvic masses
Abnormal appearance of the cervix or lower genital tract
Contact bleeding on cervical examination

The commonest causes of a pelvic mass in women of reproductive age are pregnancy, uterine fibroids and ovarian tumours (see Chapter 55). Fibroids are not usually associated with IMB unless pedunculated and arising from within the uterine cavity. They may then prolapse through the external cervical os and become necrotic or ulcerated.

The presence of a raised or ulcerated area, or of abnormal looking blood vessels on the ectocervix, indicates the need to exclude malignancy even if the last cervical smear was normal. Bleeding or inflammatory change may make it impossible to obtain a satisfactory negative smear. Tenderness of the uterus or cervical excitation may be present in pelvic inflammatory disease.

Investigations

Relevant investigations

Cervical smear
Swabs
Colposcopy
Hysteroscopy

Unless there is a clear and correctable cause identified on the initial history (such as non-compliance on the COCP) or examination (cervical polyp in a young woman), a woman with recurrent IMB should be referred for further investigation.

Hysteroscopy is more likely to be of value in older women and those at increased risk of malignancy. Breakthrough bleeding that occurs after more than 6 months' use of HRT should be investigated as postmenopausal bleeding (see Chapter 56). Colposcopy is indicated in the presence of abnormal cytology or where there is any doubt about the appearance of the cervix, even if cytology is normal.

Management

This depends on diagnosis, need for contraception and coexisting menstrual problems.

Where there is persistent breakthrough bleeding on the OCP, this may indicate an increased risk of failure. If this is due to poor compliance, a suitable alternative form of contraception should be sought. Where there is a possible drug interaction, a higher-dose preparation may be required. In other cases, changing to a different pill preparation such as a biphasic or triphasic pill may give better cycle control (see Chapter 48). Once pathology of the genital tract has been excluded, patients on HRT may benefit from changing to a different preparation or route of administration (see Chapter 53).

Any coexisting infection should be treated.

Benign polyps can be avulsed in the outpatient setting where they arise from the ectocervix, but a hysteroscopy should still be carried out on all post-menopausal women with these polyps to exclude other lesions in the uterine cavity.

If examination of the cervix, including cytology, is normal, a symptomatic cervical ectropion may be treated by cryocautery. The management of cervical carcinoma is discussed in Chapter 45.

Learning Points

- **Intrauterine pathology should be excluded unless a clear correctable cause for IMB is apparent from the history or initial examination**

See Also

The abnormal cervical smear test (Chapter 45)
Contraception (Chapter 48)
Postmenopausal bleeding (Chapter 56)

Further Reading

Royal College of Obstetricians and Gynaecologists. The initial management of menorrhagia. *Evidence-based Clinical Guidelines No. 1*. RCOG, London, 1998.

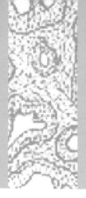
Menopausal symptoms

Definition

The menopause is the last menstrual period and the climacteric is the period of time around the menopause when ovarian function gradually ceases. The menopause is usually said to have occurred after 6 months of secondary amenorrhoea in a woman aged over 45.

Importance

The median age of the menopause has remained unchanged at 51. Increased life expectancy means that most women in the UK can expect to spend 40 per cent of their life after the menopause. Postmenopausal women make up 20 per cent of the population. The oestrogen deficiency that occurs as a result of ovarian failure is a source of morbidity and increases the chance of mortality from cardiovascular disease and osteoporosis. About 1 per cent of women will undergo the menopause before the age of 40.

Pathophysiology

From the age of 40 onwards, the pituitary responds to falling inhibin production by the ovaries by increasing plasma levels of follicle-stimulating and luteinizing hormones (FSH and LH). There is an increase in anovulatory cycles, a reduced length of the luteal phase and reduced fertility. The resulting relative progesterone deficiency leads to unopposed oestrogen effects on the endometrium, which may cause irregular heavy bleeding and increase the risk of endometrial hyperplasia and carcinoma. After ovarian failure the stroma remains active, producing androgens and a weak oestrogen, oestrone, by peripheral conversion of androgens in adipose tissue.

The decline in oestrogen levels affects other oestrogen target organs. Glycogen secretion in the vagina is reduced, with a decline in lactobacilli causing a rise in vaginal pH. This makes the lower genital tract more susceptible to infection at the same time as there is atrophy of the epithelium itself and a decrease in vascularity. There is a 30 per cent loss of skin collagen in the 10 years following the menopause. Bone mass falls by 50 per cent by the age of 70 as a result of loss of the collagen matrix with normal calcification (osteoporosis). Fifty per cent of women will have sustained a fracture by the age of 70, the commonest sites being the distal radius, neck of femur and vertebral bodies. A quarter of women at this age will die within a year of sustaining a hip fracture and a further 50 per cent will suffer a permanent loss of mobility and independence.

After the menopause there is an increase in low-density lipoprotein (LDL) concentrations and an increase in atheroma formation in the coronary arteries. At the same time the protective vasodilator effect of oestrogen on the coronary arteries is lost. As a result of these changes, the risk of ischaemic heart disease (IHD) increases to those levels seen in men.

Diagnosis and Clinical Assessment

History

Ask about:

Symptoms
- Hot flushes
- Psychological
- Urogenital tract

Menstrual history
Previous surgery
Treatment for breast and endometrial cancer
Liver disease and thromboembolic disease
Current medication
Smoking

Symptoms of the climacteric usually precede the menopause. The commonest reported symptoms will be of vasomotor instability (70 per cent), usually described as hot flushes or sweats, and psychological symptoms. Hot flushes may also present as syncopal episodes and headaches. Psychological changes include anxiety, depression, loss of concentration and irritability. These may be difficult to distinguish from depression and anxiety unrelated to hormone changes. Hot flushes and urinary frequency may disturb sleep patterns, which itself can cause tiredness. Atrophic changes in the urogenital tract may cause vaginal dryness and superficial dyspareunia. There may be an associated loss in libido due to declining androgen levels. An increase in frequency and urgency of micturition may also occur as a result of atrophic changes in the urinary tract. Unopposed oestrogen stimulation of the uterus in anovulatory cycles may lead to increasingly heavy and erratic menstruation.

Irregular bleeding will need to be investigated before starting hormone replacement therapy (HRT). Previous treatment for malignancy does not exclude the possibility of HRT, although recent breast and endometrial carcinomas are contraindications. There is an increased risk of venous thromboembolism with HRT. Liver disease may contraindicate the use of HRT.

The type of HRT used may be influenced by the length of time since the last period. Premature ovarian failure occurring spontaneously or as a result of surgery increases the long-term risks of heart disease and osteoporosis. Even where the ovaries are conserved, ovarian failure occurs 12–18 months earlier following hysterectomy. Ovarian failure may also be precipitated by radiotherapy. The risk of osteoporosis is increased in women on long-term corticosteroid therapy, smokers and those with an excessive alcohol intake.

Examination

Check for:

Anaemia
Hypothyroidism

Abnormal body mass index (BMI)
Hypertension
Breast lumps
Pelvic masses/abnormal cervix (smear)

There are no diagnostic findings of the climacteric as such, although there may be evidence of atrophic change in the genital tract. The main purpose of examination is to look for other causes of symptoms such as anaemia and hypothyroidism and to exclude any contraindications to HRT, such as breast or genital tract pathology. Hypertension itself is not a contraindication to treatment, although it will need to be monitored and controlled. After ovarian failure, peripheral adipose tissue becomes the major source of oestrogen. As a result women with a high BMI are at greater risk of endometrial hyperplasia and carcinoma, whilst those with a low BMI are at greater risk of osteoporosis.

Investigations

The diagnosis is generally made on the basis of the history but can be confirmed by an elevated FSH level. Ovulation may continue intermittently during the climacteric, so pregnancy should be excluded in any woman of reproductive age presenting with amenorrhoea. Thyroid disease and anaemia may produce some of the same symptoms (including amenorrhoea). Endometrial pathology should be excluded by hysteroscopy and endometrial biopsy in women with irregular bleeding (see Chapter 56).

Management

Priorities

Know the common clinical conditions that affect post-menopausal women
Differentiate menopausal from other causes of symptoms
Establish a plan of management for common post-menopausal problems
Assess the needs of an individual for HRT

Indications for Treatment

- Symptomatic
- Premature menopause (natural/iatrogenic)

- Gonadal dysgenesis
- High-risk of osteoporosis.

The commonest reason for treatment will be patient request because of symptoms. The first step in management must be to establish that these symptoms are in fact due to the oestrogen deficiency. The patient, or sometimes her doctor, may also be aware of the increased risk of osteoporosis after ovarian failure and request treatment to reduce this, whether she is symptomatic or not. This is especially important in women with early ovarian failure or other risk factors for osteoporosis. In both cases a decision will need to be taken as to whether or not to treat with oestrogens. This will depend on identifying those cases where oestrogens are contraindicated and balancing the advantages against the risks of such treatment in the remainder. This should be done in a way that can be understood, so that each woman can make an informed choice.

HRT has not been proven to reduce the risk of cardiovascular disease.

For some women, all that is required is an explanation of the nature of their symptoms. Lifestyle changes such as increasing exercise, stopping smoking and reducing alcohol intake will reduce the risk of IHD and osteoporosis.

Hormone Replacement Therapy

Contraindications

Active/recent cardiovascular disease
Recent/current breast cancer
Undiagnosed vaginal bleeding
Endometrial carcinoma
Pregnancy
Venous thromboembolism
Acute liver disease

Hypertension (if controlled), diabetes, endometriosis and fibroids are not contraindications to HRT. Oestrogens can be given orally, as subcutaneous implants or absorbed transdermally from patches or creams. Serum levels required for symptomatic relief are the same regardless of the route of administration, although the amount that needs to be taken depends on the route. In women with an intact uterus, oestrogen needs to be taken with a suitable progestogen to prevent endometrial hyperplasia. Unfortunately,

this may mean that the woman continues to have 'periods' and may develop premenstrual syndrome-like symptoms from the progestogen.

A third of oral oestrogen is converted to oestrone-3-gluconamide on first pass through the liver and is excreted in the urine and bile, leading to an inappropriate oestrone:oestradiol ratio and increases in sex hormone binding globulin (SHBG), cortisol and blood glucose and to a decrease in antithrombin III levels. Oral preparations use either conjugated equine oestrogens or synthetic 17-beta-oestradiol. They need to be taken daily and an oral progestogen given for part of each month, following which the patient will have a withdrawal bleed every 1 to 3 months. In women whose last period was more than 12 months before starting treatment, a continuous combined preparation can be given and the need for a withdrawal bleed avoided, but this is not suitable for women who still have some endogenous ovarian activity.

Topical treatment can be given as cream or twice-weekly patches. The patches can be placed anywhere except on the face or breasts. Compliance is easier because of the less frequent doses required, but some women will find that the adhesive causes a local skin reaction. Progestogens can be given as a combined patch for part of each month or as tablets as above. Where symptoms are predominantly lower genital tract in nature, locally applied oestrogens may be used in the form of creams or pessaries.

Oestrogen implants can be inserted at the time of operation or as an outpatient procedure under local anaesthetic into the subcutaneous fat of the thighs or lower abdomen. This has clear advantages as far as compliance is concerned, especially after hysterectomy when there is no need for a progestogen to be taken. However, serum levels of oestradiol tend to peak after 2–3 months and decline to pre-treatment levels by 6 months and some patients will experience a recurrence of symptoms even in the presence of supra-physiological oestradiol levels.

All patients should be warned about short-term side-effects of HRT, including breast tenderness, leg cramps, fluid retention, headaches and mood changes (see Table 53.1). Most symptoms will improve on their own or respond to changes in dose or type of HRT. Excessively heavy withdrawal bleeds can be treated in the same way as dysfunctional bleeding, but any irregular bleeding occurring more than 6 months after starting or changing HRT should be investigated as postmenopausal bleeding (see Chapter 56).

Table 53.1 Advantages and disadvantages of combined hormone replacement therapy

Disadvantages	Advantages
↑ Risk of endometrial cancer	Abolishes vasomotor symptoms
Cramps, breast tenderness	Reverses genital atrophy
↑ Risk of breast cancer	↑ Skin thickness
↑ Risk of venous thrombosis	↑ Bone density 2–8% per year
	50% ↓ hip fracture after 5 years

More serious side-effects are rare. The most important of these are an initial increase in the risk of venous thromboembolism (VTE) by 41 per 10 000 women per year. If VTE does not occur within 6 months of starting treatment, the long-term risk is the same as that of the rest of the population. There is an increase in the risk of breast cancer after taking HRT of 6 extra cases per 1000 women after 10 years' use. However, there is an excess in oestrogen receptor-positive tumours that develop in women taking HRT with a better prognosis.

The risk of endometrial cancer is increased by 42 cases per 1000 women treated with oestrogen-only HRT. This risk is reduced but not eliminated by the addition of progestogen. Against these complications and side-effects has to be weighed the advantages of improved quality of life with control of menopausal symptoms and long-term health benefits of HRT. Most significantly these include a reduction in fractures. HRT may also be of benefit in reducing the risk of non-infarctive dementia such as Alzheimer's.

Alternatives to oestrogen

Progestogens
Gonadomimetics (tibolone)
Selective oestrogen receptor modulators (SERMs)
α-Adrenergics
Bisphosphonates
Hypnotics/sedatives
Diet/exercise
Alternative therapies

For those women who are unwilling or unable to take oestrogen-containing HRT, progestogens can be given alone and will give some protection against bone loss and hot flushes, but long-term use may adversely affect lipoprotein levels. Tibolone is a synthetic androgen with oestrogenic properties. It does not cause endometrial proliferation so there is no withdrawal bleed, but it is only suitable for women more than a year after the menopause. It is effective at reducing vasomotor symptoms and osteoporosis.

Since it is known that different tissues express different oestrogen receptors, attempts are being made to develop drugs that will act on receptors in bone without affecting the breast or endometrium. One of these selective oestrogen receptor modulators (SERMs) currently available is effective at reducing bone loss without stimulating breast or endometrium, but does not relieve vasomotor symptoms and is associated with the same increased risk of VTE as conventional oestrogen therapy.

Clonidine is an antihypertensive that has some effect on vasomotor symptoms but no effect on other symptoms or long-term health. Biofeedback techniques, acupuncture and selected use of anxiolytics or sedatives may help to control psychological symptoms of insomnia and anxiety. Cyclical bisphosphonate therapy increases bone mass and reduces the rate of fracture and provides an effective alternative for women at risk of osteoporosis who are unwilling or unable to take HRT. Calcium supplements alone do not appear to prevent bone loss.

Follow-up

Patients on HRT should be seen 3 months after starting treatment and then annually. Ask about improvement in menopausal symptoms. Breast examination should be performed if no recent mammogram has been carried out and blood pressure checked.

Learning Points

- Oestrogens are produced by peripheral conversion of androgens after ovarian failure
- 25 per cent of women die within 1 year of hip fracture
- Depressive illness and hypothyroidism may mimic menopausal symptoms
- Progestogen needs to be given with oestrogen if the uterus is intact

- HRT increases the risk of venous thrombosis
- HRT increases the risk but not the mortality from breast cancer

See Also

Postmenopausal bleeding (Chapter 56)
Premenstrual syndrome (Chapter 57)

Further Reading

Studd JW, Baber R. The menopause. In: Shaw RW, Soutter WP, Stanton SL, eds. *Gynaecology*. Churchill Livingstone, Edinburgh, 1992, ch. 24

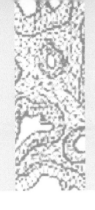

Chapter 54

Painful intercourse

Definition

Dyspareunia is pain or discomfort associated with intercourse. It is described as superficial when associated with penetration or deep when there is pelvic or abdominal pain during or after intercourse. It may be primary (i.e. having been present since the first attempt at intercourse) or secondary (a problem arising after previously satisfactory intercourse). In vaginismus there is involuntary contraction of the pelvic floor muscles closing the vaginal introitus, making any attempt at penetration painful. Inability to achieve orgasm may or may not be associated with inability to become aroused. Hypoactive sexual desire or loss of libido is the commonest presenting complaint. Inability to achieve arousal may occur as part of loss of sexual desire and contribute to inability to achieve orgasm. However, even when sexual desire is normal, anxiety and fear of interruption may interfere with normal arousal.

Importance

Problems with sexuality may present with a variety of gynaecological symptoms, although this may not always be immediately apparent. Discomfort with intercourse may be a symptom of organic disease of the genital tract or a manifestation of a more general physical or emotional problem or relationship difficulty. The true incidence of sexual problems is unknown. Up to a third of women aged 40 report some sexual problems, and sexual problems account for up to 1 in 14 referrals to gynaecological outpatients. If all women attending clinics are asked about sexual dysfunction, the apparent incidence of problems doubles. Five to 10 per cent of women have

not experienced orgasm by the age of 40. Vaginismus affects between 1 and 3 per cent of women aged 15–50.

Causes

Disorders of female sexual function

Loss of desire
Failure of arousal
Orgasmic dysfunction
Dyspareunia
Vaginismus

Sexual dysfunction may present as a secondary problem associated with contraception, pelvic pain, infertility, premenstrual syndrome or the menopause.

It will usually be possible to distinguish likely organic and psychological causes of sexual dysfunction from the history. Although there may be components of both in all types of sexual dysfunction, organic causes are more likely to be present in patients with dyspareunia.

Causes of loss of libido

Childbirth
Menopause
Depression, anxiety
Drugs

Neuropathy associated with diabetes or multiple sclerosis may interfere with sexual response. Sexual drive is linked to mood and can be suppressed by anxiety and depression. Up to a third of partners of women presenting with sexual dysfunction will themselves have problems. Changes in libido that occur at the time of the menopause, in the puerperium and premenstrually may be linked in part to hormonal changes but are often multifactorial. Although drugs with anxiolytic effects, including alcohol, may increase sexual desire in small doses, most drugs will either have no effect or reduce libido.

Causes of dyspareunia

Atrophic change
Vulvovaginitis
Vulval dystrophies
Pelvic inflammatory disease
Endometriosis
Previous surgery (including episiotomy)
Psychogenic

Gynaecological surgery for malignancy or vaginal prolapse may cause narrowing of the introitus or shortening of the vagina. Hysterectomy as such does not normally result in loss of libido or dyspareunia (unless part of the upper vagina is removed). Radiotherapy for cervical cancer may cause vaginal stenosis and reduce lubrication. Organic causes of dyspareunia (such as infection) may cause vaginismus or loss of libido and arousal (because of anxiety about pain) which persists even after the original organic lesion has resolved.

Diagnosis and Clinical Assessment

To identify problems with intercourse, ask about:

Frequency of intercourse
Patient satisfaction with quality of sexual relationship
Difficulties with arousal
Pain during intercourse
Difficulty achieving orgasm

Having identified that a problem exists, start by concentrating on the presenting complaint before going to a more general sexual history. Ask when the problem first occurred and whether the onset was gradual or sudden. Does the problem relate to a particular partner or sexual position? Are there any factors (such as time of the menstrual cycle) that make it worse or better?

For dyspareunia ask about:

Whether superficial or deep
Onset and duration

Situation
Precipitating or relieving factors
Previous gynaecological surgery (including episiotomy)

Examination

On general examination, look for signs of systemic illness or abnormalities of secondary sexual development. Severe vaginismus may make any attempt at vaginal examination impossible. Careful inspection of the external genitalia is essential to look for areas of tender scar tissue, infection or swelling. If pelvic infection is suspected, appropriate swabs should be taken for culture. Pelvic masses (including malignancy) may present with discomfort during intercourse. Retroversion of the uterus may be as a result of pathology such as endometriosis, which itself causes pain or may lead to discomfort during intercourse because of prolapse of the ovaries into the pouch of Douglas. In cases of dyspareunia, it may be possible to reproduce the pain on pelvic examination.

Investigations

Cases of deep dyspareunia should be investigated as for chronic pelvic pain (see Chapter 47), including if necessary the use of diagnostic laparoscopy.

Management

Principles of management

Permission
Limited information
Specific instructions
Intensive therapy

Superficial dyspareunia due to narrowing of the introitus or the presence of tender scar tissue may be treated surgically by excision of the scar tissue or a Fentom's procedure. There is a risk of further scar tissue formation after surgery and this should be delayed if there is evidence of spontaneous improvement. In vaginismus it is important to explain the involuntary nature of the contractions of the pelvic floor muscles. If pelvic floor exercises and simple relaxation techniques are unhelpful, desensitization may be achieved by encouraging the patient to insert progressively larger dilators into her vagina. Other organic causes of superficial or deep dyspareunia are treated according to the underlying diagnosis (see Chapters 47 and 65). Both oestrogen and testosterone appear to have a role in female sexual response. Where loss of libido is a feature of menopausal symptoms this will occasionally respond to testosterone therapy along with conventional oestrogen hormone replacement therapy.

Once organic disorders have been excluded or treated, an appropriate level of response can be selected for each problem. At its simplest this may be reassurance from the doctor that changes in sexual activity are acceptable (permission). In other cases women may need information about what constitutes a normal sexual response and how this can change at different times during their life. Specific suggestions may be in the form of where to get further information or advice on alternative positions or stimulatory techniques. Intensive therapy usually involves a more structured series of sessions, typically at 2-weekly intervals over 6 months.

By their nature general gynaecological outpatient clinics are not the most suitable places to manage sexual problems and any couple requiring intensive treatment should be referred to a specialist psychosexual clinic. Such treatments adopt a patient-centred approach with a stepwise approach to sexual activity, usually starting with a ban on penetrative sex. Progress in these steps is examined in the context of the couple's relationship.

The success of treatment depends largely on the state of the relationship between the couple but will also be affected by age and general health; 60–65 per cent of couples who stay in therapy will report improvement or complete resolution of their sexual problem, although the long-term prognosis is less clear.

Learning Points

- Sexual problems are a common secondary symptom in gynaecological clinics
- The commonest presenting symptoms are loss of sexual desire and dyspareunia
- Psychosexual disorders may occur in one relationship but not another
- Once organic causes have been excluded, sexual dysfunction is usually better managed in a specialist psychosexual clinic
- Even where there is an underlying organic cause, the prognosis is dependent on the attitude and expectations of the couple

See Also

Chronic pelvic pain (Chapter 47)
The swollen or painful vulva (Chapter 65)

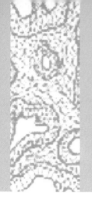

Chapter 55

The pelvic mass

Importance

A mass arising from the pelvis is the commonest presenting symptom for ovarian cancer, most patients presenting with advanced disease. Benign tumours of the ovaries and uterus (fibroids) are both commoner, however, and also asymptomatic in up to 50 per cent of cases. Pregnancy should be excluded in any woman of reproductive age.

Ovarian cancer is the fourth commonest cause of death from cancer in women in the UK, with more than 4000 new cases per year. The lifetime risk of developing the disease is 1.3 per cent. There are 17 new cases per 100 000 women each year.

Causes

Causes of a pelvic mass

Ovarian tumours
- Benign
- Malignant
- Endometriosis

Tubo-ovarian
- Pelvic inflammatory disease

Uterine
- Pregnancy
- Fibroids
- Malignancy
- Haematometra

Full bladder

Bowel
- Faeces
- Malignancy
- Diverticular disease

Ovarian cancer is rare under the age of 35. The peak incidence occurs in the sixth decade. Eighty-five per cent of primary ovarian tumours arise from the epithelium of the ovary. The remainder arise from the stroma and cells in follicles (sex-cord stromal tumours) or the germ cell themselves (teratomas and dysgerminomas) (Table 55.1). The ovary is a common site for metastatic tumours, particularly from the breast and gut. Epithelial tumours are associated with nulliparity, early menarche and late menopause. Use of the combined oral contraceptive pill (COCP) reduces the risk by up to a half. Infertility treatment with drugs to induce ovulation may be associated with an increased risk if pregnancy does not occur. A minority of tumours produce oestrogens or androgens and present with irregular bleeding or amenorrhoea, respectively.

Table 55.1 Classification of primary ovarian tumours

Epithelial	Sex-cord stromal	Germ cell
Serous	Granulosa	Dysgerminoma
Mucinous	Androblastoma (Sertoli–Leydig cell)	Teratoma
Endometrioid	Gynadoblastoma	Choriocarcinoma
Clear cell		Yolk sac
Brenner		
Undifferentiated		

Diagnosis and Clinical Assessment

Ask about:

Menstrual history
Contraception
Pain
Previous surgery
Gastrointestinal or urinary symptoms
Family history of breast or ovarian cancer

Tumours arising from the uterus and ovaries, both benign and malignant, can grow to a large size without causing pain and therefore present relatively late with symptoms of abdominal distension. The presence of pain suggests infarction as a result of torsion of the tumour on its pedicle, bleeding into an ovarian cyst or occasionally rupture. Endometriomas may be associated with a longer history of cyclical pain that is worse at the time of menstruation. Weight loss is suggestive of malignancy.

A history of primary amenorrhoea associated with a pelvic mass and cyclical pain suggest a congenital abnormality of development of the lower genital tract such as an imperforate hymen leading to distension of the uterus with blood (haematometra). This may also occur as an acquired problem in later life following surgery to the cervix (cervical stenosis). The commonest cause of secondary amenorrhoea in a woman of reproductive age with a pelvic mass is pregnancy, although androgen-secreting ovarian tumours and abnormalities of the lower genital tract may also produce this combination (see Chapter 46). Abnormal uterine bleeding occurs in 50 per cent of women with fibroids. Postmenopausal bleeding (see Chapter 56) is more likely to be associated with uterine malignancy in a woman with a pelvic mass but may occasionally be due to a hormonally active ovarian tumour.

Pressure on adjacent organs from a pelvic mass may produce urinary symptoms such as frequency and hesitancy. Changes in bowel habit may also occur but are more likely to be associated with a primary bowel lesion. Occasionally such a mass may present with acute urinary retention or renal failure. In patients who have had previous treatment for gynaecological malignancy or cancer of the gastrointestinal tract or breast, recurrent or metastatic disease should be suspected. Women with two or more relatives with breast and/or ovarian cancer are at greater risk of ovarian malignancy.

Examination

Check for:

Pallor
Breast lumps
Lymphadenopathy
Ascites/pleural effusions
Size of mass on abdominal palpation
Cervical lesions
Whether mass is separate from uterus on bimanual examination

Anaemia may be due to increased menstrual blood loss associated with fibroids or any malignancy. The ovaries are a common site for metastases from the breast. The presence of palpable supraclavicular or inguinal lymph nodes suggests stage IV malignancy. Ascites is most commonly found with ovarian cancer, although pleural effusions may occasionally be associated with fibroids (Meig's syndrome). Masses arising from the pelvis are normally described in terms of the number of weeks of pregnancy that a gravid uterus of equivalent size would be, and it is not normally possible to feel the lower edge of the mass. An imperforate hymen can be diagnosed as a bulging membrane across the introitus with a slight bluish colour. Primary cervical cancer presenting as a pelvic mass is unlikely to be suitable for surgical treatment (see Chapter 45) and should be excluded by cervical examination and, if necessary, biopsy. A pelvic mass separate from the uterus or fluid filled is more likely to be an ovarian cyst.

Investigations

Relevant investigations

Pregnancy test
Ultrasound
Full blood count
Tumour markers

Once pregnancy and non-gynaecological causes have been excluded, the commonest differential diagnosis will be between an ovarian tumour and fibroids. It is usually possible to differentiate these on ultrasound scan. The presence of solid areas and multiple loculations is associated with malignant change in an ovarian cyst. Other forms of imaging such as barium studies and intravenous urography may be necessary to exclude involvement of the bowel or ureters by the mass prior to surgery. Tumour markers are glycoproteins shed into the circulation by ovarian malignancies. They may help to distinguish benign from malignant tumours but are not sufficiently specific to avoid the need for laparotomy and their major role is in monitoring for recurrence after treatment.

Management

Ovarian Tumours

Unilocular cysts less than 5 cm in size with no solid areas in a premenopausal woman are likely to be functional (i.e. corpus luteum or follicular cysts), associated with normal ovulation and require no treatment. Larger or persistent cysts should be removed surgically. The risk of malignant change in an ovarian cyst increases with age and is relatively uncommon under 40. The commonest solid tumour in young women is the mature cystic teratoma (benign dermoid cyst). Because of this and the greater importance of preserving reproductive hormonal function, the usual treatment will be removal of the cyst (ovarian cystectomy) alone or unilateral oophorectomy. This can be done either laparoscopically or through a small abdominal incision. In older women, especially where there are features suggestive of malignancy, the management is that for ovarian cancer (see below).

Ovarian Cancer

Where possible, all patients with suspected ovarian cancer should be referred to specialist gynaecological cancer centres for treatment.

Surgery

Laparotomy is required to confirm the diagnosis and stage of the disease (see Table 55.2). The aim is to remove all macroscopic disease and to sample other areas for evidence of microscopic disease. This normally means removing the uterus, both ovaries and the infracolic portion of the omentum. Washings or ascites from the peritoneal cavity are sent for cytology. Samples of peritoneum and the retroperitoneal lymph nodes may also be sent. There is no contraindication to hormone replacement therapy.

Table 55.2 FIGO staging of ovarian cancer

Stage	Description
Stage I	Tumour limited to the ovaries
Stage II	Tumour involves one or both ovaries with pelvic extension
Stage III	Tumour involves one or both ovaries with peritoneal metastasis outside the pelvis and/or regional lymph node metastasis
Stage IV	Distant metastases

Chemotherapy

Surgery alone may be curative for patients with stage I disease. Patients with more advanced disease are given chemotherapy to treat any remaining tumour or to reduce the risk of recurrence where surgical excision appears complete. This is given on an outpatient basis by intravenous infusion, the principal drugs being carboplatin or cisplatin. The addition of other drugs appears to confer little further improvement in 5-year survival and the role of the drug paclitaxel in particular remains controversial. The most important side-effects are nausea and bone marrow suppression.

Follow-up

Patients are normally followed up for 5 years in combined outpatient clinics at 3-monthly to 12-monthly intervals. Symptoms of recurrence include abdominal distension, weight loss and pain. Examination should include both pelvic and rectal examination. Blood is taken for tumour markers and imaging with computerized tomography or magnetic resonance can be used to monitor disease response to treatment. A rising tumour marker level is highly suggestive of recurrence. Recurrence may be treated by further chemotherapy but the response rate is significantly less than for primary disease (see Figure 55.1).

Fibroids

Although there is a risk of malignant change occurring in uterine leiomyomata, treatment is usually given because of symptoms. The presence of asymptomatic fibroids, especially where the uterus

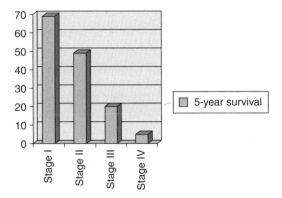

Prognosis depends on:
- Stage at diagnosis
- Residual disease after surgery
- Response to chemotherapy
- Age and general health

Figure 55.1 Prognosis for ovarian cancer

is less than 12 weeks in size, is not normally an indication for surgery (see Figure 55.2). Associated menorrhagia can be treated symptomatically (see Chapter 49). Selective embolization of the blood supply to fibroids is an alternative to surgical treatment but is not yet widely available.

Surgery

Hysterectomy is curative and is the treatment most commonly offered to women who have completed their families. Removal of the fibroids with conservation of the uterus (myomectomy) can be performed where the patient wishes to preserve her fertility, but is associated with an increased risk of bleeding and of uterine rupture during subsequent pregnancies. Fibroids may recur after myomectomy. The procedure can be carried out by laparotomy or endoscopically.

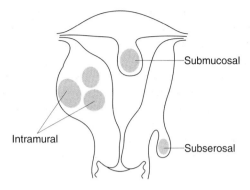

Figure 55.2 Types of uterine fibroid

Other Masses

Malignant tumours of the uterus may present as a pelvic mass, although sarcomas may not be diagnosed until hysterectomy. Tubo-ovarian inflammatory masses as a complication of pelvic inflammatory disease (see Chapter 67) may require surgical drainage or salpingo-oophorectomy. Endometriosis involving the ovaries may be associated with the development of cysts filled with altered blood (chocolate cysts) causing a mass (for treatment, see Chapter 47).

Learning Points

- **The common causes of pelvic masses are pregnancy, fibroids and ovarian cysts**
- **Laparotomy is required for ovarian tumours**

See Also

Intermenstrual bleeding (Chapter 52)
Chronic pelvic pain (Chapter 47)
Postmenopausal bleeding (Chapter 56)
Amenorrhoea and oligomenorrhoea (Chapter 46)

Postmenopausal bleeding

Definition

Postmenopausal bleeding (PMB) refers to genital tract bleeding occurring more than 12 months after the menopause.

Importance

70%

Seventy per cent of cases of endometrial carcinoma present with PMB. It is also a presenting symptom of cervical and vulval malignancy. The prognosis for endometrial carcinoma is better if diagnosed at an early stage.

Causes

Causes of PMB

✓Atrophic changes ± infection
✓Malignancy
- Endometrial
- Cervical
- Ovarian
✓Endometrial hyperplasia
✓Benign cervical or endometrial polyps
✓Iatrogenic
✓Hormone replacement therapy (HRT)

Benign Lesions

The commonest cause is atrophy of the lower genital tract. Oestrogen deficiency following the menopause results in a decline in glycogen levels, causing vaginal pH to rise and increasing the risk of superimposed infection. The epithelium of the lower genital tract is thinner and more likely to bleed if traumatized or infected. Other benign lesions, including endometrial and cervical polyps, occur in approximately 10 per cent of cases of PMB.

Malignancy

Endometrial carcinoma affects 13 per 100 000 women per year in the UK. One per cent of women will develop the disease by the age of 75, with a peak incidence at 61; 30 per cent of cases occur in premenopausal women but it is extremely rare in women under the age of 40. The aetiology is unknown, although it is more likely to occur in conditions where there is exposure of the endometrium to oestrogen in the absence of progesterone.

The ovarian stroma continues to produce androgens after the menopause, which are converted to the oestrogen oestrone in adipose tissue. As there is no corresponding increase in progesterone to oppose the effects of excess oestrogen on the endometrium, this results in endometrial hyperplasia and malignancy in obese patients. This also occurs in some anovulatory cycles, polycystic ovarian syndrome (PCOS) and in women given unopposed oestrogen treatment. Anti-oestrogens such as tamoxifen used in the treatment of breast cancer have oestrogenic effects on the endometrium and may cause hyperplasia and bleeding. A minority of ovarian tumours produce oestrogen and this may present as PMB because of stimulation of the endometrium. This is most commonly associated with granulosa cell tumours where it is a favourable prognostic feature.

In premenopausal women, endometrial carcinoma usually presents with intermenstrual bleeding or heavy periods (see Chapters 52 and 49).

Table 56.1 FIGO staging of endometrial carcinoma

Stage	Description
I	Tumour confined to the corpus uteri
	a) limited to the endometrium
	b) invades less than half the myometrium
	c) invades more than half the myometrium
II	Tumour invades the cervix but does not extend beyond the uterus
III	Local/regional spread to the serosa of the uterus, vagina or lymph nodes
IV	Tumour invades the bladder or bowel mucosa or distant metastases

The staging is based on surgical and pathological examination (see Table 56.1).

The commonest histological type is the endometrioid endometrial carcinoma. Other uterine malignancies occur less commonly and include leiomyosarcoma and mixed mesodermal tumours.

Diagnosis and Clinical Assessment

History

Ask about:

Age
Time since menopause
Last cervical smear
Current medication
- Tamoxifen
- HRT
Risk factors for endometrial cancer
- Diabetes
- Hypertension
- Obesity
- PCOS

It is important to distinguish rectal bleeding and haematuria from PMB. Where there is still doubt about this, it may be necessary to carry out additional investigations.

Withdrawal bleeds occur whilst on cyclical combined HRT (see Chapter 53). Irregular bleeding may also occur in continuous combined preparations, particularly if started within 12 months of the last period. Abnormal bleeding occurring more than 6 months after starting HRT should be investigated as for PMB.

The risk of malignancy increases with age. At 65, less than 10 per cent of women with PMB will have endometrial carcinoma, but at 85 this will be the diagnosis in 60 per cent of cases.

Cervical neoplasia is very unlikely to occur for the first time in a woman in her 60s who has previously had regular, normal cervical cytology. Women who have used the oral contraceptive pill in the past have up to a 50 per cent lower risk of developing the disease.

A small number of patients belong to families with a history of endometrial carcinomas.

Examination

Check:

Weight and height (body mass index)
Blood pressure
For signs of anaemia
For abdominal masses
For signs of atrophy
Appearance of the cervix
Uterine size

The association with older age and conditions such as morbid obesity, diabetes and hypertension means that a significant number of women presenting with PMB will have major risk factors for anaesthesia and be difficult to assess clinically.

Evidence of genital tract atrophy does not remove the need to exclude abnormalities of the uterus.

Investigations

Relevant investigations

Cervical smear
Full blood count
Ultrasound TVS
Hysteroscopy
Endometrial biopsy
Cystoscopy/sigmoidoscopy

Transvaginal ultrasound can be used to measure endometrial thickness. If this is less than 5 mm, the risk of endometrial pathology is less than 5 per cent. Ultrasound may also help to identify any adnexal pathology such as an oestrogen-producing ovarian tumour.

Abnormal endometrial (glandular) cells in a post-menopausal smear may be an indication of endometrial hyperplasia.

Hysteroscopy is inspection of the endometrial cavity using a rigid or flexible fibreoptic endoscope passed through the cervix (Figure 56.1). It is more invasive but is more likely to detect endometrial lesions than ultrasound or curettage alone. It can be performed under general or local anaesthetic as an outpatient procedure.

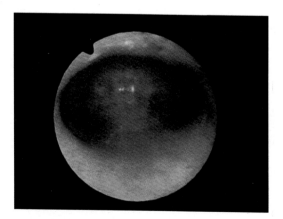

Figure 56.1 View of a normal endometrial cavity as seen at hysteroscopy

Cystoscopy and proctoscopy are usually only carried out if the origin of the bleeding is unclear from the history.

Management

Where no abnormality is found, the patient can be reassured and discharged. However, recurrent episodes of PMB may be due to a missed endometrial, tubal or ovarian pathology (such as an oestrogen-producing ovarian tumour) and are an indication for further investigations such as ultrasound.

Benign structural lesions such as endocervical polyps should be removed.

Endometrial Hyperplasia

Endometrial hyperplasia is found in 15 per cent of women with PMB. It may be associated with structural and cytological abnormalities and in the latter case carries a risk of malignant change. For this reason, so-called atypical hyperplasia may be an indication for hysterectomy, although lesser degrees can be treated by oral progestogens.

Endometrial Carcinoma

Removal of the uterus and ovaries is the mainstay of treatment. The disease spreads by local or lymph node metastases. As most cases present early, complete surgical removal can usually be achieved, although coexisting medical problems and obesity in some cases may complicate surgery. Lymph node spread can either be determined by sampling at the time of operation (with increased morbidity) or estimated indirectly from the histological examination of the uterus. Radiotherapy is used as adjuvant treatment for stage Ib and above and for palliative treatment of more advanced disease.

Hormone therapy using high doses of progestogens such as medoxyprogesterone acetate can be used to slow disease progression but is of no proven value as routine adjuvant treatment.

The prognosis depends on the stage at diagnosis, tumour type and grade and lymph node involvement (Figure 56.2).

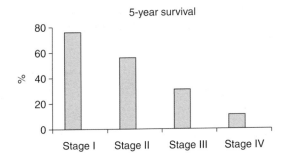

5-year survival

Adverse features:
- Node involvement
- G3 differentiation
- Clear cell/serous type
- Oestrogen receptor negative

Figure 56.2 Prognosis for uterine cancer

Atrophic Changes

- Topical oestrogens
- Systemic HRT
- Antibiotics

Superimposed infections such as bacterial vaginosis should be treated. Oestrogen deficiency can be treated with topical oestrogen creams or pessaries or by systemic HRT. There is some systemic absorption from topical oestrogen, which may cause endometrial hyperplasia.

Learning Points

- **The commonest presenting symptom of endometrial cancer is PMB**
- **Adequate assessment of the uterine cavity by ultrasound or hysteroscopy should be carried out in all cases of PMB**

See Also

The abnormal cervical smear test (Chapter 45)
Intermenstrual bleeding (Chapter 52)
Menopausal symptoms (Chapter 53)
The pelvic mass (Chapter 55)

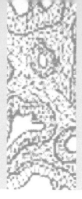

Chapter 57

Premenstrual syndrome

Definition

Premenstrual syndrome (PMS) is characterized by non-specific somatic, psychological and behavioural symptoms, severe enough to disrupt social, family or occupational life, occurring in the premenstrual phase which resolve completely (primary) or improve markedly (secondary) by the end of menstruation.

Importance

Only 5 per cent of women have no premenstrual symptoms at all. PMS affects 1.5 million women in the UK severely enough to affect their quality of life and interpersonal relationships. More than a third of these will seek medical treatment.

Cause

The aetiology is unknown. PMS is related to the ovarian cycle but there is no clear evidence of progesterone deficiency or an abnormal ratio in the levels of oestrogen and progesterone. Possible explanations include β-endorphin deficiency, prolactin excess, and abnormalities in fatty acid and prostaglandin synthesis.

The differential diagnosis includes psychological disorders wrongly attributed to PMS, menopausal changes, other medical causes of lethargy and oedema, and organic breast or pelvic diseases.

Diagnosis and Clinical Assessment

History

Symptoms of PMS

Somatic

- Bloating
- Breast tenderness
- Clumsiness
- Headache
- Weight gain

Psychological

- Aggression
- Anxiety
- Depression
- Loss of concentration

Although the commonest presenting symptoms are given above, it is the cyclical nature of the symptoms that is the key to distinguishing PMS from other underlying psychological or organic conditions which may be exacerbated premenstrually. Psychiatric disorders, especially depressive illness, psychosexual problems and family discord, may all present as PMS. In order to meet the criteria for PMS, symptoms must occur in the premenstrual (luteal) phase of the cycle, disappear during menstruation, be sufficiently severe to disrupt the woman's life and have been present in at least four of the last six cycles. It may not be possible to establish which, if any, of the presenting symptoms fulfil these criteria at the initial consultation and patients should be asked to keep a record of their symptoms using a menstrual calendar (Figure 57.1).

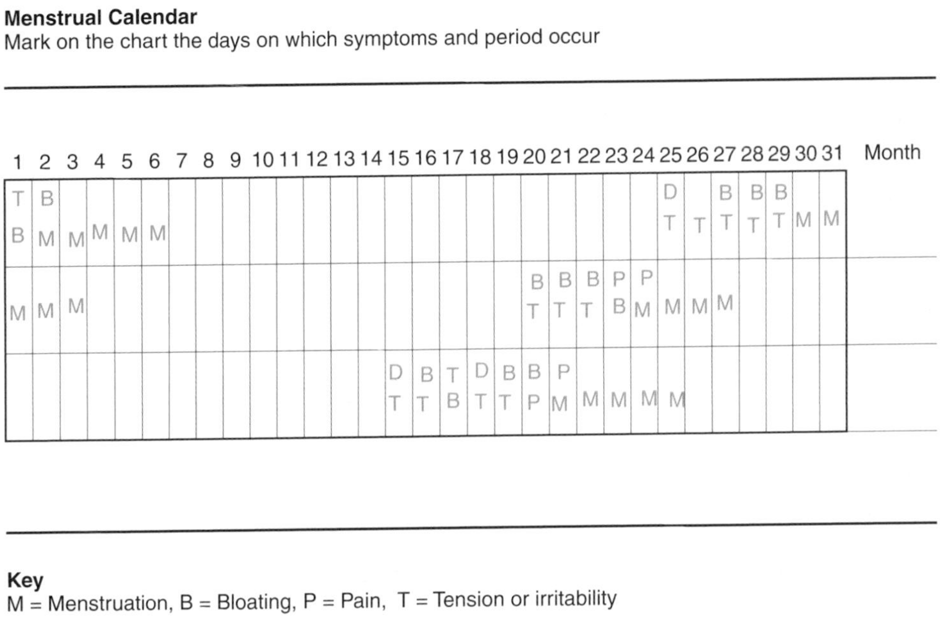

Menstrual Calendar
Mark on the chart the days on which symptoms and period occur

1	2	3	4	5	6	7	8	9	10	11	12	13	14	15	16	17	18	19	20	21	22	23	24	25	26	27	28	29	30	31	Month
T	B																							D		B	B	B			
B	M	M	M	M	M																			T	T	T	T	T	M	M	
																				B	B	B	P	P							
M	M	M																		T	T	T	B	M	M	M	M				
																D	B	T	D	B	B	P									
																T	T	B	T	T	P	P	M	M	M	M	M				

Key
M = Menstruation, B = Bloating, P = Pain, T = Tension or irritability

Figure 57.1 Example of a menstrual calendar

Examination

There are no specific clinical findings in PMS but other conditions that may mimic the somatic symptoms of PMS should be excluded. Lethargy and tiredness may be due to anaemia or disorders of thyroid function. Breast examination should be carried out to exclude non-cyclical causes of pain, including malignancy. Pelvic and abdominal examination should be performed to exclude organic causes of bloating and pelvic pain.

Investigations

In most cases, the diagnosis will be made on the basis of the history. The role of further investigations, as with examination, is mainly to exclude other conditions that may mimic some of the symptoms. Menopausal symptoms and thyroid disease can be excluded by measurement of follicle-stimulating hormone (FSH) and thyroid-stimulating hormone (TSH), respectively, and pelvic pathology such as endometriosis by laparoscopy. Symptoms of bloating or weight gain should only be treated with diuretics where there is measured weight increase or demonstrable oedema. Where doubt remains, ovulation can be suppressed by administration of a gonadotrophin-releasing hormone (GnRH) antagonist. Any symptoms that persist after 3 months will not be due to PMS.

Management

Outline management for PMS

First line
- Counselling and explanation
- Dietary and lifestyle changes
- Pyridoxine
- Essential fatty acids
- *Agnus castus*

Second line
- Oral contraceptive pill
- Bromocriptine

Third line
- Danazol
- Oestradiol implants or patches
- GnRH analogues
- Bilateral oophorectomy

Treatment depends on establishing the correct diagnosis, and the menstrual calendar may help both the patient and her doctor in gaining insight into which symptoms are likely to respond to treatment. Underlying psychopathology should be treated appropriately and reassurance given that there is no breast or genital tract cancer. The main principles of treatment are a combination of increasing the ability to cope with symptoms and alteration of hormone status.

Controlled studies of the efficacy of different treatments for PMS are characterized by very high levels of placebo responses.

Dietary changes involve eating little and often and taking plenty of carbohydrates to keep blood sugar levels up, whilst reducing salt and alcohol intake during the premenstrual phase. Psychotherapy, counselling, discussion in self-help groups and education augmented by exercise help to increase tolerance to premenstrual symptoms and reduce mild underlying psychological problems.

Vitamin B_6 and evening primrose oil are frequently self-prescribed for PMS but, if not, they are worth trying as first-line treatment. Vitamin B_6 (pyridoxine) is a cofactor in neurotransmitter synthesis. Although there is no evidence of any actual deficit in PMS, the largest controlled study showed an 82 per cent response rate compared with 70 per cent on placebo. Peripheral neuropathy has been reported at high doses, but a dose of 100 mg is probably safe. Evening primrose oil contains the unsaturated fatty acid precursors of prostaglandins. There is some evidence of improvement in selected symptoms but the recommended dose of eight capsules a day is difficult to sustain.

The dry extract of the *Agnus castus* fruit (20 mg daily) may also be effective in reducing symptoms of irritability, mood change, headache and breast fullness. Anti-prostaglandin pain-killers such as ibuprofen may be useful for breast pain and headaches. Diuretics such as spironolactone may be of benefit in the small group of women who experience true water retention but should be avoided in women with bloating without measurable weight gain.

Users of the combined contraceptive pill report lower levels of PMS than those using barrier contraception, but individual response varies and is unpredictable. Progestogens and progesterone supplements (given as pessaries or injections) have been used extensively on the basis of the theory that PMS is related to a progesterone deficiency in the second half of the cycle. There is no evidence to suggest they are more effective than placebo. Bromocriptine (5 mg on days 10–26) relieves cyclical breast symptoms but has no effect on other systems.

The most effective treatments are those that suppress normal ovulation, but these are also the treatments associated with the most significant side-effects. Danazol is effective in reducing breast symptoms and some psychological symptoms even at doses lower than those required for suppressing ovulation. Androgenic side-effects are common but may be acceptable in a low-dose regimen. There is a risk of masculinization of a female fetus if pregnancy occurs whilst taking the drug.

Oestradiol implants or patches are effective in PMS but cannot be given alone because of the risk of endometrial hyperplasia and cancer (see Chapter 56) and a significant number of women will continue to get PMS symptoms when they are used in combination with a progestogen.

GnRH agonists suppress symptoms during treatment but these recur when treatment is stopped. They are unsuitable for long-term use because of osteoporosis but they may be of value in identifying those who would benefit from oophorectomy, for short-term relief or in the perimenopausal patient.

As a last resort, bilateral oophorectomy (usually with hysterectomy) will provide a surgical cure for symptoms if these are true PMS. This should only be undertaken after treatment with GnRH agonists has shown that the symptoms are abolished by suppression of ovulation.

Learning Points

- **Most women experience some psychomotor or psychological changes in the premenstrual phase of the cycle**
- **It is essential to distinguish true PMS from underlying psychiatric or psychosocial problems that are merely exacerbated in the second half of the cycle**
- **Symptoms of PMS should either disappear or substantially improve during menstruation and do not occur in the absence of ovulation**

- **There is a very high level of placebo response to treatment for PMS**

See Also

Menopausal symptoms (Chapter 53)

Further Reading

O'Brien PMS. Premenstrual syndrome. In: Shaw R, Soutter WP, Stanton SL, eds. *Gynaecology*. Churchill Livingstone, Edinburgh, 1992, pp. 325–39.

Wyatt K, Dimmock P, Jones P, Obhrai M, O'Brien S. Efficacy of progestogens in management of premenstrual syndrome systematic review. *British Medical Journal* 2001; 323: 776–80.

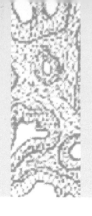

C h a p t e r 5 8

Prolapse

Definition

Prolapse is the protrusion of organs or structures beyond their normal anatomical confines occurring as a result of faults in the mechanisms for vaginal and uterine support. Prolapse of the anterior vaginal wall and bladder is known as cystocele, of the posterior wall with the rectum as rectocele, and of the posterior wall and pouch of Douglas as enterocele (Figure 58.1). Grade 1 uterine prolapse is descent of the uterus within the vagina, grade 2 is descent to the introitus, and grade 3 (also known as procidentia) is descent beyond the introitus.

Importance

Genitourinary prolapse accounts for about 20 per cent of gynaecological surgical workload and is the commonest reason for surgery in the over-50s. It is estimated to affect 12–30 per cent of multiparous women, with 1 in 10 women undergoing one or more operations.

Causes

The pelvic floor muscles of levator ani normally support the pelvic viscera. The uterosacral and cardinal (transverse cervical) ligaments support the cervix and the upper third of the vagina. The middle third of the vagina is attached to the pubocervical fascia, and the lower third to the urogenital diaphragm comprising the perineal body and the levator ani fascia.

Damage to these structures occurs as a result of trauma (childbirth), especially after prolonged labour and instrumental delivery. There is an increased risk of vault prolapse after hysterectomy if the divided uterosacral ligaments are not attached to the vault. Congenital connective tissue disorders and changes after the menopause also predispose to prolapse. Prolapse may occur as a result of increased abdominal pressure due to chronic respiratory disease or intra-abdominal neoplasms.

Diagnosis and Clinical Assessment

History

Ask about:

Vaginal discomfort
✓Urinary incontinence   PU
✓Difficulty with defecation BM
✓Sexual activity pain ?
Abnormal vaginal bleeding
Obstetric history
Medical history

Mild prolapse may be asymptomatic. The commonest presenting complaint is a feeling of fullness in the vagina or 'something coming down'. If the prolapse extends beyond the introitus, the patient may be able to see a bulge protruding from the vagina. Symptoms are typically worse towards the end of the day or after a prolonged period of standing. Discomfort or altered sensation with intercourse may occur but this is more likely to be due to vaginal atrophy in the postmenopausal age group. It is important to know whether the patient is sexually active, however, as this may influence the surgical approach (see below).

Urinary symptoms such as stress incontinence (see Chapter 63), recurrent urinary tract infections, incomplete emptying and poor stream are more

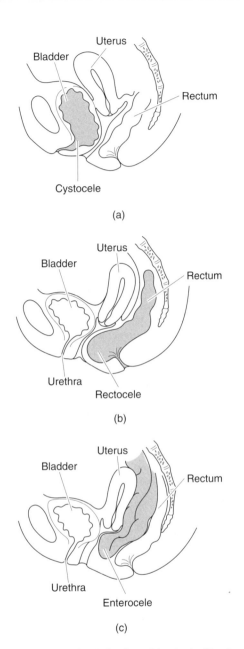

Figure 58.1 Types of vaginal prolapse: (a) cystocele, (b) rectocele, (c) enterocele

likely to occur in association with cystocele. Rectocele may cause difficulty in defecation relieved by pushing the prolapse back with a finger in the vagina. A non-specific dragging sensation and backache are associated with uterine prolapse. If the prolapse extends beyond the introitus, the vaginal skin may become ulcerated and infected, leading to bleeding.

Examination

Key findings BMI
Body mass index and cardiovascular respiratory condition
Abdominal masses and ascites
Prolapse of vaginal walls and any ulceration
Movement of vaginal walls and stress incontinence
Size and mobility of uterus and other pelvic masses

Cystocele may be seen, by parting the labia and asking the patient to bear down, as a bulge in the anterior vaginal wall distal to the urethral meatus but it is best evaluated by examination using a Sims' speculum in the left lateral position (Figure 3.3). Prolapse may be the presenting symptom of an intra-abdominal neoplasm, so it is essential to exclude the presence of a mass or ascites.

Investigations

The diagnosis of prolapse is clinical and any investigations are most likely to be required to assess fitness for anaesthesia or to exclude coexisting neoplasia (ultrasound, cervical smear). Uterine prolapse or cystocele may lead to impairment of the flow of urine, predisposing to urinary tract infection and, rarely, renal failure as a result of 'kinking' of the ureters (check midstream urine, urine and electrolytes).

Management

Any coexisting urinary tract infection or underlying neoplasia should be treated first and, where possible, factors predisposing to prolapse, such as obesity or chronic respiratory disease, should be controlled. The mainstay of treatment is surgical correction of the prolapse, but it is important to remember that this entails a certain degree of risk (especially in the age group most likely to be affected), whereas the condition itself is usually benign. Minor degrees of prolapse without symptoms do not require treatment and others with minimal symptoms may respond to pelvic floor exercises, physiotherapy and hormone replacement therapy. (HRT)

Vaginal Pessaries

Vaginal pessaries made of inert plastic can be used to control vaginal prolapse whilst awaiting surgery or where surgery is contraindicated. The commonest type used is the ring, fitting between the posterior fornix and the symphysis pubis (Figure 58.2). Pessaries can cause erosion of the vaginal mucosa and should be changed every 6–12 months. Shelf pessaries (Figure 58.3) are used where the ring will not stay in, or to control uterine prolapse or enterocele, although they tend to be more difficult to insert and remove.

Indications for vaginal pessaries

Unfit for anaesthesia
As a diagnostic test to determine whether surgical treatment would help symptoms
Pregnant
Awaiting surgery
Patient preference

Surgery

Surgical procedures used for prolapse

Cystocele – anterior repair
Rectocele – posterior repair
Enterocele – enterocele repair
Uterine prolapse – vaginal hysterectomy, Manchester repair
Vault prolapse – sacrocolpoplexy, sacrospinous fixation

The aim of surgery is to correct the prolapse whilst preserving continence and sexual function. Over-aggressive or repeated surgery may lead to narrowing of the vagina, making intercourse difficult. Vaginal hysterectomy is the usual treatment if uterine prolapse is present. Suturing the uterosacral and cardinal ligaments into the vault after removal of the uterus

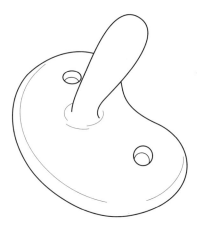

Figure 58.3 Shelf pessary

supports the vault. The uterus can be preserved, if desired for fertility, by amputating the cervix and then suturing the ligaments in front of the cervical stump (Manchester repair). Anterior and posterior vaginal repairs (also know as colporrhaphy) are the main operations performed for vaginal prolapse and can be combined with hysterectomy. Both procedures can be associated with difficulty with micturition postoperatively. Sacrocolpoplexy involves suturing the vaginal vault to the sacral promontory using a non-absorbable mesh. In sacrospinous fixation, the vaginal vault is sutured to the sacrospinous ligament vaginally.

Complications of surgery

Anaesthetic
Bleeding
Damage to bladder/rectum
Pain – urinary retention
Vaginal stenosis/dyspareunia
Recurrence

Learning Points

- **Asymptomatic vaginal prolapse does not require treatment**
- **Prolapse may be a presenting symptom of intra-abdominal neoplasia**
- **Sexual activity should be taken into account when planning management**
- **Urinary incontinence is not necessarily due to coexisting prolapse**

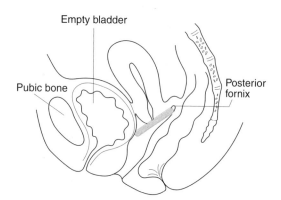

Empty bladder
Pubic bone
Posterior fornix

Figure 58.2 Ring pessary *in situ*

See Also

Urinary incontinence (Chapter 63)

Further Reading

Jackson S, Smith P. Diagnosing and managing genitourinary prolapse. *British Medical Journal* 1997; 314: 875–80.

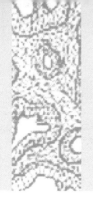

Chapter 59

Recurrent miscarriage

Definition

Recurrent miscarriage is characterized by three or more successive early pregnancy losses (miscarriages).

Importance

Recurrent miscarriage affects approximately 1 per cent of all women, about three times the rate that would be expected by chance alone. A proportion of women have a persisting underlying cause.

Causes

Important causes

Antiphospholipid antibody syndromes
Cervical incompetence
Hormonal factors
Parental chromosomal abnormalities

Although up to 50 per cent of sporadic miscarriages are associated with fetal chromosomal abnormalities, only 3–5 per cent of couples with recurrent miscarriage will have an abnormal karyotype. Cervical incompetence is a cause of late second trimester miscarriage or early preterm delivery. It may be congenital but commonly occurs as a result of damage to the cervix caused by mechanical dilatation or cone biopsy. Other structural abnormalities of the uterus, including uterine septa, occur in a similar proportion of women with normal reproductive histories as in those with miscarriage. Bacterial vaginosis has been reported as a risk factor for preterm labour and second but not first trimester miscarriage. Other infections tend to be a cause of sporadic rather than recurrent miscarriage.

Well-controlled endocrine disorders such as diabetes and thyroid disease are not associated with an increased risk of miscarriage. The prevalence of polycystic ovarian syndrome (PCOS) is significantly higher in women with recurrent miscarriage than in the general population. Antiphospholipid antibodies (lupus anticoagulant and anticardiolipin antibodies) are present in up to 25 per cent of women with recurrent miscarriage compared with 2 per cent of the general population.

Diagnosis and Clinical Assessment

History

Ask about:

Confirmation of pregnancy
Gestation at time of miscarriage
History of pain or bleeding in second trimester miscarriages
Other pregnancies
History of diabetes and thyroid disease

Conditions causing oligomenorrhoea followed by a heavy withdrawal bleed may be confused with recurrent miscarriage. Cervical incompetence should only be considered as a cause in second trimester miscarriage that occurs after painless cervical dilatation or spontaneous rupture of the membranes. The prognosis for future pregnancies is significantly better where there is a previous history of live birth.

Investigations

Relevant investigations

Lupus anticoagulant
Anticardiolipin antibodies

Blood for karyotyping from both partners
Karyotyping of products of conception
Ultrasound

Ultrasound may be of value in identifying women at increased risk of pregnancy loss from uterine malformations or PCOS. Routine use of hysterosalpingography is not recommended. Lupus anticoagulant and anticardiolipin antibodies need to be confirmed with two tests at least 6 weeks apart. Testing for other autoantibodies is of no clinical value. An abnormal fetal karyotype in the presence of normal parental chromosomes suggests a diagnosis of sporadic miscarriage on that occasion. Routine testing for diabetes and thyroid disease is not indicated in otherwise asymptomatic women. If no cause can be identified after careful investigation, there is a significantly better prognosis in any subsequent pregnancy (75 per cent chance of ongoing pregnancy).

Management

Couples with karyotypic abnormalities should be referred for genetic counselling. It is important to remember when assessing any treatment that even after three miscarriages the chances of a successful pregnancy with no treatment are still better than 50 per cent. Psychological support (in the form of attendance at a dedicated early pregnancy unit) alone may be beneficial. Thyroid disease and diabetes should be controlled, but at present there are no treatments of proven benefit for other endocrine causes of miscarriage.

The value of surgery for uterine defects is unproven and needs to be considered against the risk of such surgery for subsequent pregnancies. Treatment of bacterial vaginosis may reduce the risks of preterm delivery but has not been shown to be of benefit in miscarriage. Cervical cerclage (the insertion of a purse-string suture in the cervix at 14–16 weeks) is associated with a decrease in preterm birth but no improvement in overall survival.

In the presence of antiphospholipid antibodies, treatment with low-dose aspirin (75 mg) from the diagnosis of pregnancy until 34 weeks improves the live birth rate from 10 to 40 per cent, with a further improvement with subcutaneous heparin. Treatment with corticosteroids is not of value. There is some evidence that in women who do not have antiphospholipid antibodies, treatment with injections of human chorionic gonadotrophin (hCG; 10 000 units/week) during the first trimester may be of benefit.

Learning Points

- Genetic factors are mainly a cause of sporadic rather than recurrent miscarriage
- Empirical treatments of unproven value should be avoided in women with no identified cause
- Antiphospholipid antibody syndrome is the most important cause to identify and treat

See Also

Small for gestational age (Chapter 21)
Bleeding in early pregnancy (Chapter 68)

Further Reading

Royal College of Obstetricians and Gynaecologists. The management of recurrent miscarriage. *RCOG Guideline No. 17*. RCOG, London, 1998.

Sterilization

Importance

Sterilization is the commonest method of contraception used by women over 40.

Clinical Assessment

History

Ask about:

Age
Whether family complete
Other forms of contraception including vasectomy
Menstrual history
Last menstrual period

It is important that the permanent nature of this form of contraception and the implications for situations such as change of partner are discussed. Sterilization may be perceived as the 'only alternative' so it is important to discuss other forms of contraception. The reported failure rate for third-generation/levonorgestrel intrauterine devices, for example, is comparable to that of sterilization.

Vasectomy can be carried out under local anaesthetic and with a lower risk of serious complications.

Examination

Check for:

Body mass index
Previous abdominal surgery
Anaesthetic risk factors
Pelvic masses

Obesity increases both the anaesthetic risk and the difficulty of safely entering the peritoneal cavity with a laparoscope. The risk of laparoscopic complications is also increased in very thin patients. Previous abdominal surgery may be associated with adhesions and increase the risk of bowel perforation during laparoscopy.

Investigations

Pregnancy should be excluded and a full blood count checked prior to surgery.

Management

Counselling

Essential topics

Nature of procedure
Irreversibility
Failure rate
Risk of ectopic pregnancy after failure
Complications of laparosocpy
Need for contraception beforehand

The nature of the procedure, including the type of anaesthetic and the potential for complications, must be discussed. These are the same as for diagnostic laparoscopy (see Chapter 67).

The risk of failure depends on the method used, but for clip sterilization it is approximately 0.5 per cent over 5 years. Patients need to be aware of the possibility of failure because of both the social implications of any future pregnancy and the increased risk of a tubal pregnancy. In comparison, the failure rate after vasectomy is 0.1 per cent.

Failure may occur because of incorrect placement of the clips or recanalization of the tube and may occur several years after the operation. Sterilization will not prevent implantation if fertilization has already occurred and the operation is performed in the second half of the cycle. Couples should be advised to use adequate contraception before admission. If an intrauterine device is present, this should be removed following the next period.

Patients using hormonal contraception should be aware that the pattern of their menstrual cycle may change after sterilization because they will no longer be using it (and not because of the operation itself). Sterilization does not cause weight gain or affect ovarian function.

Methods of Sterilization

Sterilization is usually performed laparoscopically under general anaesthetic as a day-case operation. Metal/plastic self-locking clips are usually used to occlude the Fallopian tubes, although diathermy may also be used to destroy part of each tube.

Sterilization performed at the time of another procedure which requires a laparotomy, such as Caesarean section, can also be carried out with clips but may be performed by removal of a segment of the tube (partial salpingectomy). An open approach using a small abdominal incision may be required if laparoscopy is contraindicated, or if access to pelvic organs is difficult.

Sterilization following pregnancy is usually carried out as an interval operation 2–3 months later, because this is associated with a lower long-term failure rate and lower operative risk.

Learning Points

- There is an increased risk of ectopic pregnancy when conception occurs after sterilization
- Vasectomy has a significantly lower failure rate than female sterilization and can be carried out under local anaesthetic
- The pregnancy rate associated with levonorgestrel intrauterine devices is comparable to that following laparoscopic sterilization

See Also

Contraception (Chapter 48)

Further Reading

Royal College of Obstetricians and Gynaecologists. Male and female sterilization. *Evidence-based Clinical Guidelines No. 4.* RCOG, London, 1999.

Termination of pregnancy

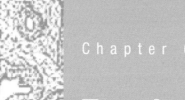

Importance

There are more than 150 000 terminations of pregnancy per year in the UK, approximately the same number as pregnancies lost through spontaneous miscarriage. This corresponds to a rate of 9–14 per 1000 women aged 15–45 per year.

Indications

Indications for termination

A   Risk to the life of the mother would be greater if the pregnancy continued

B   To prevent permanent harm to the mental or physical health of the mother

C   Risk to mother's health would be greater if the pregnancy continued (only if less than 24 weeks)

D   Risk to other children in the family (only if less than 24 weeks)

E   Risk of serious disability in the child

Therapeutic termination is regulated in the UK by the 1967 Abortion Act (modified 1984). In cases A–D above, the risk of continuing the pregnancy must be greater than that of termination.

The majority of first trimester terminations (70 per cent of the total) are performed because of the risk of anxiety or depression (clause C). A higher proportion of second trimester procedures, especially after 16 weeks, are performed because of fetal abnormality identified on ultrasound or karyotyping (see Chapters 9 and 10).

In the UK, all terminations must be registered and supported by at least one (normally two) medical practitioner.

Clinical Assessment

History

Ask about:

Reason for requesting termination
Last menstrual period
Positive pregnancy test
Previous contraception
Last cervical smear

Pregnancy is not the only cause of missed periods (see Chapter 46). It is essential to discuss the woman's reasons for not wishing to continue with the pregnancy and to determine if this is her wish or a decision she is being pressurized into taking by other family members or a partner.

The GP may be in a better position to assess social and personal circumstances, but many doctors are not prepared to support termination on personal ethical grounds.

Examination

A full cardiovascular and respiratory examination should be performed to identify any anaesthetic problems. A pelvic examination should be carried out to confirm the clinical size of the pregnancy and swabs taken for *Chlamydia* and gonorrhoea. A cervical smear should be taken if due.

Investigations

Relevant investigations

Full blood count
Blood group

Cervical swabs

Ultrasound

Rhesus-negative women will require an injection of anti-D immunoglobulin at the time of termination to prevent isoimmunization affecting subsequent pregnancies, so it is essential to determine the blood group of all women who undergo this (see Chapter 4).

There is a risk of introducing pathogens from the lower genital tract into the uterus and Fallopian tubes at termination, causing subsequent infertility. For this reason, all women undergoing termination should either be offered antibiotic prophylaxis or be tested for infection prior to termination and treated accordingly.

Ultrasound can be used to determine gestation as this will have a bearing on the method of termination.

Management

Counselling

Discuss the alternatives available, including adoption and possible support, that could be put in place to help with the pregnancy and child. Explain what is involved, any alternatives to the method recommended and the risks of the method recommended. Allow time to consider any new information, particularly if the woman appears to be equivocal about the decision, and if necessary arrange further counselling.

Methods of Therapeutic Termination

Methods

First trimester
- Suction evacuation
- Mefipristone and prostaglandins

Second trimester
- Prostaglandins
- Dilatation and evacuation

Suction evacuation is normally carried out under general anaesthetic. It involves dilatation of the cervix and removal of the pregnancy with a suction curette. The cervix can be made easier to dilate (and hence the risk of damage to it and uterine perforation reduced) by the prior oral or vaginal administration of a prostaglandin such as misoprostol. The failure rate of termination is greater when carried out at less than 7 weeks' gestation.

Prior to 9 weeks' gestation, pregnancy may also be terminated using a combination of the antiprogesterone mefipristone given orally, followed 36–48 hours later by a prostaglandin given vaginally. This will induce abortion in more than 95 per cent of women without the need for surgical evacuation.

After 13 weeks, termination is usually carried out using prostaglandins to induce uterine contractions and expulsion of the fetus. These are increasingly being used in combination with mefipristone (as for first trimester medical termination). Prostaglandins can be administered as vaginal pessaries or as an infusion (usually with Syntocinon) into the extra-amniotic space through a Foley catheter passed through the cervix. Exploration of the uterus under anaesthetic may be required to remove the placenta.

Surgical removal of the fetus (by dilatation of the cervix and piecemeal removal of the fetus) can be performed under general anaesthetic up to 20 weeks but requires an operator with experience in the technique.

Complications of termination

Early
- Bleeding
- Uterine perforation and possible damage to other pelvic organs
- Cervical trauma
- Retained products
- Infection

Late
- Infertility
- Depression

Sterilization can be performed at the same time but is associated with a higher regret rate for both procedures and a higher failure rate. An intrauterine contraceptive device can be inserted at the same time as termination. Patients should be advised to check that the device remains in place before resuming sexual intercourse (see also Chapter 48).

Injectable contraceptives can be given at the same time as termination but increase the risk of irregular bleeding. Oral contraception can be started on the same day as termination.

Learning Points

- **In the UK, approximately the same number of pregnancies end in therapeutic termination as in spontaneous miscarriage**
- **All women undergoing termination should be screened and/or treated for sexually transmitted infections**
- **Ensuring adequate arrangements for contraception after termination of an unplanned pregnancy is an essential part of management**

See Also

Contraception (Chapter 48)
Sterilization (Chapter 60)

Further Reading

Royal College of Obstetricians and Gynaecologists. Induced abortion. *RCOG Guideline No 11*. RCOG, London, 1997.

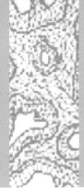
Urinary frequency

Definition

Frequency of micturition is more than seven times a day. Nocturia is having to get up in order to pass urine on more than one occasion at night. Urgency is an overwhelming desire to void.

Importance

Symptoms of urgency or frequency affect 20 per cent of women aged 30–64.

Causes

Causes of frequency

Detrusor instability
Infection
Pregnancy
Diabetes, renal failure
Diuretics
Excess fluid intake

Detrusor instability is a condition in which bladder contractions occur during bladder filling whilst the subject is attempting to inhibit micturition. Detrusor instability may occur following surgery, particularly colposuspension (see Chapter 63), or as a result of neurological abnormality, but most cases are idiopathic.

Clinical Assessment

History

Ask about:

Duration of symptoms
Associated urgency and nocturia
Incontinence
Fluid intake
Medication
Glaucoma and ischaemic heart disease

Urgency and frequency are present in approximately 80 per cent of women with detrusor instability. The prevalence of nocturia increases with age and occurs to some degree in 70 per cent of women. It is normal to void twice a night over 70 and once a night for younger adults. Remember that women with stress incontinence may increase the frequency of micturition to reduce the volumes leaked.

Anticholinergic treatment is contraindicated in patients with ischaemic heart disease or closed-angle glaucoma.

Examination

Check for:

General health and mobility
Prolapse, urethral caruncle
Atrophic changes
Neurological changes in S2, 3, 4

Investigations

Relevant investigations

Midstream urine
Frequency–volume chart
Bladder pressure studies
Cystoscopy

Urinary infection may cause or worsen the symptoms of frequency and urgency. Ask the patient to keep a record of the frequency of micturition and fluid intake. This provides a more objective measure of excessive fluid intake and the severity of frequency and incontinence. The chart may also be used as an adjunct to bladder training. The definitive diagnostic test of detrusor instability is the presence of systolic or unprovoked detrusor contractions, which the patient cannot suppress, during the filling phase of subtraction cystometry (see Chapter 63).

Conditions causing a reduction in functional bladder volume, such as radiotherapy, bladder stones and tumour, may occasionally present with frequency and can be diagnosed by cystoscopy or intravenous urography.

Management

Treat any associated urinary infection and control any associated medical conditions that cause polyuria such as diabetes. Review current medication, especially diuretics, and reduce to the minimum required or try alternative methods of treatment. Reduce the intake of caffeine-containing drinks and alcohol, especially towards the end of the day.

Detrusor Instability

Management

Explanation
Bladder drill
Anticholinergics
• Probantheline
• Oxybutynin
• Tolterodine
• Amitriptyline
Surgery

Detrusor instability tends to be a chronic condition although spontaneous remissions may occur. There is a high placebo response to treatment. Behavioural therapy such as bladder drill aims to help the woman to 're-learn' how to inhibit the voiding reflex. Patients are encouraged to pass urine at timed intervals starting at 1 hour and gradually increasing as greater control is obtained. Initial response rates are up to 70 per cent improvement, although 40 per cent relapse within 3 years.

Drug therapy uses anticholinergic drugs to block the parasympathetic nerves activating the detrusor. Oxybutynin hydrochloride is the most widely used of these and also has a direct smooth muscle relaxant effect. Tricyclic antidepressants act by potentiation of the bladder relaxant effect of the sympathetic system as well as by their anticholinergic effect. They are most useful where nocturia is the major problem because of their sedative side-effects. The use of these drugs is limited by their systemic side-effects. Newer anticholinergics such as tolterodine, which are more specific for the type of receptor found in the detrusor, are as effective with a lower side-effect profile.

Surgical treatments such as transcervical phenol injection and bladder distension appear to give poor long-term responses.

Side-effects of anticholinergics

Dry mouth
Constipation
Blurred vision
Glaucoma
Tachycardia

Learning Points

• **The commonest cause of urinary frequency is idiopathic detrusor instability**

See Also

Urinary incontinence (Chapter 63)

Further Reading

Bidmead J, Cardozo L. *Detrusor Instability in PACE Reviews*, vol. 2. RCOG Press, London, 1999.

Urinary incontinence

Definition

Urinary incontinence is characterized by involuntary loss of urine causing social or hygienic problems and which is objectively demonstrable.

Importance

Urinary incontinence affects up to 20 per cent of women. The average time from onset to presentation is 5 years, reflecting the embarrassment felt by many women and the social isolation this can lead to.

Mechanisms of Normal Urinary Continence

During bladder filling, continence is maintained by a combination of inhibition of detrusor activity and closure of the internal urinary meatus by tonic contraction of the rhabdosphincter and the tone of urethral mucosa. At 200 mL volume there is subconscious inhibition of detrusor from the hypothalamus. Voluntary inhibition is normally required at approximately 300 mL, and at 500 mL with symptoms of urgency continence is maintained by contraction of the muscles of the pelvic floor.

Continence during coughing is normally maintained by the rise in intra-abdominal pressure transmitted to the proximal urethra and an increase in levator tone.

Causes

Common causes of incontinence

Genuine stress incontinence
Detrusor instability
Fistula
Infection

Genuine stress incontinence occurs when intra-vesical pressure exceeds maximal urethral pressure in the absence of detrusor activity. Detrusor instability is an uninhibitable systolic detrusor contraction at less than normal volumes causing a rise in intra-vesical pressure that exceeds maximal urethral closure pressure.

Fistula formation is most commonly between the bladder or the ureters and the vagina. This is a relatively rare cause of incontinence in the developed world, where it mostly occurs as a complication of either surgery to the female genital tract (hysterectomy, Caesarean section) or radiotherapy or as a result of malignancy. It is commoner in developing countries as a result of prolonged or obstructed labour or infections such as schistosomiasis, tuberculosis or actinomycosis.

Most causes are acquired but incontinence may also be due to congenital defects in development of the urogenital tract such as ectopic ureters and urethral diverticulae.

Diagnosis and Clinical Assessment

History

Ask about:

Pattern of incontinence
Frequency of incontinence and effect on lifestyle
Associated urgency, frequency and nocturia
Symptoms of prolapse (see Chapter 58)
Diabetes, back trauma, multiple sclerosis
Previous pelvic surgery or radiotherapy

There are three commonly seen clinical patterns of incontinence:

- *Stress incontinence* is the involuntary passing of urine associated with movement and a rise in intra-abdominal pressure such as with coughing or sneezing. This is the pattern most commonly associated with underlying genuine stress incontinence but can also occur in detrusor instability.
- Urinary incontinence preceded by a strong desire to void (*urge incontinence*) is typical of detrusor instability, although detrusor contractions may also be provoked by coughing or sneezing, causing incontinence indistinguishable from stress incontinence. Women with stress incontinence tend to leak on penetration and those with detrusor instability tend to leak at orgasm.
- A history of continuous leakage is more typical of *urinary fistula* or *overflow incontinence*.

Examination

Check for:

General condition
Palpable bladder
Abnormal neurological examination S2, 3, 4
Prolapse
Leakage of urine on coughing

The patient's general condition may determine her suitability for surgical treatment. Urinary retention is relatively uncommon in women but may occur after surgery or childbirth or as a result of focal neurological disorders and present as overflow incontinence.

About 50 per cent of cases of genuine stress incontinence are associated with prolapse, although the presence of prolapse does not exclude other possible causes. Stress incontinence may only occur in some women whilst standing.

Investigations

Always request:
Midstream urine sample
Volume/void chart

Depending on history:
Methylene blue dye test
Bladder pressure studies
Intravenous urogram/cystoscopy

A midstream urine sample should be sent for culture in all cases of incontinence. Other investigations will depend on the results of the examination and history.

Fistula formation is unlikely in the absence of a history of malignancy or surgery and can be confirmed by intravenous urography if ureteric or, if vesical, by instillation of methylene blue dye into the bladder with a pack or pad in the vagina. Bladder pressure studies (cystometry) (Figure 63.1) are indicated where there are mixed symptoms, voiding difficulties and a history of previous unsuccessful surgery.

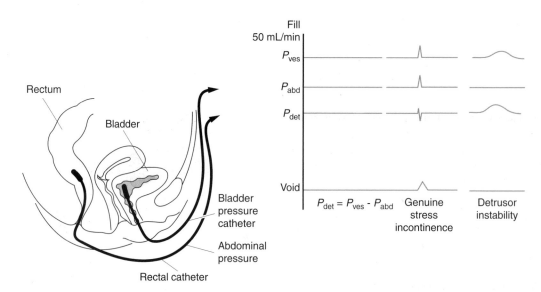

Figure 63.1 Bladder pressure studies. P_{det} = detrusor pressure; P_{ves} = intravesical pressure; P_{abd} = intra-abdominal pressure

The patient is asked to void and the rate of flow measured. Pressure transducers are placed in the rectum and bladder and the detrusor pressure calculated by subtracting the intra-abdominal (rectal) pressure from the intravesical pressure. The bladder is filled (16–100 mL/min) using a catheter and any symptoms of urgency recorded. The patient is asked to interrupt a void, cough and stand and any leakage of urine is recorded.

Normal values for cystometry

Capacity of 400 mL
Flow > 15 mL/s
Residual < 50 mL
First desire at 150–200 mL
No systolic detrusor contractions
Maximum voiding pressure < 70 mL H_2O
No leakage on coughing

Management

Treat any urinary tract infection. Management will otherwise depend on the diagnosis of the underlying cause, but it is important to bear in mind that there may be a mixture of more than one cause and that treatments are not without their own potential side-effects or complications that need to be balanced against the severity of the symptoms.

The management of detrusor instability is discussed in Chapter 62.

Genuine Stress Incontinence (GSI)

Diagnosis is made on the basis of a history of demonstrable stress incontinence without other symptoms or by exclusion of detrusor instability on cystometry.

Non-surgical

Satisfactory control of mild to moderate stress incontinence can be achieved by strengthening of the pelvic floor muscles using pelvic floor exercises. This may be supplemented by biofeedback techniques such as the use of weights or vaginal cones under the supervision of specialist physiotherapists or continence clinics. Vaginal pessaries or tampons may provide temporary improvement by elevation of the bladder neck.

Surgery

More severe or refractory symptoms may require surgery. It is essential to treat any concomitant detrusor instability first. Most surgical treatments involve procedures to elevate the bladder neck. In abdominal operations such as Burch colposuspension, this is achieved by pulling up the vagina adjacent to the proximal urethra to the iliopectineal ligament (Figure 63.2).

In sling operations, the bladder neck itself is elevated to the iliopectineal ligament with a synthetic mesh or a graft of homologous or heterologous tissue.

Endoscopic procedures include the Stamey operation, where a curved needle is inserted either side of the bladder neck and a length of suitable suture is passed from the pubocervical fascia to the rectus sheath.

A major difficulty is achieving enough elevation of the bladder neck to prevent incontinence without preventing normal voiding. Because of this, a suprapubic catheter may be inserted at the end of the operation and the volume of urine remaining in the bladder after voiding measured. The catheter is then removed only when this residual volume is less than 100 mL.

Bladder neck elevation can also be achieved by tension-free tape instead of a conventional Stamey suture. As this can be carried out under local anaesthetic, the amount of bladder neck elevation can be adjusted until it is just sufficient to prevent leakage when the patient bears down. The long-term effectiveness of this treatment is not yet known.

Approximately 70 per cent of patients will remain dry after colposuspension. Vaginal (anterior) repair is relatively ineffective in the treatment of urinary symptoms, having a 50 per cent response rate, and is of no value in the absence of prolapse.

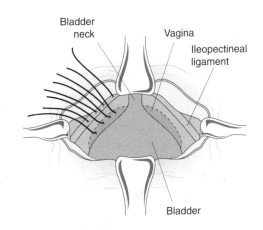

Figure 63.2 Burch colposuspension

Complications of surgery for GSI

Damage to bladder or ureters

Bleeding

Infection

Detrusor instability

Urinary retention

Prolapse

Fistula

Fistula

Some fistulas will heal spontaneously provided the bladder is kept empty by catheterization. If there is an underlying condition such as malignancy, the priority is to treat this.

General health and tissue healing should be optimized and any inflammatory response allowed to settle (2–3 months) unless the injury is recognized at the time it occurs. Surgical repair usually involves excision of fistulous tract and repair in layers with absorbable sutures. Meticulous haemostasis, control of infection and free bladder drainage are essential. If surgical repair is not possible, or is unsuccessful (10 per cent), urinary diversion may be necessary.

Learning Points

- The surgical correction of stress incontinence may lead to detrusor instability
- Incontinence is commonly due to a mixture of genuine stress incontinence and detrusor instability

See Also

Prolapse (Chapter 58)

Urinary frequency (Chapter 62)

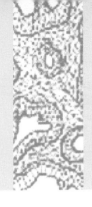

Chapter 64

Vaginal discharge

Importance

Vaginal discharge is one of the commonest gynaeco-logical complaints and occurs in up to a third of women referred to the outpatient department. Intractable vaginal discharge is the main presenting complaint in 1 per cent of referrals.

Causes

Common causes of vaginal discharge

Physiological
Atrophic vaginitis
Infective
- Candida
- Bacterial vaginosis
- Tricomonas vaginalis
- Chlamydia
Foreign bodies

The commonest cause of vaginal infection is bacterial vaginosis (BV). Whilst *Trichomonas vaginalis* (TV) and gonorrhoea have declined, the incidence of candidiasis has increased. Candidiasis is more common in pregnancy and in immunosuppressive conditions. The modern low-dose oral contraceptive pill (OCP) is not thought to be a predisposing factor. Less common causes are various Gram-positive and Gram-negative organisms, *Chlamydia*, herpes and human papilloma virus (HPV).

The commonest reasons for intractable or recurrent discharge are cervicitis, recurrent vulvovaginitis and atrophic vaginitis. Cervicitis occurs where a cervical ectropion becomes infected. Vaginitis can also occur as an allergic or chemical irritative response.

Atrophic changes can occur during breast-feeding and in prepubertal females as well as following the menopause. Note that asymptomatic atrophic change does not itself require treatment.

Diagnosis

History

Ask about:

Onset
Colour or blood-staining and odour of discharge
Associated pain or irritation
Treatments
Sexual history
Diabetes, steroid or immunosuppressive history

Examination

Check for:

Inflammation of the vulva
Colour of exudate
Appearance of vagina and cervix
Vaginal pH
Evidence of infection by immediate direct examination of wet smear

Physiological discharge is usually white or clear, tends to increase at ovulation and is non-irritant. Both *Candida* and *Trichomonas* may cause inflammation of the labia, while BV rarely does but is often associated with a homogenous greyish discharge. The pH of the discharge can be measured using simple pH paper. BV is unlikely in the presence of a low pH (<5).

The motile trichomonates of TV can be seen by scanning a simple slide prepared with normal saline solution from the discharge at low power. Clue cells (epithelial cells with bacteria adherent to cell membrane) indicate BV. If available, a couple of drops of 10 per cent potassium hydroxide will elicit a characteristic fishy odour when mixed with discharge from BV.

Investigations

Swabs should be taken from the vaginal fornices and cervix and put into a suitable transport medium (e.g. Stuart's) for culture and from the endocervix for *Chlamydia*. A cervical swab should be taken if this has not been done within the last 3 years.

Colposcopy is indicated where there is obvious cervicitis or an abnormal smear.

Management

Screen for other sexually transmitted diseases (STDs) and treat contact traced partners as appropriate. Remember that gonorrhoea and *Chlamydia* are notifiable diseases. (Treatment of *Chlamydia* and *Neisseria gonorrhoea* is discussed in Chapter 67.)

Bacterial vaginosis and *Trichomonas* respond to systemic treatment with metronidazole 400 mg t.d.s. for 7–10 days. Patients should be warned to avoid alcohol because of the 'antabuse' type of reaction that is produced with this.

Candida normally responds to topical treatment with clotrimazole 500 mg p.v. Recurrent disease may occur as a result of colonization with non-*albicans*

species and can be treated with pessaries a week before and after menstruation for 6 months or by systemic anti-candidials such as fluconazole 150 mg on the first day of each period for 6 months. Concurrent treatment of sexual partners does not appear to reduce the number of recurrences.

Atrophic vaginitis is treated with topical oestrogens for 4–6 weeks.

Learning Points

- **The cause of vaginal discharge can be determined by simple means in the clinic**
- **Where appropriate, contact tracing and treatment of partners may be required to eradicate infection**
- **Treatment for *Chlamydia* should be followed up by a further test to confirm cure**

See Also

Acute abdominal pain (Chapter 67)

Further Reading

Emens M. *Intractable Vaginal Discharge. PACE Review 95/07.* Royal College of Obstetricians and Gynaecologists, London, 1995.

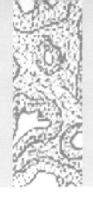

Chapter 65

The swollen or painful vulva

Importance

Vulval pain can be acute or chronic and requires careful evaluation, as the causes may not be obvious on examination. When pain of any type becomes chronic in nature, it can lead to disturbances in mood. This is especially true for chronic vulval pain, which in the young woman can cause significant problems in relationships and psychological disturbance. Swelling of the vulva may be either discrete or generalized and the causes are somewhat easier to elucidate.

Causes

Causes of vulval pain

Generalized vulval infection
Localized infection of the Bartholin's or Skene's glands
Dermatological conditions
Some systemic diseases
Hormonal changes
Trauma
Neoplastic changes
Vulvodynia

Infection affecting the majority of the vulva is usually due to herpes simplex or *Candida*. Herpes simplex occurring for the first time causes a systemic illness characterized by malaise, flu-like symptoms and severe vulval ulceration. Type 2 has been the most common genital infection, although type 1, which has previously been associated with perioral herpes (cold sores), now accounts for over 40 per cent of genital infection in many populations. The vulval pain of a first attack can be severe enough to cause urinary retention. Recurrent infections often have a

short prodromal period of burning pain, before more localized vesicles appear.

Candidiasis can cause burning vulval pain. It is implicated in a small number of women who go on to experience chronic vulvodynia. It is more common when the normal vaginal flora is disturbed, e.g. during pregnancy and after systemic antibiotic treatment. Recurrent infections should prompt screening for diabetes. It must also be remembered that immune deficiency may present with recurrent infection, and screening for human immunodeficiency virus (HIV) may be appropriate.

Other less commonly seen infections can cause localized ulceration of the vulva, which is generally painless, unless it becomes secondarily infected. These include primary syphilis, chancroid (*Haemophilus ducreyi*) and lymphogranuloma venereum (subtype of *Chlamydia trachomatis*). HIV is commonly associated with ulcerative sexually transmitted diseases in countries with a high prevalence.

The glands of the vulva are shown in Figure 65.1. The Bartholin's gland is particularly prone to duct blockage. This produces a non-tender swelling of the gland. If this becomes infected, a painful abscess can form. Occasionally this is bilateral. *Gonococcus* is sometimes responsible for these infections. Infection of Skene's glands is less common.

Many dermatological conditions can affect the vulva. Eczema of both atopic and allergic (contact) origin can cause a raw, red swelling of the vulva.

Two dermatoses, lichen sclerosus and lichen planus (Chapter 66), can cause significant changes in vulval architecture and may lead to fissuring and soreness, especially after intercourse. Psoriasis can also affect the vulva, leading to soreness if secondary infection occurs. Less commonly, bullous dermatoses, which can be precipitated by drug reactions or viral infections, will cause vulval ulceration.

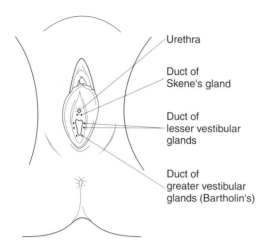

Urethra

Duct of
Skene's gland

Duct of
lesser vestibular
glands

Duct of
greater vestibular
glands (Bartholin's)

Figure 65.1 Normal vulval anatomy

Two systemic diseases can cause severe anogenital ulceration: Crohn's disease and Behçet's syndrome. Oral ulcers may also be present, and in acute Crohn's disease, other gastrointestinal symptoms may become apparent. However, vulval ulceration often precedes these.

The hormonal changes, which occur at the menopause, lead to thinning of the vulval epithelium. This can lead to irritation, especially after intercourse. Neoplastic changes may be preceded by itching. The ulceration of vulval carcinoma is usually painless, but secondary infection will lead to pain and swelling. Very rarely, neoplastic changes can occur within the Bartholin's gland, leading to unilateral swelling of the gland.

Vulvodynia refers to a specific type of vulval pain occurring on stretching or pressure.

Features of vulvodynia

Burning
Stinging
Irritation
Rawness

Some women experience cyclical symptoms associated with menstruation or coitus, and are asymptomatic in the intervals. The aetiology may be cyclical changes in vaginal pH leading to recurrent infections such as bacterial vaginosis or *Candida*. In other women, inflammation of the vestibular glands (Figure 65.1) can be demonstrated, leading to severe dyspareunia. In most of these cases, women will not have experienced previous problems with intercourse.

In a small number of women, the vulvodynia will be part of a wide somatization of psychological distress related to prior experiences.

Diagnosis

History

This must differentiate between problems of an acute or chronic nature.

Ask about:

Duration of pain/swelling
Localization
Type of pain
Associated discharge
Relieving or exacerbating features
Other systemic illnesses or symptoms
Sexual history

Examination

Look for:

Ulceration
Unilateral swelling
Discharge
Groin lymphadenopathy

A systems examination should include examination of the skin, to look for other dermatological signs, and the mouth. Many of the dermatological and systemic causes of vulval pain will manifest signs elsewhere.

Careful inspection of the vulva should be performed to assess the site of pain.

Investigations

Relevant investigations

Swabs for microbiology
Full blood count and C-reactive protein
Blood glucose
Vulvoscopy and biopsy

Where infection is suspected, swabs should be taken for microscopy, virology and bacteriology. Inspection of the cervix may be impossible in the acute stages of infection, especially herpes.

A full blood count and C-reactive protein are helpful in the assessment of systemic disease. A random blood sugar level should be taken if recurrent *Candida* is suspected and HIV testing should be considered for recurrent infection (after appropriate counselling).

Vulvoscopy (examination of the vulva using the colposcope) can be helpful in the diagnosis of vulvodynia, especially if vulvar vestibulitis is present. Vulval biopsy may be needed to differentiate the dermatoses when these are not clinically obvious. Suspected malignancy requires a full examination, including colposcopy of the cervix, and a wide biopsy of the whole lesion.

Management

Once a diagnosis has been established, the treatment options will be clear.

Infective Lesions

Genital herpes is treated with oral acyclovir. This can reduce the severity and length of the attack, although once the lesions are fully developed it is usually too late to produce much reduction in symptoms. The pain of the attack should be treated with analgesics. Sometimes, in a first attack, parenteral analgesia is needed, and if urination is excessively painful a short period of catheterization may be needed, suprapubic catheterization being less painful. Recurrent attacks can be averted by oral acyclovir treatment. Topical treatment is not effective.

Candidiasis is usually amenable to topical therapy with antifungals. Treatment must also eradicate the vaginal load, as reinfection of the vulva will occur if only topical vulval treatment is given. Occasionally oral therapy can be helpful, using a single-dose regimen in the first instance.

If infection does not improve or is recurrent, the possible reasons include:

- unusual strain of *Candida* with some resistance to standard therapy
- diabetes
- immune suppression (HIV, drugs).

These should be investigated as appropriate.

The other infective conditions are treated with appropriate antibiotic therapy.

Bartholin's Abscess

Acute painful swelling of the Bartholin's gland usually implies infection. If in the very early stages, treatment with a broad-spectrum antibiotic after swabs are taken may avert the attack. If an abscess has formed, then incision and drainage are needed. If *Gonococcus* is confirmed, contact tracing must be undertaken.

Treatment of the dermatoses is discussed in Chapter 66. They are all managed by topical steroids in reducing doses, with advice on avoiding irritating factors.

Systemic Disease

The systemic diseases that present with vulval ulceration and pain are also usually managed with steroids. They will require systemic treatment initially to bring the disease process under control. Behçet's disease may then be managed with topical steroids as necessary. Crohn's disease may sometimes require the addition of antibiotics (metronidazole or ciprofloxacin) to reduce the severity of fissuring, and surgery may be necessary if fistula formation has occurred.

Trauma

Vulval pain from trauma, due to difficult intercourse, is often associated with the changes in the vulval skin during and after the menopause. Hormone replacement therapy (HRT) will improve the collagen content of the skin and restore some of the elasticity. The newer combinations are suitable for women who have been period-free for at least 6 months and are designed to avoid the monthly bleed. Where systemic HRT is not acceptable, or poorly tolerated, topical oestrogens can be used. These should be used sparingly, as they do become absorbed and can produce uterine effects.

Neoplastic changes will require surgery and are discussed in Chapter 66.

Vulvodynia

Vulvodynia is the most difficult of these conditions to treat. This is at least in part because the underlying cause is often not apparent.

Topical steroids

Antifungals

Topical oestrogens

Surgical excision of the vestibular area

Intralesional alpha interferon injections

Amitriptyline

Local anaesthetic nerve blocks

None of the above treatments will guarantee a cure and many women will obtain only partial or temporary relief with these. Sometimes, when the features of the vulvodynia do not fit the diagnostic criteria, careful counselling may reveal other underlying psychological problems that must be addressed before improvement can be seen.

Surgery to remove normal vulval tissue must be avoided at all costs, as symptoms can recur in the newly refashioned vulva. Occasionally, in cases where treatment fails, a lesion in the lower back can be implicated and a search using magnetic resonance imaging can be fruitful.

Symptom control rather than cure may be the best solution for many women with vulvodynia. Avoidance of exacerbating problems, sympathetic treatment and providing coping strategies will help most women to keep the problem under control.

Learning Points

- Vulval pain can be caused by a wide range of infective, systemic and localized diseases
- The causes of vulvodynia are poorly understood
- Careful history and investigation are needed to arrive at the correct diagnosis
- Steroids are the mainstays of initial treatment of the systemic and dermatological conditions
- Vulvodynia is difficult to cure, with symptom control being the long-term aim

See Also

Vulval pruritus (Chapter 66)

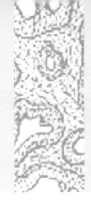

Chapter 66

Vulval pruritus

Importance

Pruritus is the commonest presenting symptom for vulval malignancy, as well as being a cause of considerable morbidity in its own right. Approximately 800 new cases of vulval cancer are registered in the UK in each year. Early diagnosis is associated with significantly better survival and lower morbidity from treatment.

Causes

Causes

Systemic
- Diabetes
- Liver or renal failure
- Drug reactions
- Eczema
- Psoriasis

Infection
- *Candida*
- *Tinea*
- Bacterial vaginosis

Vulval dermatoses
- Lichen sclerosus
- Squamous cell hyperplasia
- Other dermatoses (lichen simplex)
- Vulval intraepithelial neoplasia (VIN)

Vulval carcinoma

Contact dermatitis

Vulval cancer occurs most commonly in post-menopausal women. It may be asymptomatic or associated with pain or burning as well as pruritus. Ninety per cent of vulval cancers are squamous in origin. The remainder are adenocarcinomas, basal cell carcinomas and malignant melanomas. Lymph node involvement is present in 50 per cent of cases at the time of presentation and is bilateral in 30 per cent of cases. Spread occurs locally and through the lymphatic system. The nodes involved are the superficial and deep inguinal and femoral nodes. VIN and lichen sclerosus are recognized risk factors for vulval cancer, although the risk of progression is less than that for cervical intraepithelial neoplasia (CIN) to cervical cancer.

Diagnosis

History

Ask about:

Duration of symptoms
Other symptoms
Treatment
Hygiene
Systemic illness

A history of acute onset and white discharge are features of candidiasis, while the dermatoses tend to have a chronic history. The itching of lichen planus may be worse in times of stress. Where the vulval symptoms are a local manifestation of a systemic disorder, there may be a history of lesions elsewhere or of atopy for eczema. In cases of contact dermatitis, it may be possible to identify a potential irritant such as a change in soap used for washing. Inappropriate treatments can exacerbate symptoms. Diabetes, liver and renal failure should be excluded.

Examination

Check for:

Systemic skin disorders
Signs of infestation (pubic hair)
Loss of normal vulval anatomy
Induration/thickening of vulval skin
Ulceration

A brief general examination, including the mouth and nails, should reveal any other areas of systemic skin disorders such as psoriasis or eczema, although the vulval form of the disease may look different (e.g. psoriasis appears as well-defined red plaques without the characteristic skin scales). Infestations such as crab louse and scabies typically involve the pubic hair. A loss of normal vulval anatomy is associated with lichen sclerosus and atrophy. This results in narrowing of the introitus, loss and/or fusion of the labia minora with burying of the clitoris. The skin appears thin and may show signs of trauma from scratching or bluish spots from small subcutaneous bleeds.

Induration or thickening of the skin is found in VIN, lichen sclerosus and lichen simplex, but in practice a biopsy is usually required to make a diagnosis. Itchy, rather than painful, ulceration can be a feature of herpes simplex, scabies and traumatic ulceration. Erythema is associated with *Candida* (with fissuring) and *Tinea*, where there may be a defined edge with clearing within the lesions. Skin scaling is a feature of *Tinea* but is also seen with eczema. More generalized erythema with oedema, weeping and excoriation is typical of contact dermatitis.

Investigations

Swabs should be taken from any discharge for culture and sensitivity. In cases of suspected fungal disease, a wet smear prep or skin scrapings may show hyphae. Contact dermatitis is usually diagnosed clinically but it is important to exclude secondary infection. Twenty-five per cent of cases of lichen sclerosus are associated with coexisting autoimmune disease such as pernicious anaemia – check a full blood count and autoantibody screen. Vulval biopsy can be carried out with local anaesthetic using a round Key's punch biopsy.

Indications for biopsy

Persistent ulceration
Pigmented lesions
Indurated lesions
Suspected neoplasia
No diagnosis from history and examination

Management

Priorities

Try to establish an underlying cause
Decide if biopsy is required
Explain diagnosis and give general advice
Initiate appropriate treatment
Arrange appropriate surveillance for premalignant conditions

This depends on the diagnosis. Emollients such as simple aqueous cream may be helpful for symptomatic relief and are unlikely to irritate. Hygiene measures to avoid irritation include advice to avoid the use of soaps, shampoos, bubble baths and antiseptics, and to wash in water only once per day. Topical or systemic antifungals should be used where a diagnosis of candidiasis or *Tinea* has been made and secondary infections treated with appropriate antibiotics.

Vulval Dermatoses

Topical steroids are the mainstays of treatment for most of the non-neoplastic dermatoses. A typical regime for lichen sclerosus or lichen simplex, for example, might involve the twice-daily application of a pea-sized amount (1–2 g) of a very potent steroid cream to the affected area for 6 weeks followed by a lower-strength cream for maintenance. It should be remembered that steroids could themselves cause irritancy and a rebound of symptoms when treatment has finished, as well as predisposing to secondary infection.

Topical steroids

Mild – hydrocortisone 1 per cent
Moderately potent – clobetasone butyrate 0.05 per cent
Potent – betamethasone 0.1 per cent
Very potent – clobetasol propionate 0.05 per cent

Table 66.1 FIGO staging of vulval cancer

Stage	Description
Stage I	Confined to the vulva and <2 cm in size with no palpable groin nodes
Stage II	Lesions >2 cm but still confined to the vulva with no suspicious nodes
Stage III	Lesions extending beyond the vulva without suspicious nodes, or lesions of any size confined to the vulva with suspicious nodes
Stage IV	Grossly positive groin nodes or involvement of bladder or rectal mucosa, urethra or bone. All cases with pelvic or distant metastases

Steroids are generally ineffective in neoplastic lesions. Treatment is by surgical excision of areas that are particularly irritating or where there is a clinical suspicion of malignant change.

Patients with VIN are at risk of both squamous carcinoma of the vulva and of similar changes in the rest of the lower genital tract (CIN, see Chapter 45) and anal mucosa. All such patients should have a complete examination, including cervical cytology and colposcopy. Lichen sclerosus also appears to increase the risk of carcinoma. Such patients should be warned to report any changes in their symptoms or appearance of the vulval skin, although the value of routine examinations in the early detection of these changes is unproven.

Vulval Cancer

There is no screening procedure for vulval carcinoma. The diagnosis should be confirmed by biopsy prior to treatment. For lesions less than 2 cm, this may be in the form of a wide local excision biopsy which should include at least a 1 cm margin of normal tissue. Patients with suspected or confirmed disease should be managed in gynaecological cancer centres. The staging is surgical (see Table 66.1).

Surgery
Lesions with less than 1 mm invasion (stage Ia) can be treated by local excision alone. All other cases will also require dissection of the groin nodes. This can be undertaken through separate incisions. For laterally placed stage I and II tumours only, the nodes on the same side need to be removed initially. Other lesions will require wide local excision (including radical vulvectomy for some cases) and bilateral lymphadenectomy. Thirty per cent of operable patients will have node involvement.

Complications of vulvectomy

Wound breakdown
Venous thromboembolism
Incontinence
Lymphoedema
Psychosexual

Radiotherapy and Chemotherapy
Adjuvant radiotherapy is indicated after surgery if the disease-free margin is less than 8 mm or two or more lymph nodes are involved with metastatic disease. Preoperative radiotherapy may also permit less destructive surgery to be carried out in advanced disease by reducing tumour volume. Chemotherapy with 5-fluorouracil is usually used in combination with radiotherapy.

Prognosis and Follow-up
The 5-year survival is 80 per cent if there is no lymph node involvement, 50 per cent if the groin nodes are involved and 10–15 per cent if there is spread to the pelvic nodes. The size of the primary lesion and node status are the only factors that determine prognosis. Local relapse usually occurs as a result of inadequate local excision. Patients should be seen at 3-monthly intervals during the first year after treatment, 6-monthly in the second and third years and annually thereafter.

Learning Points

- **Vulval pruritus may have a systemic cause**
- **Accurate diagnosis is essential for effective treatment**

- Indurated or erosive lesions require biopsy
- Lichen sclerosus and VIN are associated with an increased risk of malignancy

See Also

The abnormal cervical smear test (Chapter 45)

Further Reading

Royal College of Obstetricians and Gynaecologists. *Clinical Recommendations for the Management of Vulval Cancer.* RCOG Press, London, 1999.

On the gynaecology wards

67. Acute abdominal pain 271
68. Bleeding in early pregnancy 276
69. Postoperative complications 283
70. Vomiting in early pregnancy 287

Chapter 67

Acute abdominal pain

Importance

Lower abdominal pain is one of the commonest reasons for admission to the gynaecology ward. By taking a good history and using a logical approach, it is possible to arrive at a short list of differential diagnoses that may then necessitate further investigation or intervention. Often the boundaries between general surgical problems and gynaecological problems are blurred, and it may not be possible, in many cases, to make a true diagnosis until definitive intervention is carried out. Many causes of acute abdominal pain will have no long-term sequelae, but because conditions such as pelvic inflammatory disease (PID) can be so disastrous in the young woman, accurate diagnosis and treatment must always be employed.

Causes

Causes of low abdominal pain (can be divided amongst the three major systems involved)

Pelvic organs
- Ectopic pregnancy and miscarriage
- PID
- Ovarian cyst accidents (including torsion, bleeding and rupture)
- Torsion of uterine fibroids

Gastrointestinal causes
- Acute appendicitis
- Diverticular disease
- Inflammatory bowel disease
- Irritable bowel disease
- Incarcerated/strangulated herniae
- Mesenteric adenitis

Urinary tract system
- Lower urinary tract infection
- Ureteric colic
- Acute retention of urine

Early pregnancy complications are discussed in Chapter 68.

Malignancy of any of these systems can produce pain, but this is usually not of acute onset unless another process occurs, such as torsion of a malignant cyst. Ovarian cyst accidents usually produce severe, often colicky, unilateral pain. This can be as severe as torsion of the testis and is mediated by similar pain pathways. Sudden vomiting is not uncommon, and a low-grade pyrexia can occur, especially if there is a torsion.

PID usually presents as generalized pelvic pain, although if the condition persists, abscess formation can be more one-sided. Usually, but not always, there is pyrexia. This is true of *Gonococcus* and the multi-microbial secondary infections that can follow a chlamydial infection. Acute chlamydial PID may simply present as pain, without obvious signs of infection. Joint pains are sometimes seen in young women.

Clinical Assessment

Because all three major systems can cause acute pain, it is important to ensure that, where possible, a full history and examination are performed. Adequate analgesia must not be withheld from a patient in pain. Opiate analgesia will not mask the signs of peritonitis, and to withhold analgesia pending investigation or senior review is unnecessarily cruel. Often a complete history and examination can only be performed once the patient is more comfortable.

History

Ask about:

Nature of the pain
Date of last menstrual period and cycle length
Type of contraception
Previous gynaecological/urinary or gastrointestinal problems
Pre-existing vaginal discharge

The history must include a careful elucidation of the type and site of pain, relieving and exacerbating factors, radiation and duration. A careful and tactful sexual history should be elicited if appropriate. Sometimes this may entail interviewing young people away from other family members, with a nurse to provide support and advocacy. Pelvic infection and pregnancy may be associated with abnormal vaginal bleeding. A history of vaginal bleeding within the last 4 weeks does not exclude the possibility of pregnancy. If pregnancy is suspected, details of risk factors for ectopic pregnancy should be sought (see Chapter 68).

Examination

Key findings

Appears unwell
Tachycardia
Pyrexia
Abdominal scars, tenderness or masses
Uterine tenderness and excitation

A general assessment of the patient's immediate well-being and need for pain relief should be the first step. Temperature, pulse and blood pressure measurement will also help to identify the acutely sick woman.

Abdominal examination should initially include an inspection for scars, abdominal distension and obvious masses. Palpation for localized or generalized guarding, rebound tenderness and site of maximal pain should be performed. The hernial orifices should be checked.

If considered appropriate following the history, a pelvic examination should be performed. This should initially include a speculum examination to visualize the cervix and perform swabs for bacteri-

ology, when PID is suspected. A bimanual examination can then be performed. This provides information on the size of the uterus and ovaries, and the presence of localized or generalized tenderness. This must be done with great care and compassion. When pelvic irritation is present, as a result of pus or blood in the pelvis, or tubal or ovarian distension, this examination can be immensely painful. Even slight movement of the cervix alone can produce severe pain (cervical excitation).

Investigations

Initial investigations should be directed at the suspected cause.

Relevant investigations

Pregnancy test
Full blood count (looking for an elevated white cell count)
C-reactive protein or erythrocyte sedimentation rate
High vaginal swab (for bacterial vaginosis, *Trichomonas vaginalis* and *Candida*)
Endocervical swab (for *Gonococcus* into Stuart's medium)
Endocervical swab (for *Chlamydia*)
Urine sample for bacteriology
Ultrasound
Laparoscopy

Even if pregnancy is not suspected, in the relevant age group a test should be performed (remember that a positive test does not rule out another cause, but it makes acute PID extremely unlikely). The diagnosis of ectopic pregnancy and other complications of early pregnancy are discussed in Chapter 68.

Ultrasound can be useful if a pelvic mass is suspected. Sometimes fluid in the pouch of Douglas can be seen when an ovarian cyst has bled, and in acute PID, abscess formation may be seen.

Ultrasound is only rarely helpful in cases of acute appendicitis. It may help to rule out other causes. In the mid-cycle, an obvious corpus luteum may be seen at the site of maximal tenderness.

Laparoscopy is particularly helpful when a diagnosis of ectopic pregnancy, acute PID or appendicitis is questioned. It is not without complications but, when used judiciously, it can be an extremely useful investigation. Missed ectopic pregnancy may rupture and cause a life-threatening bleed. Ectopic pregnancy is the commonest cause of pregnancy-related death in the first trimester of pregnancy. Undertreated or untreated PID can lead to long-term fertility problems and chronic pelvic pain syndromes. Missed appendicitis usually becomes apparent with time, but early diagnosis can prevent widespread peritonitis, with its attendant risks and sequelae.

Laparoscopy allows careful inspection of the pelvic organs, the appendix, the peritoneal cavity, the inferior surface of the liver and gall bladder. Samples for bacteriology can be taken from the pouch of Douglas, and blood can be aspirated, if found. It can also be combined with further treatment if the cause is then apparent, such as laparoscopic salpingectomy, appendicectomy or ovarian cystectomy.

Laparoscopy

Adequate anaesthesia is usually provided by general anaesthetic. The patient is placed in the Lloyd-Davies position with the legs elevated but not completely flexed at the thigh, allowing access to the abdomen, and the bladder is emptied. A 15–20° head-down tilt allows the abdominal contents to move out of the pelvis.

A pneumoperitoneum with carbon dioxide is obtained either by using a guarded Veress needle inserted at the umbilicus or by insertion of the sheath of the trochar under direct vision. Usually 2–3 L of CO_2 are needed to lift the anterior abdominal wall.

A trochar and sheath are inserted through an incision just below the umbilicus, if a Veress needle has been used. Once these are in place, the trochar is removed and the laparoscope inserted. A second port can be inserted to allow manipulation of the pelvic organs.

Complications include anaesthetic problems, bowel perforation and vascular injury.

Diagnosis and Management

Priorities

Full resuscitation of the acutely unwell patient
Provide adequate pain relief
Use appropriate investigations
Plan appropriate treatment and follow-up

The management of ectopic pregnancy and miscarriage is discussed in Chapter 68.

Pelvic Inflammatory Disease

A diagnosis of acute PID will usually be made by a combination of history, examination and investigation. The history is typically one of bilateral lower abdominal pain of a constant nature, which is often worse on moving. There may be an associated vaginal discharge. Use of a non-hormonal intrauterine contraceptive device slightly increases the risk of PID, as does a history of PID. Younger women who are not in a stable relationship are the highest risk group.

On examination, there may be an elevation in temperature, mild tachycardia and generalized lower abdominal tenderness, sometimes even guarding and rebound tenderness. Vaginal examination may reveal an obvious vaginal discharge, and on bimanual examination cervical excitation and bilateral adnexal tenderness, but usually no obvious masses.

Initial investigations may show a leucocytosis on full blood count, a raised C-reactive protein and negative urine microscopy. If a Gram stain of the genital swabs can be obtained, a definitive organism such as Gonococcus may be seen. Cultures are usually helpful, but may be delayed, and treatment must not be deferred if PID is strongly suspected. An ultrasound can be helpful in ruling out other causes, but cannot make the diagnosis. Laparoscopy is the gold standard. The finding of bilateral swollen, red tubes with frank pus in the pelvis leaves no doubt. However, very early PID, especially chlamydial (the commonest cause), may not be easy to spot, and sometimes treatment must be started empirically whilst culture results are awaited.

Treatment will encompass a number of elements.

Antibiotics

Whilst waiting for culture confirmation, antibiotics that cover all the common organisms must be used. In severe cases, these should be given parenterally in the first instance. Most public health laboratories will know whether there is a high rate of penicillin-resistant Gonococcus locally.

Antibiotic therapy for clinically diagnosed PID should be effective against *Chlamydia trachomatis*, *Neisseria gonorrhoeae* and the anaerobes causing bacterial vaginosis. The currently recommended regimes are as follows:

- Cefoxitin 2 g i.v. 6-hourly plus doxycycline 100 mg i.v. (or orally) 12-hourly (continued for a minimum of 48 hours after the patient demonstrates substantial clinical improvement), followed by doxycycline 100 mg orally, twice daily up to a total of 14 days' treatment; or

- Clindamycin 900 mg i.v. 8-hourly plus gentamicin 2 mg/kg as i.v. or i.m. loading dose, then 1.5 mg/kg 8-hourly (continued for a minimum of 48 hours after the patient demonstrates substantial clinical improvement), followed by doxycycline 100 mg orally twice daily, or clindamycin 450 mg orally four times daily up to a total of 14 days' treatment; or
- Oflaxacin 400 mg orally twice daily plus clindamycin 450 mg orally four times daily or metronidazole 500 mg orally twice daily, all for 14 days (an oral regime more suitable for outpatient administration).

Bed Rest

Some suggest that bed rest is an important part of the healing process in acute PID. It appears rational in that limitation of movement of the pelvic organs will probably limit pain and inflammation.

Analgesia

Opiates and non-steroidal anti-inflammatory agents are the mainstay of treatment. Anti-inflammatory agents may also reduce soft tissue inflammation and long-term damage.

Contact Tracing and Treatment

Before the patient is discharged, steps must be taken to ensure partner notification, making sure that sexual partners are treated empirically with regimens effective against both *Chlamydia* and *Gonococcus*.

Ovarian Cysts

Ovarian cyst accidents can occur in women of any age, but the type of cyst is dependent on the age of the patient, timing of the cycle and type of contraception.

Types of ovarian cyst

Corpus luteum
Follicular cyst
Mature cystic teratoma
Benign epithelial tumours
Malignancies

The corpus luteum forms after ovulation. It is a physiological cyst that can only occur in women who are ovulating. Thus the combined oral contraceptive pill will suppress this, and only if a woman misses pills can this occur. It is a very vascular entity, and if bleeding into the cyst occurs, rupture and intra-abdominal bleeding can be torrential, leading to collapse. More usually, bleeding occurs into the cyst, causing sudden onset of unilateral pain, but without rupture. Ultrasound will almost always make the diagnosis in the context of a history of acute-onset mid-cycle pain. The treatment is conservative, unless the bleeding is excessive, when occasionally removal of the ovary may be needed.

Follicular cysts are also physiological in nature. They are lined with granulosa cells and represent a persistent enlarging and unruptured follicle. They can persist over several menstrual cycles, and because of their hormone-producing potential can cause lengthening of the cycle and even periods of amenorrhoea. Occasionally they will spontaneously rupture or lead to a torsion of the ovary or whole adnexum. If the cyst has ruptured, no further treatment apart from analgesia is needed. If torsion has occurred, then laparoscopy to inspect the adnexum, leading on to untwisting with cyst aspiration if still viable, or removal if not, will be needed. Torsion of the adnexum/ovary is a surgical emergency, the same as torsion of the testis.

Mature cystic teratomas (dermoid cysts) are germ cell tumours. They are benign. Torsion is the most common complication, especially in pregnancy when the cyst may be elevated out of the pelvis as the uterus enlarges. These can occur in young women, and rarely exceed 15 cm. On ultrasound, they have a characteristic appearance due to the fact that they often contain epithelial contents such as hair and teeth. Treatment must aim to relieve torsion of the adnexum and remove the intact cyst. The cyst contents cause intense peritoneal irritation, and aspiration must not be attempted.

Benign and malignant epithelial tumours are commoner in women over 40. They may be large in size, and when encountered in the acute setting demand definitive surgical treatment. The type of procedure will be dictated by many parameters, including suspected risk of malignancy, age of the patient, presence of other pathology etc. Fortunately these cysts rarely present with acute abdominal pain, allowing a full work-up to be done before surgery is planned (see Chapter 55).

Other Surgical Causes

Other surgical causes of acute pain, such as strangulated or incarcerated herniae, ruptured diverticulum or appendicitis, may be apparent from the history and diagnosis. The surgical approach used will depend on the condition.

Irritable Bowel Syndrome

Irritable bowel syndrome (IBS) is a diagnosis of exclusion, although it characteristically affects young women who may be going through a period of anxiety or stress. It is often associated with periods of loose stools followed by constipation, with faecal urgency. The pain can be continuous or intermittent and occasionally excruciating. Abdominal bloatedness is often reported. It can be difficult to differentiate from chronic PID, except on laparoscopy, which is normal in IBS. The management is discussed in Chapter 47.

Learning Points

- Acute abdominal pain in the non-pregnant woman can herald an illness that may have a profound effect on her future
- Appropriate investigation should be determined by the history and examination findings
- Prompt investigation and treatment can limit the sequelae of both PID and ovarian torsion
- Suspected causes will overlap with other specialties, and advice should be sought from these when needed

See Also

Abdominal pain in pregnancy (Chapter 24)
Chronic pelvic pain (Chapters 47)
Bleeding in early pregnancy (Chapter 68)

Bleeding in early pregnancy

Importance

Bleeding in early pregnancy complicates as many as 25 per cent of all pregnancies. Approximately half of the cases will settle without further problems, but the remaining 50 per cent of pregnancies will end in miscarriage, ectopic pregnancy or late pregnancy problems.

Causes

Causes of bleeding in early pregnancy

Threatened or actual miscarriage
Ectopic pregnancy
Gestational trophoblastic disease
Local causes (ectropion, infection, polyps etc.)

Miscarriage

Miscarriage (which is the preferred term, rather than abortion) complicates a large number of pregnancies. The earlier a pregnancy test is performed, the higher the quoted rate of miscarriage, with rates of up to 60 per cent being reported for pregnancies with very early testing. The majority of these miscarriages will be of chromosomally abnormal conceptuses, but it is rare for this to be related to parental karyotypic abnormality (usually balanced translocations). The major causes of recurrent miscarriage are discussed in Chapter 59. For all women with a wanted pregnancy, miscarriage is a devastating blow, and women need to be treated with care and sympathy. The fact that miscarriage is common is little consolation to individual women.

Most women in whom early bleeding settles are at little increased risk for the rest of pregnancy, but a small number may have later problems of intrauterine growth restriction (IUGR) and pre-eclampsia. This is particularly true of women who have bleeding in the early second trimester, or recurrent bleeding.

Miscarriage presents with bleeding and usually central period-like crampy abdominal pain. The bleeding may be very heavy and can lead to volume depletion. In addition, if products of conception are partially expelled and lie within the cervical canal, a profound vasovagal reflex can occur, exacerbating the degree of shock. With improved services many women present for investigation with only mild bleeding, which can precede a spontaneous miscarriage. In many of these women, there will not be a viable fetus seen.

Types of miscarriage

Threatened
Inevitable
Complete
Incomplete
Early embryonic demise
Anembryonic pregnancy

Threatened miscarriage is the presence of bleeding from the uterus in the presence of a viable intra-uterine pregnancy and a closed cervix. The bleeding tends to be light and painless.

Inevitable miscarriage occurs when the cervical canal opens to allow the uterus to expel the products of conception. The cervical os will admit a fingertip on vaginal examination. If the process of miscarriage leads to an empty uterus, it is a complete miscarriage. If products are still within the cavity and bleeding continues, this is an incomplete miscarriage. This is usually a clinical diagnosis, and ultrasound may not add additional information. (Indeed, the demonstration of a beating fetal heart on scan, which is inevitably going to miscarry as the cervix is open, will only add to the distress of the patient).

Early embryonic demise occurs when a pregnancy is identified within the uterus on ultrasound, but despite a fetus being visible no fetal heartbeat is seen. When scans are performed in very early pregnancy, it is vital that the assumption of a miscarriage is not made too early when a viable fetus is present but too small to see. If the gestational sac measures more than 2 cm, a fetal heart should be visible. This stage will progress to a spontaneous miscarriage in almost every case, but the time taken to do this will be very variable. Occasionally a gestational sac is seen on ultrasound, but there is no evidence of a fetus or fetal parts. This is due to an anembryonic pregnancy. Again, care must be taken in diagnosis when the sac is small, as a fetus may be too small to see.

Ectopic Pregnancy

Ectopic pregnancy is becoming increasingly common. It is defined as a pregnancy that implants outside the cavity of the uterus. The commonest sites for implantation are shown in Figure 68.1.

In many areas, ectopic pregnancy occurs in between 1 in 100 and 1 in 150 pregnancies. The reason for this is probably increased diagnostic sensitivity, but there is also an increasing incidence of pelvic inflammatory disease (PID), the major risk factor (see Table 68.1). This is especially true of chlamydial infection, which affects many women without symptoms, but which causes synechiae in the Fallopian tubes, increasing the risk of ectopic pregnancy. In the teenage population of many inner cities, the infection rate for *Chlamydia* is 10 per cent.

The increased risk for the intrauterine contraceptive device (IUCD, see Table 68.1) applies only to

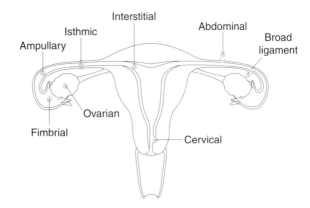

Figure 68.1 Sites of implantation of ectopic pregnancies

pregnancies that occur despite the presence of an IUCD. Because of their effectiveness as contraceptives, ectopic rates per year in IUCD users are lower than in women not using contraception.

Many ectopic pregnancies end in spontaneous resolution or tubal abortion and clinical findings alone are a poor predictor of ectopic pregnancy, with only 50 per cent of clinical diagnoses being correct.

Gestational Trophoblastic Disease

This is an uncommon condition that also is termed molar pregnancy or hydatidiform mole. It occurs in between 1 in 400 and 1 in 2000 pregnancies, depending on the region and the age of the population. It is commoner in young women and in oriental countries. In this strange condition, a conceptus is formed which carries two paternal complements of chromosomes, both containing an X chromosome. The role of the paternal X chromosome is unclear, but it does seem to have an impact on trophoblast development. This causes problems in two cases.

Table 68.1 Risk factors for ectopic pregnancy

	Relative risk
Previous history of pelvic inflammatory disease	4
Failed sterilization	9
Previous ectopic pregnancy	10–15
Tubal surgery (e.g. reversal of sterilization)	4.5
Intrauterine contraceptive device *in situ*	10

Partial Hydatidiform Mole

This occurs when two sperm carrying X chromosomes fertilize the egg. This leads to a conceptus with 69 chromosomes, and has an XXX complement. This conceptus may form a fetus, but the placenta overgrows and the fetus is not viable. The placenta becomes hydropic and may bleed. Although the trophoblast may persist, this condition does not become malignant.

Complete Hydatidiform Mole

In this case, the ovum is fertilized by two X-bearing sperm, or by one X-bearing sperm which then divides. The female complement does not persist, and the conceptus thus carries 46 chromosomes but two paternal X chromosomes. No fetus is formed, but the placenta grows in a rapid and pathological way, forming hundreds of tiny vesicles. The trophoblast can be pathologically invasive and can metastasize to other sites. Persistently invasive and metastatic disease leads on to a condition called choriocarcinoma in 11–25 per cent of cases. Approximately 25 per cent of women will have marked ovarian enlargement.

> **Presenting features of molar pregnancy**
>
> Bleeding ranging from light to torrential
> Passage of vesicles *per vaginum*
> Hyperemesis gravidarum (because of hugely elevated human chorionic gonadotrophin, hCG)
> Large-for-gestational-age uterus (although 50 per cent will be normal or small)
> Very early onset pre-eclampsia
> Symptoms of thyrotoxicosis

Local Causes of Bleeding

> **Commonest local causes**
>
> Infection, particularly *Chlamydia* and *Trichomonas vaginalis*
> Trauma to a cervical ectropion, especially after intercourse
> Cervical polyps

The cause of local bleeding may become apparent on a speculum examination. Swabs for infection should always be submitted.

Diagnosis and Clinical Assessment

An initial assessment is vital. Early resuscitation and recourse to surgery will be required for women who are hypotensive on admission. If the pulse rate is low, suspect products in the cervical os. Removing these gently can remedy the hypotension. With most patients, there is time to take a full history and examination before moving on to investigations. By the time you have taken a history and examined the patient, you should have a clear list of differential diagnoses in the order of suspected likelihood.

History

The history will include a number of important pieces of information.

> **Ask about:**
>
> The age of the patient
> Her past obstetric history (especially previous miscarriages or ectopic pregnancies)
> Involuntary subfertility
> Past episodes of confirmed PID or abdominal pain of unknown cause
> Date of last menstrual period
> Date of first positive pregnancy test
> Duration and type of bleeding
> Duration and type of pain (abdominal, shoulder tip)
> Heavy or offensive vaginal discharge
> General state of health and fitness for surgery

Examination

Remember that some of your patients will require surgery and that a general examination is important in these cases.

> **Key things to check**
>
> Abdominal examination
> * Fundal height (is it larger or smaller than expected?)
> * Tenderness (generalized or local)
> * Rebound and guarding
> * Distension
>
> Speculum examination
> * Local causes
> * Products obvious in the vagina or cervix
> * Vesicles
> * Take swabs for bacteriology
>
> Bimanual examination
> * Cervical os open or closed?
> * Uterine size
> * Cervical excitation
> * Adnexal mass or tenderness?

Vaginal examination should be deferred if an ectopic pregnancy is suspected until facilities are available for surgical treatment.

These occur when the pregnancy distends the tube causing smooth muscle contractions and a small amount of bleeding, which tracks down through the uterus and out of the fimbrial end of the tube. The small amount of blood in the pelvic cavity can produce mild to moderate abdominal discomfort, like a heavy period. Clinical findings are of a uterus that is small for the expected dates, pain on moving the cervix (cervical excitation, occurring because of moving an inflamed peritoneal surface), and unilateral tenderness in one adnexum.

Some women with a moderate amount of intraperitoneal blood will complain of shoulder-tip pain. This occurs when the blood tracks up under the diaphragm and gives rise to pain referred to the dermatome of the same origin, which lies over the shoulder.

As the pregnancy enlarges, the risk of tubal rupture and torrential bleeding increases. Tubal rupture can occur from 2 weeks after conception (i.e. at any time after the first missed period). Pregnancies that implant in the ampullary portion of the tube tend to expand more and can establish a large blood supply before rupture.

Investigations

Relevant investigations

Urinary pregnancy test

Ultrasound scan

Quantitative hCG

Full blood count

Blood group and cross-match

Laparoscopy

A negative urinary pregnancy test will exclude pregnancy in 97 per cent of cases and provides a useful method of rapidly assessing the possibility of early pregnancy causes of abdominal pain or vaginal bleeding.

Ectopic pregnancy is associated with an ultrasound finding of an empty uterus and in some cases an adnexal mass or free fluid in the pouch of Douglas.

When the gestation is early (i.e. 4–7 weeks) the gestational sac may not be visible in the uterus and other investigations can be useful. In 90 per cent of ongoing pregnancies, the hCG level will rise by at least 60 per cent over 48 hours. A suboptimal rise may be indicative of an ectopic pregnancy or a failing intrauterine pregnancy. However, some caution is needed, as 5 per cent of ongoing pregnancies will show a suboptimal rise. If the hCG level is >1500 IU/mL, the gestational sac should be visible on transvaginal scanning.

Laparoscopy remains the most reliable method of diagnosing an ectopic pregnancy; although small ectopics can be missed, the majority are seen.

Management (Figure 68.2)

Priorities

Rapid assessment and resuscitation of the shocked mother
   to elucidate the cause and manage accordingly

Establish the site of the pregnancy

Examine the cervix in the case of intrauterine pregnancy to
   determine whether miscarriage is inevitable

Decide whether pregnancy is ongoing

Manage according to findings

Administer anti-D if Rhesus-negative (see Chapter 4)

Confirmed Miscarriage

There are three options if a miscarriage is confirmed:

- surgery
- medical treatment
- conservative management.

Which is chosen will depend on the gestation of the pregnancy and the wishes of the mother.

Surgical Management

This is the modality of choice when there is heavy bleeding or there is a very bulky uterus suggesting a

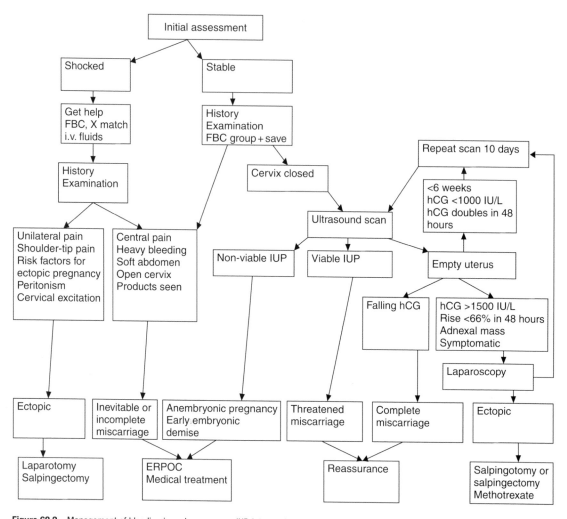

Figure 68.2 Management of bleeding in early pregnancy. IUP, intrauterine pregnancy; ERPOC, evacuation of retained products of conception.

large residuum of retained products of conception. Some women will choose this option for missed miscarriages or blighted ovum, because it is a self-limiting procedure which allows women to put behind them the emotional trauma of the miscarriage quickly.

Surgical evacuation of retained products of conception involves dilatation of the cervix and gentle curettage to remove the products. It is not without risk to the patient. The major risks are of uterine perforation (especially if the cervix remains tightly closed, or the products are very adherent) and curettage of the underlying decidual layer to the myometrium. Curettage of the surface of the uterus can lead to a condition called Asherman's syndrome. The exposed myometrium fuses with that on the opposite side, obliterating the uterine cavity. It is more

common when there is infection associated with retained products. After the curettage, periods do not resume, and at hysteroscopy the uterine adhesions can be visualized. This is a serious condition, with a low rate of subsequent successful pregnancy.

Medical Management

When the uterine contents have not begun to be expelled naturally, the process can be expedited by the use of a combination of the anti-progesterone mefipristone with a prostaglandin analogue such as misoprostol or dinoprostone. Successful passage of the products will be accomplished in 95 per cent of cases. This takes approximately 48–72 hours and many women find the uncertainty and the fact that they miscarry at home disturbing. The major problems are of persistent bleeding in a small number, necessitating evacuation under general anaesthetic. This is not common. The advantages are that a general anaesthetic is avoided, as are the potential complications of evacuation.

Conservative Management

This is the favoured option for incomplete miscarriages when the uterus is small, or when, on scan, there is minimal evidence of retained products. It is acceptable management in women with missed miscarriages who do not wish to undergo either of the former options.

Whichever method is chosen, products should be sent for histological examination, as a small number will prove to be gestational trophoblastic disease.

Ectopic Pregnancy

A ruptured ectopic pregnancy, which presents with collapse, a tender abdomen and a positive pregnancy test, requires immediate resuscitation and laparotomy.

Medical Treatment with Methotrexate

Medical treatment involves giving methotrexate to arrest trophoblast growth and to allow the ectopic pregnancy to regress. It has a 95 per cent success rate if the mass is <3 cm, does not contain a viable fetus, and the measured hCG is <10 000 IU/L. It is important to follow the hCG levels sequentially until they reach normal levels (<2 IU/L).

Surgical Management

Once the diagnosis is confirmed, the options for treatment are:

- removal of the ectopic pregnancy and tube (salpingectomy);
- opening the tube and removing the ectopic pregnancy (salpingotomy).

Both can be carried out as an open procedure or laparoscopically. The laparoscopic approach is associated with quicker recovery time, shorter stay in hospital and less adhesion formation and is the method of choice if the patient is stable.

Conservative surgery also carries a 5 per cent risk of persistent trophoblast, and monitoring with serial hCG levels must be instituted. If the levels do not fall, methotrexate can be given or the tube removed by a second surgical procedure.

After an ectopic pregnancy treated by any method, 90 per cent of subsequent pregnancies will be intrauterine, but only 60 per cent of women will manage to conceive spontaneously, reflecting global tubal disease.

Trophoblastic Disease

Gestational trophoblastic disease can be diagnosed by ultrasound, with histological confirmation. The ultrasound generally shows the hydropic vesicles, and usually the absence of a fetus.

The treatment of choice is surgical evacuation of the uterus. This is a hazardous procedure and the risks of torrential bleeding are high. Syntocinon infusions help to maintain haemostasis.

Following surgical treatment, all women must be registered with one of the three trophoblastic disease follow-up centres. Follow-up is initially by blood samples, but if an adequate fall in hCG is seen, urine samples are sufficient. After a partial mole, follow-up with complete resolution is usually for 6–8 months. After a complete mole, 12 months is needed. During this time women must be advised not to become pregnant, and should be given adequate contraception. This is often the most difficult part for women, as a pregnancy was often their aim. Consequently, the commonest reason for a sudden rise in hCG during follow-up is a pregnancy.

Learning Points

- **Bleeding in early pregnancy is very common**
- **Miscarriage is a devastating event for women with a wanted pregnancy, and demands careful and sympathetic management**
- **Gradually, treatment modalities are becoming more medically biased, allowing women to avoid anaesthesia and surgery**
- **Conception rates after ectopic pregnancy are lower, but pregnancies are likely to be intrauterine**

See Also

Recurrent miscarriage (Chapter 59)
Acute abdominal pain (Chapter 67)

Further Reading

Royal College of Obstetricians and Gynaecologists. The management of tubal pregnancies. *RCOG Guideline No. 21*. RCOG, London, 1999.

Royal College of Obstetricians and Gynaecologists. The management of early pregnancy loss. *RCOG Guideline No. 25*. RCOG, London, 2000.

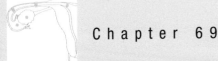

Chapter 69

Postoperative complications

Importance

Minor complications as a result of surgery (including Caesarean section) occur in as many as 10–20 per cent of patients. Without good postoperative care minor problems can escalate. Major complications are rarer, but can be life-threatening if undiagnosed or ignored. As patients are discharged from hospital earlier than ever nowadays, it is vital that doctors are vigilant for the early signs of impending trouble, as it may be many days before a patient realizes that all is not completely well and calls for medical help.

Early Postoperative Problems

Causes

Problems related to the surgery itself
- Bleeding
- Visceral damage

Anaesthetic problems
- Delayed recovery from anaesthesia leading to respiratory problems
- Excessive opiate response leading to respiratory problems
- Reaction to drugs given (nausea and vomiting)
- Retention of urine, with continued regional blockade (usually epidural anaesthesia)
- Exacerbation of pre-existing medical problems by the surgery or anaesthetic
- Myocardial dysfunction (infarction, left ventricular failure)
- Chest infection

Most serious complications in the immediate postoperative period present with features of cardiovascular compromise. Complications occurring in the first few hours after surgery are usually due to bleeding, exacerbation of medical problems, such as asthma, cardiac disease or inappropriate fluid management leading to overload. Differentiating these requires knowledge of the operation, the patient's medical background, and a careful history from the patient if possible. If the patient is unconscious due to anaesthesia, or too unwell, the recovery staff or ward staff are usually able to provide important information.

Cardiovascular Compromise

Problems often occur together, making the diagnosis difficult. Advice from anaesthetic and medical colleagues can be invaluable in these situations. The main findings will usually be:

- low blood pressure
- tachycardia
- peripheral vasoconstriction.

Often the oxygen saturation on pulse oximetry will be low (<95 per cent).

Haemorrhage

Bleeding may be revealed or concealed. Intra-abdominal bleeding can lead to distension, but large amounts of blood will be lost before this is obvious. Percussion of the flanks can be helpful. If blood pressure is low, pulse rate is raised, oxygen saturations are normal or slightly low and there are no signs of cardiac failure, then treatment for bleeding should be instituted, with fluid replacement, and re-operation if it is thought to be continuing. Where the picture is unclear, as may often be the case with the very frail or elderly, central venous pressure monitoring can be useful.

If bleeding is severe, resuscitation may be unsuccessful until loss is corrected surgically.

Myocardial Infarction

This may be associated with the typical pain, but is often silent, particularly in the elderly. There may be signs of left ventricular failure, such as a raised jugular venous pulse, crepitations in the lung bases, reduced saturations and, in severe cases, pink frothy sputum. When suspected, an electrocardiogram (ECG) should be performed, with cardiac enzyme analysis. Management will need to be coordinated with the medical team, as recent surgery will complicate the treatment as fibrinolysis becomes much more difficult.

Left Ventricular Failure

In the elderly, many factors can contribute to a short-term decrease in myocardial function, leading to left ventricular failure (LVF). These include intraoperative fluid overload, drugs used during anaesthesia and accidental omission of previously prescribed drug therapy. The signs are as above, but there is no evidence of ischaemia on ECG. Treatment will include facial oxygen and diuretics (usually frusemide 20–40 mg in the first instance). Severe LVF will need admission to the intensive therapy unit, continued ventilation, and may lead on to adult respiratory distress syndrome.

Opiate Overdose

Poor oxygen saturations and mildly depressed blood pressure without tachycardia may be signs of excessive opiate dosage. If the respiratory rate is low, this may provide a clue. Although naloxone will quickly reverse the effects of opiates, it will also rapidly restore pain. Care must be taken, therefore, not to leave the patient in extreme discomfort. Facial oxygen and careful supervision should be instituted whilst the opiate wears off.

Nausea and Vomiting

Nausea and vomiting occurring in the immediate postoperative period are usually due to a combination of drug effects and surgery. Opiates, if given without antiemetics, are particularly emetogenic. Treatment with standard antiemetics such as metoclopramide is usually effective. Newer antiemetics such as ondansetron are very effective in resistant cases (see also 'Ileus' below).

Late Postoperative Complications

Common causes

Infections

Ileus

Thromboembolism

Altered mental state

These are usually directed at a particular system or problem. Again a full account of the problem, a review of the operating note and postoperative management are imperative.

Postoperative Pyrexia

Pyrexia is one of the commonest postoperative findings. A transient low-grade pyrexia is not usually a cause for concern, but a sustained pyrexia needs investigation. A pyrexia of $>37.8\,°C$ generally implies infection. A sustained or recurrent low-grade pyrexia can be a sign of inflammation from other causes, including venous thromboembolism and atelectasis.

Classic sites for infection

Wound

Pelvis

Chest

Urinary tract

Samples taken from the appropriate sites must be sent prior to commencing antibiotic therapy. These will include wound swabs, high vaginal and endocervical swabs, midstream or catheter urine and sputum samples.

If the surgery involved the lower gastrointestinal tract, or there was the possibility of visceral damage (e.g. difficult laparoscopy or possible uterine perforation), intra-abdominal sepsis must be considered.

Pelvic infection can be precipitated by uterine manipulation during surgery. Ascending infection can occur after termination of pregnancy or evacuation of the uterus.

Wound

Problems with the wound are of three major types:

- erythema/tenderness
- pain and discoloration
- dehiscence.

Infection is the most commonly encountered problem with wounds. It presents as increasing redness and tenderness and, if infection leads to abscess formation, drainage of pus through the wound can occur. Signs of systemic illness may also be present, i.e. pyrexia, tachycardia, general malaise. Infection may be preceded by the formation of a haematoma, which subsequently becomes infected. Haematomas may cause pain, swelling and discoloration at the wound edges.

In the early stages, if identified, evacuation of a large haematoma may prevent the onset of infection. Small haematomas are usually treated conservatively, with careful observation for any infection. Often these will discharge spontaneously through the wound, which can be frightening for the patient if unexpected.

Infection can be localized, in terms of abscess formation, or become cellulitic, with spread into the abdominal wall. Abscesses are best treated by drainage. Cellulitis requires appropriate high-dose antibiotic treatment. This is a dangerous condition and necrotizing fasciitis is a real risk. Necrotizing fasciitis requires radical debridement to the edges of the healthy tissue.

Wound dehiscence is a major complication with significant morbidity. It occurs when the wound partially or completely separates, allowing the intra-abdominal contents to spill out. Risk factors include long-term steroid therapy, diabetes and infection. The management is surgical repair, utilizing strategies to increase wound strength, such as tension sutures.

Urinary Tract Infection

This can be precipitated by catheterization. The classical symptoms of cystitis are not often present. Treatment is with antibiotics. Many hospital-acquired urinary tract infections are multiresistant. A broad-spectrum cephalosporin is usually a good first-choice antibiotic.

Chest Infection

Chest infection is commonest in those with an underlying chest complaint, smokers, and after extensive abdominal surgery.

Examination may reveal generalized signs of wheeze or inspiratory crackles or localizing signs of consolidation. Investigation should include a sputum sample and, if severe infection is considered, a chest X-ray.

Treatment should be by broad-spectrum antibiotic and at least daily physiotherapy. Atelectasis requires physiotherapy and good pain relief, to encourage breathing exercises to reinflate collapsed segments of lung. A low-grade pyrexia with chest pain or cough should also prompt investigation for pulmonary embolism (see Chapter 44).

Abdominal Distension

The important differential diagnoses will be:

- ileus
- intra-abdominal bleeding
- urinary retention.

Clinical Assessment

Ask:

Is the distension associated with pain?
Has the patient passed a bowel motion since surgery?
Are there any urinary symptoms, and has urine been passed?
Is there any nausea or vomiting?

Palpate the abdomen for areas of tenderness that may point to a collection. Listen for bowel sounds and percuss for bladder and dullness in the flanks.

Investigation should include:

- electrolytes
- full blood count (white cell count is particularly important)
- plain abdominal X-ray
- ultrasound to identify collections.

Ileus

Gut motility is restored very soon after surgery, and simply handling the bowel will not stop it from functioning. Thus, after elective Caesarean section in women having spinal anaesthesia, a cup of tea can be given in recovery without problems.

Gut motility can be impaired by:

- metabolic derangement
- intra-abdominal collections (blood or pus)
- mechanical kinking or obstruction.

The commonest metabolic disturbances seen are hyponatraemia and hyperkalaemia and hypokalaemia. Gut motility may also be reduced by magnesium sulphate, which is commonly used in severe pre-eclampsia and eclampsia. Bowel sounds will be reduced or absent.

Localized collections within the abdominal cavity can cause gut motility dysfunction. The ileus seen a few days postoperatively is usually a transient adhesional problem. Generally, this is self-limiting. Bowel sounds will be present.

Treatment will be aimed at correcting any electrolyte imbalance. Prevention of overdistension is achieved by passing a large-bore nasogastric (NG) tube. Oral intake should be limited to sips of water, if an NG tube is present, until function is restored. Adhesional obstruction usually resolves with conservative management. Collections of blood will resolve with time, but abscesses may need to be drained.

Distension with tenderness or guarding can be signs of developing peritonitis. When visceral damage is suspected, laparotomy will be indicated for diagnosis and treatment.

Intra-abdominal Bleeding

Intra-abdominal bleeding generally occurs as an early complication. If bleeding is acute, signs of cardiovascular collapse will be apparent as above. A more chronic loss can occur if coagulation is disturbed, such as in severe pre-eclampsia, acute fatty liver of pregnancy or disseminated intravascular coagulopathy. Treatment must be aimed at correcting the coagulopathy. Laparotomy is often necessary, but does not always reveal a source, as generalized oozing is usually the cause in these cases.

Urinary Retention

> **Causes**
>
> Overdistension
> Pain
> Drugs
> Obstruction

Overdistension is only a real problem if good bladder care is not given during prolonged epidural anaesthesia. This can be a particular problem for women who undergo Caesarean section after a prolonged labour, if an indwelling catheter is not present. Disruption of the neural network of the bladder leads to loss of sensation of filling. This can be a significant problem, leading to long-term loss of sensation. Pain can lead to inhibition of urination, especially if the patient is fearful of pain on passing urine after vaginal surgery.

Drugs such as antihistamines and some antihypertensives can precipitate retention of urine. Obstruction can be due to a number of causes. A tight vaginal pack placed without an indwelling catheter will obstruct outflow. Large paravaginal haematomas may also present with acute retention. Care should be taken to identify the cause.

Treatment is to relieve the retention and to treat the cause. Overdistension may lead to the need for catheterization for a few days, and some women will continue to require intermittent catheterization.

Altered Mental State

Confusion and agitation are quite common in elderly patients following major surgery. Younger patients are less susceptible, but certain vulnerable groups are at risk.

> **Common causes**
>
> Infection
> Metabolic disturbance
> Hypoxia
> Prescribed drugs

Occasionally other problems can be unmasked by surgery, including alcohol or drug dependence. A history may reveal a previous problem.

> **Management of altered mental state**
>
> Exclude hypoxia by measuring the P_aO_2
> Look for metabolic disturbance (hyponatraemia or hypernatraemia and hypoglycaemia)
> Look for evidence of infection
> Consider whether a cerebrovascular accident is possible
> If all these are unlikely or negative, consider acute alcohol withdrawal

Delirium tremens is treated with an infusion of chlormethiazole, titrated to the patient's condition.

Learning Points

- Postoperative complications are common
- Careful fluid balance is needed to prevent metabolic disruption, especially in the elderly
- Early identification of infection can prevent the development of major complications
- Good pain relief and physiotherapy can reduce chest complications after major surgery
- Altered mental state may be due to a serious underlying problem

See Also

Venous thrombosis (Chapter 44)

Vomiting in early pregnancy

Importance

Nausea and vomiting in early pregnancy are extremely common, with 50–85 per cent of all mothers experiencing some problems. Pregnancies in which the mother has mild or moderate symptoms of nausea or vomiting carry an improved outcome for the fetus, in terms of a lower risk of miscarriage and preterm delivery.

In a small number of women, the degree of sickness can lead to significant dehydration and even metabolic derangement. This condition, if occurring for the first time before 20 weeks, is termed 'hyperemesis gravidarum'. Approximately 5 in 1000 women will be so affected. This condition is serious and requires hospital admission and management. In general, the outcome for the fetus is good. In exceptionally rare cases, the pregnancy may need to be terminated, to allow the recovery of the patient.

Causes

Moderate or severe vomiting is more common in:

Multiple pregnancies
Trophoblastic disease
Women who had it in a previous pregnancy

The cause of the nausea is unknown. Some association with human chorionic gonadotrophin (hCG) levels is possible but unproven.

It is important to remember that other conditions, which occur in non-pregnant as well as pregnant women, will also cause vomiting. Pregnancy-induced vomiting commonly occurs between 6 and 16 weeks, and has resolved in almost all cases by 20 weeks. Vomiting of new onset after this time will almost always carry an entirely different aetiology.

Differential diagnosis of vomiting in pregnancy

Reflux oesophagitis
Peptic or gastric ulceration
Gall bladder disease
Gastrointestinal infections
Urinary tract infection
Benign intracranial hypertension
Psychogenic vomiting

Some of these, such as reflux and urinary tract infection, may be worsened by the pregnancy.

Diagnosis and Clinical Assessment

History

It is important to ask about the frequency of vomiting, trigger factors and whether any other members of the family have been affected. A history of vomiting in a previous pregnancy or outside pregnancy should be sought. Other associated features, including pain, jaundice, dysuria, urinary frequency and headaches, may be important. Smoking and alcohol can both exacerbate symptoms and should be enquired about. If this pregnancy resulted from fertility treatment, or if there is a close family history of twins, a multiple pregnancy is more likely. Early pregnancy bleeding or a past history of trophoblastic disease may point to a hydatidiform mole.

Examination

Key findings

Dry tongue
Sunken eyes

(cont.)

(cont.)
Dry or sallow skin with reduced turgor
Tachycardia
Reduced jugular venous pressure
Jaundice
Abdominal tenderness

Look initially for signs of dehydration. Palpate the abdomen for areas of tenderness, especially in the right upper quadrant, hypogastrium and renal angles. Feel for the fundus of the uterus and note its size.

Make a note of the pulse, blood pressure, temperature, colour of the urine and presence on dipstick analysis of ketones, blood or protein. It is important that the vomiting is witnessed and the vomitus is examined at least once for presence of blood. Very occasionally, psychogenic vomiting presents in pregnancy. Misdiagnosis can lead to prolonged inappropriate treatment.

Investigations

Once a full history and examination have been performed, it should be possible, at least in part, to decide whether this vomiting is pregnancy-related or incidental, possibly exacerbated by the pregnancy. Which investigations are ordered will depend on the differential diagnoses. Some investigations will be pertinent to all women.

Relevant investigations

Blood testing for urea and electrolytes
Liver function tests
Urine for culture and sensitivity
Ultrasound of the uterus to establish fetal number and exclude trophoblastic disease

Management

Mild to Moderate Vomiting

If the vomiting is mild to moderate and is not causing signs of dehydration, then usually reassurance and advice will be all that is necessary. Simple measures include:

- taking small carbohydrate meals;
- avoiding large-volume drinks, especially milk and fizzy drinks (like Lucozade);
- raising the head of the bed if reflux is a problem.

Some women find ginger very helpful. Although the commonly used antiemetics are not thought to be teratogenic in humans, these should not be considered until simple measures have been tried and failed. Antacids such as Gaviscon are safe and can be used to alleviate reflux.

Severe Vomiting

This is usually bad enough to require hospital admission.

Principles of management

Removal of the need to eat or drink
Rehydration
Drug treatment for resistant cases
Nutritional support

In order to rest the alimentary tract, removal of the need to eat and drink is an important first step. This is accomplished by siting an intravenous line by which rehydration can be given. During this time, it is important that a close check on electrolyte status is maintained. Most women will settle in 24–48 hours with these supportive measures. The psychological aspect of this condition must not be overlooked. Placebo-controlled trials have shown that 50 per cent of women will settle with placebo alone. Once the vomiting has ceased, small amounts of fluid, and eventually food, can be reintroduced. It is worthwhile doing this gently. If rushed, many women relapse and require readmission.

If vomiting continues and the history is suggestive of severe reflux or ulcer disease, endoscopy can be very valuable. It is a safe technique in pregnancy. If severe oesophagitis is confirmed, then appropriate treatment with alginates and metoclopramide can be given. Ulcer disease will require H_2-antagonist treatment (ranitidine) or, if very severe, omeprazole, although there is limited experience of this in pregnancy.

Antiemetic therapy is reserved for those women who do not settle on supportive measures or who persistently relapse. Metoclopramide and prochloperazine have not been shown to be teratogenic in humans (although metoclopramide is in animals).

Very occasionally, women do not settle with a combination of the above measures. Some of these women may improve with steroid therapy, although trials are still ongoing. Women in whom there is liver function derangement may benefit particularly. H_2 antagonists must be given in conjunction with the steroid treatment. Parenteral nutrition is necessary for some who develop severe protein/calorie malnutrition. Specialized nutrition units can be very helpful in this setting.

Thiamine must be prescribed for women with severe vomiting, as cases of Wernicke's encephalopathy have been reported. As the vomiting settles, oral intake can be gradually reintroduced. Women are often very frightened of the prospect of going home, fearing that the symptoms will recur. Advice on how to pre-empt recurrence and some home support can help to limit the need for readmission. If symptoms recur, women should be readmitted before they become significantly dehydrated, as this may limit the time needed to allow symptoms to resolve.

Reassurance that this condition is usually self-limiting should also be given.

Learning Points

- Mild or moderate nausea or vomiting is very common in early pregnancy
- Most severe cases settle with supportive measures
- Drug therapy is reserved for resistant or recurrent cases

See Also

Acute abdominal pain (Chapter 67)

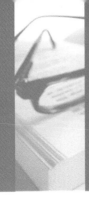

Appendices

Appendices

A. Commonly used abbreviations 293

B. Glossary of commonly used terms 296

C. Self-assessment questions 305

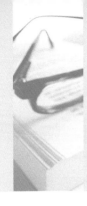

Appendix A

Commonly used abbreviations

Abbreviation	Term
AC	Abdominal circumference
ACA	Anticardiolipin antibodies
ACTH	Adrenocorticotrophic hormone
AF (AFI)	Amniotic fluid (amniotic fluid index)
ANC	Antenatal clinic
APA	Antiphospholipid antibodies
APH	Antepartum haemorrhage
ARM	Artificial rupture of membranes
ART	Assisted reproductive technique
βhCG	Beta human chorionic gonadotrophin
BBA	Born before arrival
BMI	Body mass index
BPD	Biparietal diameter
BPP	Biophysical profile
BSO	Bilateral salpingo-oophorectomy
BV	Bacterial vaginosis
CCT	Controlled cord traction
CIGN	Cervical intraglandular neoplasia
CIN	Cervical intraepithelial neoplasia
CL	Corpus luteum
CMV	Cytomegalovirus
COCP	Combined oral contraceptive pill
CPD	Cephalopelvic disproportion
CRL	Crown–rump length
CTG	Cardiotocograph
CVS	Chorionic villus sampling
D&C	Dilatation and curettage
DHAS	Dehydroepiandrosterone sulphate
DI	Donor insemination
DIC	Disseminated intravascular coagulation
DUB	Dysfunctional uterine bleeding
DVT	Deep vein thrombosis
E2	Oestrogen
EBL	Estimated blood loss
ECG	Electrocardiogram
ECV	External cephalic version
EDD	Estimated date of delivery
EDF	End-diastolic flow
EFW	Estimated fetal weight
EPAU/PAC	Early pregnancy assessment unit/centre
ERPOC	Evacuation of retained products of conception
EUA	Examination under anaesthetic
EWA	Examination in theatre not under anaesthetic
FBC	Full blood count
FBS	Fetal blood sampling
FHHR	Fetal heart rate heard
FIGO	International Federation of Obstetrics and Gynaecology
FL	Femur length

FM	Fetal movements	IUI	Intrauterine insemination
FSE	Fetal scalp electrode	IUS	Intrauterine system
FSH	Follicle-stimulating hormone	IVF	*In vitro* fertilization
FTA	Fluorescent treponemal antibody	IVH	Intraventricular haemorrhage
G	Gravida	IVU/IVP	Intravenous urogram/pyelogram
GA	Gestational age	LAC	Lupus anticoagulant
GIFT	Gamete intra-fallopian transfer	LGA	Large for gestational age
GnRH	Gonadotrophin-releasing hormone	LFT	Liver function test
GnRHa	Gonadotrophin-releasing hormone analogue (antagonist)	LH	Luteinizing hormone
GSI	Genuine stress incontinence	LLETZ	Large loop excision of the transformation zone
GTT	Glucose tolerance test	LLP	Low-lying placenta
GUM	Genitourinary medicine	LMP	Last menstrual period
HC	Head circumference	LSCS	Lower segment Caesarean section
HELLP	Haemolysis, elevated liver enzymes, low platelets	MCV	Mean corpuscular volume
HFEA	Human Fertilisation and Embryology Authority	MMR	Maternal mortality rate
HIV	Human immunodeficiency virus	MRCOG	Membership or Member of the Royal College of Obstetricians and Gynaecologists
HMG	Human menopausal gonadotrophin	MROP	Manual removal of placenta
HPV	Human papilloma virus	MSAFP (AFP)	Maternal serum alpha-fetoprotein
HRT	Hormone replacement therapy	MSU	Midstream urine sample
HSG	Hysterosalpingogram	NND	Neonatal death
HSV	Herpes simplex virus	NSAID	Non-steroidal anti-inflammatory drug
HVS	High vaginal swab	NTD	Neural tube defect
IBS	Irritable bowel syndrome	OA	Occipito-anterior position
ICSI	Intracytoplasmic sperm injection	OHSS	Ovarian hyperstimulation syndrome
IDDM	Insulin-dependent diabetes mellitus	OP	Occipitoposterior position
IMB	Intermenstrual bleeding	OT	Occipitotransverse position
IOL	Induction of labour	P	Para
ITP	Idiopathic thrombocytopenic purpura	PCB	Postcoital bleeding
IUC	Intrauterine catheter	PCOS	Polycystic ovarian syndrome
IUCD	Intrauterine contraceptive device	PCT	Postcoital test
IUFD or IUD	Intrauterine fetal death	PET	Pre-eclamptic toxaemia
IUGR	Intrauterine growth restriction	PID	Pelvic inflammatory disease

PIH	Pregnancy-induced hypertension	SVD	Spontaneous vaginal delivery
PMB	Postmenopausal bleeding	TAH	Total abdominal hysterectomy
PMR	Perinatal mortality rate	TCI	To come in (to be admitted)
PMS	Premenstrual syndrome	TCRE	Transcervical resection of the endometrium
POP	Progestogen-only pill	TORCH	Viral screen for antibodies to toxoplasma, rubella, cytomegalovirus and herpes viruses
PPH	Postpartum haemorrhage		
PRL	Prolactin	TOS	Trial of scar
PROM	Premature rupture of membranes	TPHA	*Treponema pallidum* haemagglutination assay
RBS	Random blood sugar		
RCOG	Royal College of Obstetricians and Gynaecologists	TSH	Thyroid-stimulating hormone
		TTN	Transient tachypnoea of the newborn
RDS	Respiratory distress syndrome	TV	*Trichomonas vaginalis*
RPOC	Retained products of conception	TVS (TAS)	Transvaginal (transabdominal) ultrasound scan
SA (SFA)	Semen analysis		
SB	Stillbirth	TZ	Transformation zone
SCBU	Special care baby unit	U&E	Urea and electrolytes
SCJ	Squamocolumnar junction	UAPI or PI	Umbilical artery pulsatility index
SERM	Selective oestrogen receptor modulator	USS	Ultrasound scan
SGA/SFD	Small for gestational age/dates	UTI	Urinary tract infection
SFH	Symphysis–fundal height	VBAC	Vaginal birth after Caesarean section
SHBG	Sex hormone binding globulin	VDRL	Venereal Diseases Research Laboratory test
SROM	Spontaneous rupture of membranes	VE	Vaginal examination
STD	Sexually transmitted disease	VIN	Vulval intraepithelial neoplasia
STOP	Surgical termination of pregnancy	VTE	Venous thromboembolism
		WR	Wasserman reaction

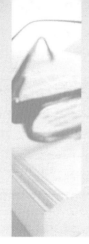

Glossary of commonly used terms

Abdominal circumference (AC) Distance around fetal abdomen at the level of insertion of umbilical vessels – used as a measure of fetal growth.

Alpha-fetoprotein (maternal serum) A 68-kDa precursor of fetal albumin produced in the yolk sac and fetal liver which crosses the placenta into the maternal circulation. It is detectable in amniotic fluid by 6 weeks, and peaks at 16 weeks. Used as a marker for neural tube defects and trisomy 21 but also reflects disorders of placental development.

Amenorrhoea Absence of menstruation. Primary when there is a failure to begin menstruation by the age of 16 and secondary where the periods have been absent for 6 months or more in a woman who has previously menstruated.

Amniotic fluid (amniotic fluid index) Formed by secretion of fluid from amnion and fetal skin and from fetal urine. The volume increases from 5–10 mL at 8 weeks to a maximum of 1000 mL at 38 weeks and then falls again, so that after 41 weeks the mean volume is less than 300 mL. Amniotic fluid volume can be estimated using ultrasound by measuring the fluid depth in four quadrants (amniotic fluid index).

Antepartum haemorrhage (APH) Bleeding from the genital tract in pregnancy after 20 weeks.

Antiphospholipid antibodies (APA) Antiphospholipid antibodies (i.e. IgG and IgM against charged phospholipids in the cell membrane) are expressed by 15–20 per cent of patients with systemic lupus erythematosus and myeloproliferative disorders. APA can cause recurrent miscarriage, thrombosis, thrombocytopenia, IUFD and IUGR.

Artificial rupture of membranes (ARM) Release of amniotic fluid by puncturing the amniotic and chorionic membranes. Usually done to induce labour.

Bacterial vaginosis (BV) An overgrowth of anaerobic organisms such as *Gardnerella vaginalis*, *Bacteroides*, *Mycoplasma hominis* and *Mobiluncus* sp. normally present in the vagina. Symptoms are usually a white or pale yellow vaginal discharge with an offensive fishy odour. It is associated with an increase in vaginal pH and the presence of clue cells on microscopic examination.

Beta human chorionic gonadotrophin (βhCG) Peptide hormone consisting of two subunits, alpha and beta. LH, FSH and TSH share the alpha subunit. The beta subunit is specific to pregnancy and is the basis for pregnancy tests. Produced by trophoblast cells and detectable in maternal blood shortly after implantation. Its role is to maintain the corpus luteum until the placenta takes over steroid hormone production. Levels peak at the end of the first trimester and then fall.

Beta-sympathomimetics Includes salbutamol, ritodrine and terbutaline. Used to relax the uterus and in the treatment of premature labour. Important side-effects are tachycardia, peripheral vasodilatation, reduced diastolic blood pressure, arrhythmias, pulmonary oedema (especially with steroids, diabetes, multiple gestation), hyperglycaemia and hypokalaemia.

Bilateral salpingo-oophorectomy (BSO) Surgical removal of both Fallopian tubes and ovaries, usually done at the same time as abdominal hysterectomy.

Biophysical profile (BPP) Antenatal assessment of fetal well-being based on fetal heart rate pattern, and ultrasound assessment of fetal movement, posture, breathing movements and amniotic fluid volume.

Biparietal diameter (BPD) Distance across the fetal head. When compared with known measurements at different stages of pregnancy it can be used to calculate gestational age in early pregnancy. Can also be used to measure fetal growth in later pregnancy but may be inaccurate in certain head shapes so head circumference tends to be used instead.

Bladder The detrusor contains large smooth muscle bundles, which act as a single unit. The mucosa is trabeculated and lined by transitional epithelium, except for the trigone which is a continuation of the ureteric smooth muscle. The nerve supply is parasympathetic from S2,3,4 via pelvic splanchnics to detrusor and urethra (cholinergic muscarinic) and sympathetic from T10 to L2 via the hypogastric plexus to bladder, blood vessels and urethra (α and β adrenergic).

Body mass index (BMI) Derived from weight and height and expressed as kg/m^2. Normal BMI for an adult female is between 19 and 26.

Booking First antenatal clinic visit. At booking, a detailed past medical and obstetric history is taken and any risk factors for the current pregnancy are identified. A general physical examination, including blood pressure, is performed. A midstream urine sample is sent for microscopy and culture. Blood is taken for blood group, hepatitis, syphilis, rubella and HIV serology, haemoglobin estimation and, depending on ethnic group, haemoglobin electrophoresis. Testing or screening for fetal abnormality is discussed. Booking usually takes place between 8 and 14 weeks.

Born before arrival (BBA) Birth of a baby booked for hospital delivery before arrival at the delivery suite.

Brow presentation A brow presents the largest diameter of the fetal head (13.5 cm) and will not fit through the normal pelvis. However, in labour, the fetal head can flex to a vertex or extend to a face. Because a brow presentation will not deliver, there is no defined denominator. Complicates 1 in 1500 deliveries. If diagnosed in labour, 2–3 hours can be allowed to see if the presentation changes. If, after this time, the head remains as a brow, a Caesarean section should be performed.

Candida A yeast, the commonest species being *Candida albicans*. It affects 75 per cent of women at some time and an estimated 20 per cent are carriers (in the gut). Predisposing factors include drugs which impair immunity, antibiotics, pregnancy, use of high-dose combined contraceptive pills, diabetes, thyroid, parathyroid and adrenal disease. Symptoms include vulval itching and soreness and a curdy white discharge (may also be thin and watery). On examination the vulva may be erythematous with fissuring and there are white plaques in the vagina which are adherent. The diagnosis can be confirmed by culture or by the presence of Gram-positive spores and long pseudohyphae on microscopy. The vaginal pH is usually normal. In recurrent infections, look for anaemia, thyroid disease and diabetes and consider acquired immunodeficiency. Asymptomatic women do not require treatment. Topical preparations such as clotrimazole 500 mg either as a single-dose pessary or as a cream for 14 days are usually effective. Recurrent or persistent infection can be treated by systemic agents such as fluconazole 150 mg (avoid in pregnancy). Treatment of the partner is usually recommended although re-infection may occur from the gut. Acetic acid jelly

(e.g. Aci-jel) may prevent or relieve mild attacks. Advice about simple hygiene measures such as wiping the vulva from front to back, avoiding chemical irritants on the vulva such as bath salts and the used of cotton underwear may help.

Caput succedaneum (caput) Oedema over the presenting part crossing the suture lines associated with long labours. Common finding after delivery.

Cephalopelvic disproportion (CPD) The relative diameter of the presenting part or the absolute smallest diameter is greater than that of the bony pelvis.

Cervical intraepithelial neoplasia (CIN) Histological diagnosis of changes in squamous epithelium of the cervix characterized by varying degrees of loss of differentiation and stratification (deepest layers up) and nuclear atypia with increased nuclear to cytoplasmic ratio. Does not extend below the epithelial basement membrane.

Cervical intraglandular neoplasia (CIGN) Changes in columnar cells of the glandular epithelium lining the endocervix, including hyperchromatic nuclei, prominent nucleoli, budding and stratification. May progress to adenocarcinoma of the cervix. Two-thirds coexist with CIN; 50 per cent have no glandular changes on smear.

Cervix Consists of vaginal and supravaginal portions; 10 per cent muscular and 80 per cent fibrous. Lined by columnar and squamous epithelium meeting at the squamocolumnar junction (SCJ). Blood supply is from the uterine artery which is a branch of the internal iliac. Lymphatic drainage is via the paracervical nodes to the internal iliac, obturator and sacral nodes draining to the aortic nodes.

Chorionic villus sampling (CVS) Removal of a sample of trophoblast from the developing placenta for karyotyping. Performed under ultrasound guidance either transabdominally or transcervically.

Climacteric The period of time before and after the cessation of menstruation (the menopause) associated with ovarian failure, rising gonadotrophin levels and falling oestrogen levels.

Clomiphene citrate (Clomid) An anti-oestrogen, which inhibits negative feedback at the hypothalamic level resulting in a rise in the frequency of GnRH release and increased LH and FSH levels. May also have direct pituitary and ovarian actions. Used in anovulatory infertility and PCOS.

Confinement Old term used for the period of time around delivery.

Controlled cord traction A technique for delivery of the placenta and membranes using gentle traction on the umbilical cord whilst guarding the uterus with the free hand placed on the lower abdomen.

Corpus luteum The structure formed from the remaining granulosa and theca interna cells of the dominant follicle after ovulation. It is yellowish in appearance, produces progesterone and, unless pregnancy occurs, undergoes a process known as luteolysis to form the corpus albicans.

Crown–rump length (CRL) Measurement of the length of the embryo used to determine gestational age prior to 10 weeks.

Crowning The baby's head is said to have crowned when the widest diameter passes through the pelvic outlet.

Denominator The part of the fetal presenting part used to denote position. For a vertex this will be the occiput.

Dilatation and curettage (D&C) Dilatation of the cervical canal using a series of metal rods (dilators) of increasing size and sampling of the endometrium using a curette.

Disseminated intravascular coagulation (DIC) Abnormality of the coagulation system characterized by increased circulating levels of fibrin degradation products, prolonged clotting times and reduced platelet levels. It occurs as a result of vascular endothelial damage, thromboplastin release and increased phospholipid levels. The main obstetric causes are amniotic fluid embolus, abruption, fetomaternal bleed, pre-eclampsia, acute fatty liver, massive haemorrhage ($>$ 25 per cent blood volume), septicaemia, transfusion reaction and following IUFD. Management is to treat the underlying cause. If antenatal, deliver the fetus vaginally if possible and minimize tissue trauma (no regional blocks). There should be prompt correction of any hypovolaemia and tissue hypoperfusion and transfusion – usually with plasma reduced blood with fresh frozen plasma (1:5 of blood) monitored with regular clotting profiles and early involvement of a haematologist.

Donor insemination (DI) Use of sperm from a donor for intra-uterine insemination.

Dysfunctional uterine bleeding Abnormal uterine blood loss occurring in the absence of any systemic or local cause.

Early pregnancy assessment unit (EPAU) A designated clinical area with dedicated ultrasound scanning facilities for women presenting with early pregnancy complications.

Effacement (of the cervix) The progressive shortening of the cervix as a result of inclusion of the length of the cervix in the lower segment of the uterus, beginning at the internal cervical os.

Engagement When the widest diameter of the presenting part has passed through the pelvic brim. This will correspond to two-fifths or less palpable on abdominal examination for a cephalic presentation.

Estimated blood loss (EBL) The amount of blood lost at the time of delivery or surgery. Normal delivery is associated with a blood loss of about 500 mL.

Estimated date of delivery (EDD) In a woman with a 28-day menstrual cycle this will be 268 days from the first day of the last menstrual period. This can be calculated by adding 7 days and 9 months to the date of the LMP but in practice a pregnancy dating wheel or calculator is usually used. For each day longer than 28 in the previous menstrual cycle, adjust the EDD by adding a day. EDD is often calculated from early ultrasound estimation of gestational age.

Estimated fetal weight (EFW) Fetal weight usually calculated on the basis of ultrasound measurements of the fetal abdominal and head circumference. There is a considerable margin of error with a range of $\pm$ 500 g for weights over 3.5 kg.

Evacuation of retained products of conception (ERPOC) A surgical procedure to remove retained pregnancy tissue (usually placenta, decidua or membranes) from the uterus.

Examination in theatre not under anaesthetic (EWA) A vaginal examination performed in theatre in order to be able to proceed to an operative procedure depending on the findings. An example would be where there is doubt about the position of the placenta in a woman in established labour and the options would be to proceed to delivery by Caesarean section or to allow labour to continue on the delivery suite.

Face presentation Face presentations occur in 1 in 500 deliveries. The face presents similar diameters to the vertex and can rotate in the same way. A face can sometimes be difficult to distinguish from a breech. Occasionally the fetus will suck the examining finger, which can be a bit alarming if unexpected! Face presentations may deliver if they rotate to have the fetal chin anterior. This diameter of 9.5 cm is the same as presents with an occipito-anterior vertex. Because delivery is possible, there is a denominator, which is the chin (mentum). Delay in the second stage can be managed with forceps but not Ventouse. Fetal scalp electrodes or fetal blood sampling in labour cannot be utilized. The mother must be warned that the baby may look very bruised after delivery, but that this resolves quickly and without problems.

Fallopian tubes These are 10 cm long, consisting of infundibular, ampullar, isthmus and interstitial sections. Made up of external serosa, circular and longitudinal muscle and lined with ciliated columnar epithelium.

Fetal movements Gross body movements of a fetus either felt by the mother or seen on ultrasound scan. Fetal movements are normally felt by 20 weeks' gestation in a first pregnancy or slightly earlier in subsequent pregnancies (this is known as the quickening).

Fetal scalp electrode (FSE) Metal clip attached to fetal scalp to record fetal ECG activity.

Follicle-stimulating hormone (FSH) Gonadotrophin produced by the anterior pituitary, which stimulates proliferation of the granulosa cells of the Graffian follicles, the production of oestrogen and LH receptor induction.

Follicular phase The part of the menstrual cycle occurring between the end of menstruation and ovulation. The length may vary. It is characterized by proliferation of endometrial glandular and stroma tissue, so is also called the proliferative phase.

Gestational age The duration of the pregnancy. This is expressed as the number of weeks since the first day of the last menstrual period (LMP) in a woman with a 28-day cycle (i.e. 2 weeks more than since ovulation). It may be abbreviated to x/40 +^{y}, where x is the number of weeks and y the number of days. Gestational age can be calculated from the date of the LMP (adding or subtracting days for women with cycles shorter or longer than 28 days) or by comparing ultrasound measurements of the fetus to growth charts.

Gonadotrophin-releasing hormone (GnRH) Decapeptide released by the median eminence of the hypothalamus, which stimulates the release of FSH and LH from the pituitary.

Gonadotrophin-releasing hormone analogue (antagonist) (GnRHa) Synthetic modified version of GnRH, which competes with GnRH for binding sites in the pituitary and causes down-regulation of gonadotrophin release. May have an initial agonist effect. Can be given as depot injection or nasal spray. Used in down-regulation prior to ovulation stimulation and in the treatment of endometriosis, menorrhagia and fibroids. The main side-effects are hot flushes (97 per cent), dry vagina (18–70 per cent), loss of libido (17–66 per cent), reduced bone density (3–5 per cent), breast atrophy, headache, acne and amenorrhoea (94 per cent).

Gravida A pregnant woman (gravidity = number of pregnancies). A woman in her first pregnancy is described as a primigravida.

HELLP syndrome Haemolysis, elevated liver enzymes and low platelets. Variant of pre-eclampsia where the major manifestations are thrombocytopenia and abnormal liver function.

Herpes gestationis Bullous skin disorder associated with pregnancy. There is C_3 deposition at the basement membrane caused by complement-fixing autoantibody to the dermis. Tends to recur.

Herpes simplex virus (HSV) A DNA virus. Types I (genital) and II (oral, cold sores); 50 per cent of genital lesions are now due to HSV I. There is an incubation period of 21 days. The first attack is the most severe, with pain, vulvitis (may be severe enough to cause urinary retention), ulceration, lymphadenopathy and discharge. Subsequent attacks are normally shorter and less severe. There may be prodromal symptoms. Asymptomatic shedding of the virus may occur. The diagnosis is made by culture of serum collected from vesicles by aspiration or by swabbing the base of the ulcers. Serum anti-HSV antibody levels are increased with both types of infection. Treatment is largely supportive with analgesia and the treatment of any secondary infections. Acyclovir 200 mg five times a day for 5 days if given within 5 days of onset of symptoms shortens the duration of the primary attack and may abort recurrent episodes if taken when prodromal symptoms occur. Condoms should be used unless both partners have a history of herpes.

High vaginal swab (HVS) Swab taken from the vaginal fornices for culture. Used as one part of triple swabs for screening and diagnosis of sexually transmitted infections. Mainly detects anaerobic and yeast infections.

Human Fertilisation and Embryology Authority (HFEA) The statutory body which oversees all units providing assisted conception treatments.

Human immunodeficiency virus (HIV) RNA retrovirus which infects T_H lymphocytes, macrophages and central nervous system. Prolonged latent phase. Transmission is by sex, infected blood products, shared needles, breast-feeding or from mother to fetus (75 per cent child cases). Risk groups are partners of bisexual and i.v. drug users, prostitutes, immigrants from (or who were transfused in) high-risk areas. Presentations include infections: *Candida* (oral, vulvovaginal), herpes simplex, warts, tuberculosis, mycobacterium, cryptosporidium, *Pneumocystis carinii* pneumonia, toxoplasma, cytomegalovirus and severe PID. Non-infective presentations include weight loss, diarrhoea, fever, dementia, Kaposi's sarcoma, lymphoma, cervical carcinoma.

Human menopausal gonadotrophin (HMG) A mixture of FSH and LH purified from the urine of postmenopausal women.

Human papilloma virus (HPV) The most important serotypes are 6, 11, 16, 18 and 31: 6 and 11 are the commonest. 16, 18 and 31 have been linked to the development of cervical cancer. There is an incubation period of weeks to months. The virus may be carried (and shed) without any visible lesions being present. Infection is sexually acquired. The lesions are usually asymptomatic (any itch is usually due to secondary infection). The appearance depends on the site. They are associated with other STDs (25 per cent). Visible lesions are treated with cryotherapy or topical application of podophyllin one to two times a week for 6 weeks. Surgical excision and ablation by laser or diathermy are alternatives. Relapse is common whatever method of treatment is used, especially in immunocompromised patients. Sexual partners should be examined for warts and other STDs. Barrier contraception is usually advised during treatment. There is no need for women with warts to have more frequent cervical screening, although patients with cervical warts should be referred for colposcopic assessment.

Hysterosalpingogram (HSG) A radiological investigation used to visualize the uterine cavity and Fallopian tubes in the investigation of patients with infertility or recurrent miscarriage. Approximately 2–3 mL of water-soluble contrast medium is instilled through the cervix into the uterine cavity. The presence of intrauterine synechiae and congenital abnormalities of the uterine cavity can also be identified. If the Fallopian tubes are patent, dye will be seen spilling into the peritoneal cavity.

In vitro fertilization (IVF) Technique for treatment of infertility. Most commonly used for patients with tubal disease, male factor and unexplained infertility.

International Federation of Obstetrics and Gynaecology (FIGO) World body of obstetrics and gynaecology. Hosts World Congress of Obstetrics and Gynaecology every 3 years. Publishes criteria for staging gynaecological cancers.

Intrauterine system (Mirena) Levonorgestrel (progestogen)-releasing intrauterine device developed primarily for contraception but also used in the treatment of heavy periods.

Intracytoplasmic sperm injection (ICSI) A type of IVF involving injection of a single sperm into the cytoplasm of a single ovum.

Intrauterine catheter Thin plastic tube inserted through the cervix alongside the fetus to measure changes in intrauterine pressure. Used in some centres to guide uterine stimulation with oxytocics.

Intrauterine contraceptive device (IUCD) Plastic framework usually with copper placed in the uterine cavity to prevent pregnancy.

Intrauterine fetal death (IUFD) Fetal demise occurring prior to delivery.

Intrauterine growth restriction (IUGR) Failure of fetus to reach its genetic potential weight. Usually due to placental failure when it is typically characterized by a relative sparing of head growth (asymmetric IUGR).

Intrauterine insemination (IUI) Assisted reproduction technique involving insertion of prepared sperm from the partner or donor directly into the uterine cavity at the time of ovulation.

Intraventricular haemorrhage (IVH) Bleeding occurring in the cerebral ventricles of the fetus or neonate. More common in preterm or difficult instrumental deliveries.

Irritable bowel syndrome (IBS) Common cause of lower abdominal pain characterized by intermittent colicky pain often associated with abdominal bloating and irregular bowel habit.

Labour The onset of regular painful contractions, more than one in every 10 minutes, with progressive cervical effacement and dilatation accompanied by descent of the presenting part.

Large for gestational age (LGA) A baby suspected antenatally, or confirmed following delivery, of having a birthweight above the 95th centile for gestational age.

Large loop excision of the transformation zone (LLETZ) Surgical excision of a shallow cone of tissue from the area of the cervix adjacent to the ectocervical os used in the treatment of CIN.

Leiomyosarcoma Malignancy arising in the smooth muscle of the myometrium. Affects 0.7 per 100 000 women per year; 5–10 per cent

arise in leiomyomas but the risk of malignant change occurring in a fibroid is thought to be only 0.2–0.3 per cent. The peak incidence is 10 years later than that for fibroids. It presents with pain, mass (rapid growth, pressure) or PMB but may be asymptomatic. The diagnosis is usually only made after removal of the uterus. Treatment is by hysterectomy and bilateral oophorectomy. Adjuvant radiotherapy and chemotherapy reduce local recurrence but do not improve survival. The prognosis is poor.

Lie The relationship of the long axis of the fetus to that of the uterus. This can be longitudinal, transverse or oblique.

Liver function tests (LFTs) Alkaline phosphatase levels may be raised on standard LFTs in pregnancy because of the presence of placental alkaline phosphatase.

Lochia The discharge/bleeding that occurs from the uterus after delivery. Normally rubra (bloody period-like loss) for 3 days, pink (leucocytes and decidua) for a further 7 days and finally alba (white) for 3–6 months (leucocytes and serous fluid).

Low-lying placenta (LLP) Placenta implanted in the lower segment of the uterus.

Lower segment The region between the reflection of the pelvic peritoneum off the anterior surface of the uterus to form the uterovesical fold and above the level of the internal cervix os.

Lower segment Caesarean section (LSCS) Delivery of the fetus through a transverse incision in the lower uterine segment.

Lupus anticoagulant (LAC) One of the group of antiphospholipid antibodies. Prolongs phospholipid-dependent coagulation. Associated with fetal loss in all trimesters. May damage platelets, inhibit prostacyclin and cause placental infarction.

Luteal phase Part of the menstrual cycle occurring after ovulation. It is associated with secretory changes in the endometrium and so is sometimes called the secretory phase. It is of fairly fixed 14-day duration.

Luteinizing hormone (LH) Oligopeptide produced by the anterior pituitary in response to GnRH from the hypothalamus. It increases slowly in the first half of the menstrual cycle then surges at day 14, stimulating ovulation. In the second half of the cycle, it supports the development of the corpus luteum in the ovary.

Malposition Unfavourable relationship between the denominator and the pelvis. Commonest example is occipitoposterior position.

Malpresentation Any presenting part other than vertex; includes breech, face, brow and shoulder.

Manual removal of placenta (MROP) Procedure to remove a retained or adherent placenta from the uterus after delivery by passing a hand through the cervix.

Maternal mortality rate (MMR) Maternal mortality is defined as the death of a woman during or within 42 days of the end of pregnancy. The maternal mortality rate is the number of maternal deaths per 100 000 maternities (i.e. live births and stillbirths after 24 weeks). The rate in the UK is 10 per 100 000 divided equally between direct and indirect causes. Direct maternal deaths are those occurring as a result of a complication of the pregnancy itself. The commonest causes of direct deaths are thromboembolism, hypertensive disorders, and haemorrhage and amniotic fluid embolism. Indirect deaths are a result of pre-existing disease or disease which develops during pregnancy and was not due to direct obstetric causes but which was aggravated by the physiological effects of pregnancy. The commonest indirect causes are cardiac disease and psychiatric disorders.

Menarche The onset of menstruation. The average age for this in the UK is 13. Initially menstruation tends to be irregular and it may take several years to establish regular ovulatory cycles.

Menopause The cessation of menstruation. The average age of the last menstrual period is 51. The term is often used incorrectly to describe the hormonal and physiological changes that occur in the years leading up to and after the last period (the climacteric).

Menorrhagia Abnormally heavy or prolonged periods.

Micturition Normal micturition is initiated by relaxation of the urethral sphincter by increased α-sympathetic and reduced β-sympathetic and parasympathetic tone. At the same time there is a reduction in the inhibition of parasympathetic spinal reflex at S2, 3, 4 which leads to sustained tonic detrusor contraction. The normal flow rate is 30 mL/s.

Miscarriage Pregnancy loss occurring before viability. The World Health Organization defines this as a fetus or embryo weighing 500 g or less. In the UK it applies to pregnancies of 24 weeks' or less gestation. Previously known as spontaneous abortion.

Mixed (Müllerian) mesodermal tumour Tumours arising in the endometrium containing malignant elements of both epithelium and stroma. Account for less than 3 per cent of uterine tumours affecting 2 per 100 000 women per year. Epithelial elements are usually endometrioid but can be squamous or a mixture. Stromal elements are either heterologous (chondroblastoma, rhabdomyosarcoma, osteosarcoma, fibrosarcoma) or homologous (leiomyosarcoma, presarcoma, ectodermal stroma). The presentation is as for endometrial carcinoma. The diagnosis is made by curettage or after hysterectomy. Treatment is hysterectomy and adjuvant radiotherapy with removal of all macroscopic disease, pelvic and para-aortic node sampling. The prognosis is similar to endometrial cancer (depending on stage) for low-grade lesions but is poor ($<$ 50 per cent 5-year survival) for others.

Neonatal death (NND) Death of baby within 7 days of delivery.

Neural tube defect (NTD) Congenital abnormality of development of fetal spine or skull.

Occipitoposterior position (OP) Commonest malposition (10–15 per cent labours, persistent in 5 per cent). More common in certain types of pelvis or where the fetal head is deflexed at onset of labour. May be suspected antenatally if the head is difficult to palpate or the umbilicus is lower than the fundus. Intrapartum diagnosis is made by vaginal examination and is typically associated with failure of the head to descend and a poorly applied cervix.

Oligomenorrhoea Infrequent periods occurring between 6 weeks and 6 months apart.

Oogenesis Primordial germ cells develop in the yolk sac by the fourth week of fetal development and migrate to the genital ridge where they undergo mitotic division. These primary oocytes undergo meiotic division to produce a single diploid secondary oocyte (the other daughter cell becoming a polar body, which degenerates) but remain suspended in prophase until ovulation. The second meiotic division commences as the oocyte enters the Fallopian tube and is finally completed after fertilization, resulting in a single haploid ovum with the remaining 23 chromosomes becoming a second 'polar body'.

Ovarian hyperstimulation syndrome (OHSS) Side-effect of drugs given to stimulate ovulation characterized by ovarian enlargement (theca lutein cysts), ascites, hypoalbuminaemia, haemoconcentration and abdominal pain.

Ovary An organ ($3 \times 2 \times 1$ cm) made up of cortex, medulla and hilum covered by a single layer of epithelium containing germinal follicles. Lies in the ovarian fossa adjacent to the obturator nerve, ureter and iliac vessels. Blood supply is from the ovarian arteries and venous drainage to the inferior vena cava (right) and renal vein (left). Lymph drains to the para-aortic nodes.

Oxytocin Hormone produced by the posterior pituitary which stimulates myometrial contraction. Also stimulates milk ejection but not secretion. Synthetic oxytocin (Syntocinon) is used to induce or augment labour.

Pelvic inflammatory disease (PID) Ascending infection of the upper genital tract usually involving either the uterus (endometritis) or Fallopian tubes (salpingitis).

Perinatal mortality rate (PMR) The number of stillbirths and deaths within the first week of life per 1000 live births. The UK rate is 9 per 1000 births. The commonest causes in order of frequency are prematurity, congenital malformation, antepartum fetal death, perinatal asphyxia and infection.

Perineum The anatomical region defined by the symphysis pubis, ischial tuberosities and coccyx. Divided by the line between tuberosities into the anal and urogenital triangles.

Placenta praevia The placenta is implanted in the lower uterine segment and lies below the presenting part of the fetus. Occurs in 1 in 200 pregnancies.

Polycystic ovarian syndrome (PCOS) An endocrine disorder of uncertain aetiology characterized by one or more of anovulation, oligomenorrhoea, subfertility, weight gain, hirsutism and insulin resistance.

Position The relationship of the presenting part to the maternal pelvis. This is described in terms of the position of the denominator of the presenting part in relation to the maternal pubic symphysis. For a cephalic presentation with a vertex presenting part this will normally be occipito-anterior at delivery.

Postcoital test An infertility investigation involving taking a sample of cervical mucus after intercourse to look for viable motile spermatozoa.

Postmenopausal bleeding (PMB) Bleeding from the genital tract occurring more than 12 months after the menopause.

Postpartum haemorrhage (PPH) Primary PPH is defined as a blood loss of more than 500 mL within 24 hours of delivery of the fetus. Secondary PPH is excessive bleeding occurring within 42 days of delivery.

Pregnancy-induced hypertension (PIH) Blood pressure of more than 140/90 mmHg on two or more occasions occurring in a previously normotensive woman in the second half of pregnancy. Usually taken to be the same as non-proteinuric hypertension of pregnancy as opposed to pre-eclampsia.

Prelabour rupture of membranes (PLROM) Spontaneous draining of amniotic fluid occurring prior to the onset of regular painful uterine contractions. Occurs in approximately 15 per cent of pregnancies. Associated with increased incidence of malpresentations and dysfunctional labour.

Premature rupture of membranes (PROM) Rupture of membranes prior to 37 completed weeks of pregnancy.

Premenstrual syndrome (PMS) Recurring physical, emotional or behavioural symptoms severe enough to disrupt social, family or occupational life occurring in the premenstrual phase which resolve or improve markedly by the end of menstruation.

Presentation The fetal part currently in the lower part of the uterus over the pelvic brim. This is cephalic (head), breech (buttocks) or shoulder. Ninety-five per cent of pregnancies at term have a cephalic presentation.

Presenting part The part of the presentation which lies immediately inside the internal os. This is determined by vaginal examination in labour. For a cephalic presentation this can be vertex, brow or face.

Preterm Before 37 completed weeks of pregnancy.

Prolactin Hormone secreted by the anterior pituitary. Stimulates milk secretion but also has a role in luteinization and progesterone production. Levels increase at mid-cycle and remain elevated during the luteal phase. Levels are increased in pregnancy and the puerperium. Secretion is regulated by prolactin-inhibiting factor (dopamine) released by the hypothalamus. Dopamine antagonists will therefore cause an increase in prolactin levels. High levels of prolactin inhibit pituitary release of LH and FSH.

Puberty A sequence of physical changes resulting in the adult fertile female occurring over 5–10 years in response to increased frequency of GnRH release from the hypothalamus. The five key stages are growth spurt, followed by breast development, then pubic hair growth, menarche and, lastly, axillary hair growth.

Puerperium The period up to 6 weeks after delivery. Oestrogen and progesterone reach pre-pregnancy levels by 72 hours. Uterine weight falls by 50 per cent in the first 7 days. By day 7–10 the endometrial surface covers the placental site and the cervix closes. Ovulation resumes on average by day 40 (4 months if lactating). By week 6 the uterus has normally returned to its pre-pregnancy size. There is relative hypo-oestrogenization if breast-feeding. Haemoglobin increases initially then falls to reach a nadir at 3–4 days. Plasma volume returns to pre-pregnancy levels by 9 days but there is increased coagulability and risk of VTE for up to 7 weeks.

Royal College of Obstetricians and Gynaecologists (RCOG) Body responsible for postgraduate training and examination in obstetrics and gynaecology (MRCOG) in the UK.

Show Bloodstained mucoid vaginal discharge from the cervix associated with cervical changes preceding labour.

Spermatogenesis Spermatogonia (diploid) develop into spermatocytes, which undergo meiosis to spermatids then spermatozoa (haploid). This takes 74 days, during which the developing sperm are nourished by Sertoli cells stimulated by FSH. LH stimulates Leydig cells to release testosterone and stimulate spermatogenesis.

Squamocolumnar junction (SCJ) The line at which the columnar epithelium of the endocervix and the squamous epithelium of the ectocervix meet.

Station The position of the presenting part relative to the ischial spines.

Stillbirth Fetus born with no signs of life after 24 weeks' gestation.

Symphysis–fundal height (SFH) Distance in cm from the top of the symphysis pubis bone to the uterine fundus. Used as an indicator of fetal growth, the height in cm $\pm$ 2 should approximate to the gestational age in weeks after 20 weeks. Recently, more accurate SFH–gestational age charts have been introduced into maternity records.

Syphilis (*Treponemum pallidum*) A treponemal infection (others include yaws and pinta). Sexual and vertical transmission occurs with an incubation period of 9–90 days. The primary infection usually presents 3–6 weeks after infection with chancre (painless genital ulceration) and inguinal lymphadenopathy. The commonest site for chancre in women is the cervix and it may therefore be relatively asymptomatic. The primary infection will resolve after a few weeks if untreated. Secondary syphilis may arise immediately after the primary disease or up to 6 months later. Signs include rash, fever, joint pains, condylomata lata (wart-like lesions), iritis and hepatitis. It can be diagnosed using microscopy of fluid obtained from the primary lesion mixed with saline. The most sensitive serological test is the fluorescent treponemal antibody test (FTA). In primary disease, serology may be negative. Intramuscular penicillin 1.2 Mu for 12 days is the treatment of choice. Contact tracing may need to involve partners from several years ago.

Term The period of gestation from 37 completed weeks to 41 weeks and 6 days.

Transformation zone (TZ) The region of the ectocervix between the current and previous SCJ.

Transvaginal (transabdominal) ultrasound scan Principal method of imaging used in obstetrics and gynaecology. Transvaginal scan (TVS) gives more information about early pregnancy. Abdominal scanning is used for most obstetric imaging.

Trial of scar (TOS) Term used to describe labour in a woman who has had a previous Caesarean section.

Trichomonas vaginalis (TV) A protozoan with four flagellae. It is sexually transmitted. Infection may be asymptomatic or present with symptoms of a mucopurulent, yellow or green offensive vaginal discharge associated with vulvovaginitis. The cervix may have a 'strawberry' appearance because of the presence of punctate haemorrhages. Flagellate organisms can be seen on wet slide preparation or cultured. Treatment is with metronidazole 400 mg twice daily for 7 days (200 mg three times a day in pregnancy) or 2 g as a single dose. Treat partners and check for other STDs (gonorrhoea).

Trisomy The presence of an additional chromosome. Trisomy 21 (Down's syndrome) is the commonest, occurring in 1 in 900 pregnancies.

Trophoblast After fertilization, the initial ball of cells (morula) is transformed into the blastocyst by the formation of a fluid-filled cavity. The outer layer of the cells of the blastocyst forms the cytotrophoblast. After implantation, the trophoblast invades the endometrium and the outer layer becomes a syncytium. This is known as the syncytiotrophoblast and induces the decidual reaction in the adjacent endometrial cells. Invading cords of trophoblast grow down to the basal layers of the decidua, forming primary villi. The area of the trophoblast which becomes the placenta is known as the chorion frondosum. The villi in the remaining trophoblast become atrophic and this area (chorion laeve) develops into the outer layer of the fetal membranes.

Trophoblastic disease An anembryonic conception characterized by hyperplastic trophoblast, with syncytiotrophoblast and cytotrophoblast elements, hydropic villi, placental vacuolation and destruction of normal stroma. Includes partial and complete molar pregnancies.

Ultrasound scan (USS) An imaging method based on the transmission of sound frequencies between 3 and 8 MHz and the detection of the echoes this generates in tissue when it meets interfaces of different densities.

Umbilical artery pulsatility index (UAPI) One of the indices of blood flow through the umbilical vessels measured using Doppler ultrasound; an increased value may indicate placental disease.

Ureter Approximately 25 cm long, this runs anterior to the psoas along the transverse processes of lumbar spines, crossed by ovarian vessels. It enters the pelvis anterior to the bifurcation of the common iliacs (SI joints) and runs anterior to the internal iliac to the ischial spines where it turns medially to the cervix. It turns anteriorly 1.5 cm from the vaginal fornix under the uterine artery to enter the posterior surface of the bladder.

Urethra The mucosa is transitional proximally and stratified squamous distally, supported by rich venous plexus surrounded by longitudinal and circular layers of smooth muscle.

Urinary tract infection (UTI) Presence of more than 10^5 organisms/mL. Usually associated with increased white cell count. More common in pregnancy.

Urogenital triangle Perforated by the urethra and vagina. The superficial part contains the vestibule, vestibular glands, bulbospongiosis, clitoris, ischiocavernosus and perineal body. The deeper layers contain the superficial transverse and perineal muscles and the sphincter urethrae.

Uterus An organ of size $9 \times 5 \times 2.5$ cm. Divided into the corpus (fundus and body) and cervix (supravaginal and vaginal). Consists of serosa, myometrium and endometrium (1–5 mm thick). It is related anteriorly to the bladder, posteriorly to the pouch of Douglas, ileum and colon, and laterally to the broad ligaments, uterine vessels, tubes, ovaries and ureters. It gets its blood supply from the ovarian and uterine vessels (which are branches of the anterior division of the internal iliac artery). Its lymphatic drainage is to the para-aortic, internal and external iliac, obturator and superficial inguinal lymph nodes. It is supported by levator ani, transverse cervical, sacrocervical ligaments and the pubocervical condensation of pelvic fascia.

Vagina Approximately 7–9 cm long. Wider laterally. Four fornices defined by the cervix. Lined by squamous epithelium with no glands. A pH of less than 4.5 is maintained by action of Döderlein's bacilli on glycogen (oestrogen-sensitive). Related anteriorly to the bladder, urethra and urogenital triangle; posteriorly to the rectum, perineal body and anal canal; and laterally to the ureters, vessels, levator ani and urogenital diaphragm. Blood supply is from the uterine and vaginal arteries. It is normally supported by transverse and sacrocervical ligaments, urogenital diaphragm and the perineal body.

Vaginal birth after Caesarean section (VBAC) The VBAC rate is the proportion of women who deliver vaginally after having a previous Caesarean section. The overall rate in the UK is 44 per cent.

Vertex The area of the fetal skull bounded by the two parietal eminences and the anterior and posterior fontanelles. This is the presenting part in normal labour.

Vulva Made up of the labia majora (hair, sweat glands and sebaceous glands) and the labia minora (no hair, sebaceous glands and erectile tissue). The blood supply is from the pudendal artery. Lymph drains to the superficial inguinal nodes (medial group) and internal iliac nodes. The nerve supply is L1 (anterior labia), S2, 3, 4 (posterior labia) and S5 (anal skin) via the ilioinguinal, pudendal and posterior femoral cutaneous nerves.

Vulval intraepithelial neoplasia (VIN) Neoplastic vulval dermatosis. Equivalent to CIN in the cervix but with a lower risk of progression to malignancy.

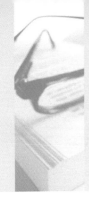

Appendix C

Self-assessment questions

Questions

Question 1

A 41-year-old woman attends the antenatal booking clinic at 12 weeks' gestation. She has had one previous pregnancy that was complicated by pre-eclampsia and culminated in the delivery of a male infant (birth-weight 1.7 kg) by elective Caesarean section at 35 weeks' gestation. **Plan the management for the remainder of the pregnancy.**

Question 2

A 27-year-old woman attends the antenatal clinic at 41 weeks' gestation in her first pregnancy. On examination, the symphysis–fundal height is 40 cm and a breech presenting part is identified. The pregnancy is otherwise uncomplicated. **Discuss the management options.**

Question 3

A 23-year-old smoker attends the antenatal booking clinic at 15 weeks' gestation. Her weight is 103 kg. An ultrasound scan reveals a twin pregnancy with two separate placentae, and her haemoglobin estimation is 8.3 g/dL. Other examination and investigation findings are unremarkable.
List the complications which she is at risk of, and detail your management of the pregnancy.

Question 4

A 17-year-old heroin addict attends the labour ward 1 hour after having lost approximately 100 mL blood vaginally. She is approximately 7 months pregnant and her HIV status is uncertain. She has had no antenatal care. Findings on general and abdominal examination are unremarkable.
Outline the management of the remainder of the pregnancy.

Question 5

A 27-year-old woman attends the antenatal clinic at 14 weeks' gestation in her second pregnancy. Her first pregnancy had ended 12 months earlier in the vaginal delivery of a stillborn baby at 33 weeks' gestation. Subsequent investigations indicated that haemolytic disease of the newborn was responsible for the still-birth; her blood group is A Rh-negative, and her husband's blood group is A Rh-positive (homozygous). Her past medical history is complicated by a road traffic accident and blood transfusion 5 years previously, and a deep vein thrombosis 3 years previously.
Discuss the management of the pregnancy.

Question 6

You are looking after a primigravida in labour. She has been fully dilated for 2 hours and pushing for an hour. The head is not visible and she is exhausted. She has had no pain relief except for Entonox.
Discuss the options available.

Question 7

A woman is admitted to the labour ward following a large ante-partum haemorrhage. This is her fourth pregnancy and she has had no previous problems. She is at 39 weeks' gestation.
How would you plan her management?

Question 8

A 24-year-old woman is admitted in her third pregnancy at 26 weeks' gestation. She has been experiencing increasingly painful tightenings and has felt a gush of fluid vaginally. Her last pregnancy ended at 32 weeks after a labour of 40 minutes. Her baby spent 29 days on the neonatal unit.
Discuss how you would investigate and manage this woman.

Question 9

A 21-year-old primigravida is admitted collapsed after a witnessed fit. She is in a postictal state and is barely conscious. She is 34 weeks' pregnant and is treated for epilepsy. Her fits are usually well controlled.
How would you investigate and treat this woman?

Question 10

A 39-year-old woman is seen in the antenatal clinic. Her midwife has told her that her baby is large and she is requesting induction of labour at 38 weeks' gestation. This is her fifth pregnancy. Her last infant weighed 3.9 kg at delivery at 41 weeks and was delivered after a spontaneous labour with no problems.
How would you advise this woman?

Question 11

A 29-year-old woman is referred to the clinic because her last three cervical smears have been reported as inadequate. She is using the pill for contraception. She has had three episodes of postcoital bleeding over the last 6 months. She is a smoker.
How would you manage her?

Question 12

A 34-year-old woman presents in the clinic with a 12-month history of infrequent periods and secondary infertility. She has noticed some weight gain. She has had one previous pregnancy, at the age of 16, and she had a therapeutic termination at 12 weeks complicated by uterine perforation requiring laparotomy. Her new partner is unaware of this and believes that her abdominal scar is due to an operation for an ovarian cyst. He has no previous children but had mumps as a child.
Describe how you establish a diagnosis and counsel this couple.

Question 13

You are asked to see a 15-year-old girl who is pregnant and requesting termination. She has come to the clinic unaccompanied and does not wish her parents to know about the pregnancy. She is uncertain when her last period was and is complaining of an offensive vaginal discharge.
How would you counsel her about the pregnancy and future contraception?

Question 14

A 54-year-old lady is referred by her general practitioner with incontinence of urine. Her doctor has performed a vaginal examination and found a moderate degree of cystocele and marked atrophic changes. She passes urine every hour during the day and has to get up at night. She has been told that she will need a vaginal repair operation.
How would you assess and advise her?

Question 15

A 43-year-old nulliparous woman presents to her GP with a 6-month history of increasingly heavy, painful periods and deep dyspareunia. On examination she has a fixed 10 cm mass arising from the pelvis.
Describe your management.

Answers

Question 1

The first step is to identify the problems:

- Increased maternal age – particular risk of fetal chromosomal anomaly
- Previous history of pre-eclampsia – risk of recurrence
- Previous history of fetal growth restriction – risk of recurrence
- Previous Caesarean section.
- The management plan must address each of these problems.

Increased maternal age (see Chapter 9, Fetal abnormality: chromosomal)

- Counsel regarding the risk of a fetal chromosomal anomaly. The risk of a fetus with Down's syndrome is approximately 1:60 on the basis of maternal age alone.
- Discuss risk predictor screening tests: biochemical and ultrasound assessments of risk.
- Discuss the invasive diagnostic tests of amniocentesis and chorionic villous sampling (CVS).

Previous history of pre-eclampsia (see Chapter 11, Hypertension)

- Confirm previous diagnosis by reviewing the medical records to ensure that the diagnosis was accurate.
- Counselling: the overall recurrence rate following a pregnancy complicated by pre-eclampsia is 25 per cent. However, the history suggests early-onset disease, thus the recurrence rate is increased, and the woman should be forewarned regarding this potential complication.
- Low-dose aspirin prophylaxis may be of some benefit and should be considered.
- Anticoagulant prophylaxis should only be considered if a thrombophilia screen performed after the previous pregnancy identified an underlying thrombotic tendency.
- Increased surveillance with hospital referral if proteinuria or hypertension occurs.

Previous history of fetal growth restriction (see Chapter 21, Small for gestational age)

- Increased surveillance to detect any recurrence. This should include serial ultrasound measurements of fetal size.
- Assessment of fetal well-being (fetal heart rate monitoring, ultrasound measurement of biophysical profile, Doppler umbilical artery waveform analysis) if growth restriction is detected.

Previous Caesarean section (see Chapter 15, Previous Caesarean section)

- Decision regarding mode of delivery. The woman's views should be sought; if the pregnancy is uncomplicated, a vaginal delivery can be planned.
- Discussion of management in labour. Later in pregnancy, if no complications have ensued, issues such as analgesia, use of oxytocics and the duration of any labour can be discussed.

Question 2

The first step is to identify the problems:

- Breech presentation in a nulliparous patient (see Chapter 7, Breech presentation).
- Prolonged pregnancy, or a pregnancy that has continued beyond the estimated date of delivery (see Chapter 17, Prolonged pregnancy). The gestational age should be consistent with an early pregnancy dating ultrasound scan.

The next step is to obtain additional information:

- The woman's views regarding the mode and timing of delivery should be sought and discussed.
- An ultrasound scan should be performed in order to confirm the presentation, determine the type of breech, exclude an obvious fetal anomaly or hyperextension of the fetal neck, estimate liquor volume and placental site, and estimate fetal weight.
- A pelvic examination will determine if the cervix is favourable; if the Bishop's score is > 4, the cervix is considered to be favourable (see Chapter 30).

The management of this case is still somewhat contentious (see Chapter 7). However, dependent on the additional information obtained, there are a number of management options which may be considered:

- *External cephalic version (ECV) (Chapter 7)*. ECV, particularly when performed with tocolysis, is a safe procedure in selected cases. If the fetal legs are extended, the uterus is irritable or the liquor volume is reduced, the procedure is less likely to be successful. If successful, the onset of labour can then be induced (particularly if the cervix is favourable) or awaited.
- *Elective Caesarean section*. Factors that would favour this option include a maternal desire for a Caesarean section, unsuitable for or failed ECV, an ultrasound estimation of fetal weight $>$ 3.8 kg or evidence of fetal growth restriction, a footling breech presentation, oligo/polyhydramnios, and an unfavourable cervix. If labour were to ensue prior to the date of the planned Caesarean section, a trial of vaginal delivery could be considered or delivery effected by emergency Caesarean section.
- *Induction of labour*. Following the publication of the term breech trial, this is now likely to be considered only where there is a maternal desire for a vaginal delivery following failed ECV. However, all patients should be counselled about this option as, although there appears to be an increased risk to the baby associated with vaginal breech delivery, the overall risk remains low and some couples will be prepared to accept this level of risk to avoid an operative delivery. A favourable cervix, an estimated fetal weight $<$ 3.8 kg and an extended breech presentation would probably be required. Labour may be induced by prostaglandin preparations or artificial rupture of membranes $\pm$ an intravenous Syntocinon infusion (Chapter 30, Induction of labour).
- *Conservative management*. Delivery could be deferred (with or without ECV) for a further 1–2 weeks, i.e. the onset of spontaneous labour awaited. If this option is chosen, there should be increased surveillance of fetal well-being: ideally this should include weekly biophysical profile measurement and Doppler umbilical artery waveform analysis (Chapter 20).

Question 3

The first step is to identify the problems:

- Twin pregnancy: as two placental sites are seen, the pregnancy is dichorionic
- Anaemia
- Smoking
- Maternal obesity.

Each of these problems is associated with particular complications.

Dichorionic twin pregnancy (see Chapter 14, Multiple pregnancy)

- Pregnancy-induced hypertension and pre-eclampsia

- Preterm labour
- Intrauterine growth restriction
- Antepartum haemorrhage
- Malpresentation
- Postpartum haemorrhage.

Increased risks of structural anomalies, twin–twin transfusions and polyhydramnios principally relate to monochorionic twin pregnancies.

Anaemia (see Chapter 5, Anaemia in pregnancy)

The complications of anaemia are largely non-specific – tiredness and fatigue, breathlessness, oedema, palpitations, and eventually fainting.

Obesity

- Gestational diabetes
- Pre-eclampsia
- Difficulty in assessment of fetal size and diagnosis of fetal malpresentation
- Increased anaesthetic and operative risk
- Thromboembolism.

Smoking (see Chapter 22, Substance abuse)

- Intrauterine growth restriction
- Preterm delivery and premature prelabour rupture of membranes (PPROM)
- Placental abruption.

Management

Booking visit. The anaemia is likely to be due to iron deficiency or an inherited disorder. Red cell indices should be checked and, if indicated, haemoglobin electrophoresis should be performed. Iron supplementation should be prescribed. Encouragement to stop or discontinue smoking should be given.

Subsequent antenatal visits. Additional measurements of blood pressure and urine dipstick testing are indicated, in an effort to detect pre-eclampsia at an early stage. Serial ultrasound assessment of fetal size will enable measurement of fetal growth. The haemoglobin concentration should be regularly checked; if there is no response to iron therapy, compliance should be ensured and other causes of anaemia considered. A glucose tolerance test should be performed at 28–32 weeks' gestation.

Careful counselling regarding the signs and symptoms of premature labour should be stressed; the need for prompt attendance at hospital if uterine activity is noted should be emphasized. A plan for delivery should be determined and will depend on fetal growth and presentation.

Intrapartum and postpartum. The intrapartum management of multiple pregnancies is discussed in Chapter 14 . Following delivery, a Syntocinon infusion should be instigated to reduce the risk of postpartum haemorrhage, and thromboprophylaxis should be prescribed (Chapter 44).

Question 4

The first step is to identify the problems:
- Antepartum haemorrhage – risk of recurrence and fetal compromise
- Opiate addiction – direct complications and lifestyle problems associated with drug dependence
- Uncertain HIV status – risk of transmission to the fetus
- Uncertain gestational age.

The management plan must address each of these problems.

Antepartum haemorrhage (see Chapter 25, Antepartum haemorrhage)
- Admission to hospital.
- Venepuncture – blood should be taken for a full blood count and for grouping and saving of serum.
- Establishment of an intravenous line in case bleeding recurs.
- Ultrasound scan to localize the placenta. No vaginal examination should be performed unless a diagnosis of placenta praevia has been excluded.
- Tests of fetal well-being – as a minimum, this should include ultrasound estimation of liquor volume and fetal heart rate monitoring.
- Further management will depend on whether a diagnosis of a placental abruption or placenta praevia is made, and is discussed further in Chapter 25.

Opiate addiction (see Chapter 22, Substance abuse)
- Tests of fetal well-being and serial ultrasound estimations of fetal growth.
- Involvement of social workers to assist with social problems.
- Involvement of drug dependency unit and consideration of methadone substitution programme.
- Screen for sexually transmitted infections.
- Involvement of anaesthetists in management plan for delivery.
- Discussion with paediatrician regarding potential neonatal withdrawal syndrome.

Uncertain HIV status (see Chapter 12, Infections in pregnancy)
Counselling regarding exposure to HIV – if appropriate, testing of HIV status should be offered; vertical transmission to the fetus is markedly reduced by zidovudine treatment (AZT), Caesarean section and avoidance of breast-feeding.

Uncertain gestational age
It will not be possible to estimate the gestational age with any accuracy and this should be explained. Ultrasound biometry in the second half of pregnancy is imprecise, particularly in cases at risk of intra-uterine growth restriction.

Question 5

The first step is to identify the problems:
- Previous history of haemolytic disease of the newborn. Assuming the father is the same as in the previous pregnancy, there is a high chance of a recurrence (her husband is Rh-positive homozygous and ABO-compatible)
- Previous stillbirth
- Previous deep vein thrombosis (DVT).

The management plan must address each of these problems.

Previous history of haemolytic disease of the newborn (see Chapter 4, Abnormal antibodies: blood group incompatibility)
- Precise details regarding the previous pregnancy must be obtained. This will include the gestation at which any abnormality was first apparent and the condition of the fetus (presence or absence of hydrops, haemoglobin) at delivery.
- The severity of the disease in the previous pregnancy and the antibody titre will determine the need for invasive tests (cordocentesis/amniocentesis).
- Serial ultrasound scans to check for fetal hydrops.
- Intrauterine transfusions if necessary (these can be combined with cordocentesis).
- Surveillance of fetal well-being (Chapters 20 and 21).
- Elective delivery at gestation, dependent on the severity of the disease.

Previous stillbirth (see Chapter 16, Previous fetal loss)
The history of fetal loss provides a further reason for:
- serial ultrasound scan estimations of fetal growth
- tests of fetal well-being
- elective delivery.

Previous deep vein thrombosis (see Chapter 44)
- Ensure that an objective diagnosis (venography, ultrasonography, MRI) was made.
- Determine the degree of risk of a recurrence on the basis of whether additional factors (family history or a thrombophilia) are present.
- Simple prophylactic measures – early mobilization, elastic stockings, calf stimulation if delivery is by Caesarean section.
- Plan appropriate anticoagulant prophylaxis (depending on the risk).

Question 6

The first step is to make a diagnosis as to why the second stage is prolonged. This will include:
- an assessment of the whole labour (Chapter 27, Failure to progress in the first stage)
- abdominal palpation to assess the size of the fetus and the engagement of the presenting part
- a vaginal examination to identify position, station, moulding
- an assessment of the frequency of uterine activity.

The other factors that must be ascertained are:

- the status of the fetus (Chapter 29, Abnormal fetal heart rate patterns in labour)
- the need for analgesia (Chapter 36, Pain relief in labour).

Management

The management options will depend on the finding at examination. The questions that must be answered are:

- Are the contractions efficient? This is the commonest cause of failure to progress in primigravida (Chapter 27).
- Is this a problem caused by a malposition? Malposition is commonly associated with epidural analgesia. It is less common when Entonox is used, but if contractions are inefficient, it can occur. Malposition increases the diameter of the presenting part.
- Is this a problem caused because the fetus is too large? This is true cephalopelvic disproportion. It is rare and only occurs when the head is fully rotated into an occipito-anterior position, when there is significant moulding, and when uterine activity is efficient. The diagnosis can only be made in a primigravida when effective uterine activity has been ensured. This usually requires a short trial of Syntocinon.
- Is the fetus tolerating labour adequately? Only if fetal well-being is not a concern can the labour be allowed to continue. Concerns about fetal well-being should prompt further assessment, e.g. fetal scalp sampling, or delivery without delay.

The options for management can be divided now into:

- delivery by assisted means by instrumental vaginal delivery or Caesarean section
- short trial of Syntocinon.

If delivery by instrumental means is considered, the requirements outlined in Chapter 28 must be met (failure to progress in the second stage). Analgesia must be provided by either local infiltration or spinal/epidural anaesthesia. If the fetus is thought to be large, consideration of the risk of shoulder dystocia (Chapter 40) must be taken into account, and help must be available quickly should difficulty delivering the shoulders be encountered.

Caesarean section would be considered if the fetal condition necessitated and vaginal delivery was not deemed safe and also if true cephalopelvic disproportion was suspected.

A short trial of Syntocinon would generally need improved analgesia for the mother in terms of epidural or opiates.

There should be progress during the next hour and delivery should be expedited if the fetal condition deteriorates. Delivery should be accomplished usually within the next hour. A full explanation should be provided for the mother and her partner.

Question 7

The important features are:

- Assessment of the maternal condition and resuscitation (Chapter 25, Antepartum haemorrhage; Chapter 32, Maternal collapse)
- Assessment of the fetal condition and the need for urgent delivery (Chapter 29)
- Diagnosis of the cause of bleeding.

The first steps are:

- Assess and stabilize the maternal condition (blood pressure, pulse rate, quick assessment of the degree of continuing bleeding).
- Venous access should be obtained.
- Blood should be taken for full blood count, clotting screen and cross-match 4 units.
- A fetal heart rate recording should be performed to assess fetal well-being.

A history of the degree of bleeding and association with any pain should be taken. The mother may have knowledge of predisposing features such as a low-lying placenta on scan. Examination of the abdomen may reveal signs of abruption (tense, tender uterus). A high presenting part may point towards a placenta praevia.

A vaginal examination to assess the cervical dilatation can only be safely performed if the placental position is known.

The next step is to decide whether immediate delivery is needed, and by what route.

Delivery must be expedited if the fetus is in jeopardy. This usually requires a Caesarean section, although occasionally the cervix will be almost fully dilated and a vaginal delivery is possible. If the fetus is compromised, a placental abruption is the most likely cause and heavy bleeding must be expected. Strategies to avoid severe postpartum haemorrhage (Chapter 37) must be utilized, e.g. Syntocinon infusion for 4 hours.

Severe continuing bleeding from a suspected or confirmed placenta praevia will also require delivery. Again, strategies to avoid heavy bleeding must be undertaken. The paediatric staff should be alerted to ensure that full neonatal resuscitation can occur.

If immediate delivery is not required, a plan must be made for the subsequent management. Generally, heavy bleeding at 39 weeks is an indication for planned delivery soon. Further investigations, e.g. ultrasound assessment of placental site, fetal size and liquor volume, may be undertaken before planning the timing and method of delivery.

If the placenta is praevia, an elective Caesarean section with senior staff available should be planned for the near future. Heavy marginal bleeding is an indication for induction of labour. This should also be planned electively.

Only under exceptional circumstances should delivery not be undertaken within a short time. If the mother is not amenable to delivery, then steps must be taken to ensure continuing fetal well-being. These will include:

- ultrasound for fetal growth
- biophysical profile
- regular fetal assessments until labour ensues.

Question 8

The first stage is to establish whether labour is advanced. Only if labour is in the early stages or has not begun will there be the opportunity to intervene.

It is important to establish the history of contractions and the gush of fluid. Examination of the abdomen should be performed to assess:

- contractions/uterine irritability
- fetal size
- presentation and engagement of the presenting part.

The maternal pulse, blood pressure and temperature must be taken. A CTG should be performed to assess fetal well-being.

A vaginal examination should be performed in two stages. A sterile speculum examination should be done first to see whether the membranes are ruptured. A high vaginal swab should be taken. If liquor is seen, visualization of the cervix is helpful as a digital examination can be avoided if the cervix is seen to be closed. If there is no liquor seen, or the cervix cannot be visualized, a digital examination may be performed to assess dilatation, effacement and station of the presenting part.

The situation can now be divided into two likely scenarios:

The woman is indeed in labour, either with or without confirmed rupture of the membranes. This means that the cervix is more than 4 cm dilated and there is regular uterine activity. Suppression of labour at this stage is unlikely to be successful. In this case, the aims of management are to ensure the safe delivery of the fetus in the best possible condition.

The important factors are:

- To assess the presentation.
- To look for and treat immediately any signs of chorioamnionitis.
- It remains contentious as to whether a breech presentation is more safely delivered by Caesarean section, but is it now common practice. Cephalic-presenting fetuses derive no benefit from Caesarean section if they are coping with the stress of labour.
- Infection is the commonest cause of preterm labour. Signs of chorioamnionitis will include:
  - maternal pyrexia
  - maternal tachycardia
  - fetal tachycardia
  - offensive liquor.

Treatment with antibiotics should not be delayed, as the fetus derives significant benefits from aggressive treatment, especially if group B *Streptococcus* is implicated.

Labour is not advanced, in which case strategies to improve fetal outcome can be instituted. These strategies include:

- steroids for fetal lung maturity
- suppression of uterine activity until 24 hours has elapsed
- consideration of antibiotics.

The remainder of the pregnancy can be planned once the immediate danger of labour is passed. The main features are:

- Treatment of any confirmed infection (HVS, urinary).
- Conservative management of ruptured membranes until 34 weeks with careful surveillance for developing chorioamnionitis, looking for the above features.
- Full assessment of fetal well-being, including fetal size, liquor volume and, if small, umbilical artery Doppler velocity measurement.

If labour does not ensue in the following 48 hours, the immediate danger is passed. The role of oral tocolytics is not established, neither is it clear that steroid doses need to be repeated if the risk is thought to continue. Women with confirmed rupture of membranes should be advised to remain in hospital for at least 3–4 days, when the risks of infection and labour are highest. If labour does not ensue in this time, some would elect to manage as an outpatient. In-patient management is the safest, but prolonged periods of time in hospital are difficult for many women to tolerate. If the woman goes home at least weekly, maternal and fetal assessment should be organized and the mother advised to return immediately if any signs of uterine activity or infection occur.

Question 9

The first step is to ensure the safety of the mother (see Chapter 32, Maternal collapse):

- Airway
- Breathing
- Circulation.

A full team is needed to assist in the resuscitation. Once the condition of the mother appears stable, every effort must be made to establish whether this is a fit due to epilepsy or eclampsia. Although the woman has epilepsy, it must not be assumed that this is the cause (see Chapter 32).

Features of eclampsia must be sought:

- blood pressure
- urinalysis
- hyperreflexia
- papilloedema
- blood for full blood count, clotting, renal and liver function.

Other factors may help to clarify the situation, including:

- an examination of the pregnancy record, if available, as previous hypertension or proteinuria may be documented
- evidence of fetal growth restriction
- problems with medication (missed pills, vomiting etc.).

The presence of hypertension and proteinuria makes eclampsia likely. Stabilization of the mother and delivery are the mainstays of management:

- Magnesium sulphate should be commenced.
- Fetal status should be confirmed.
- Maternal haematological and renal function should be ascertained.

- Delivery should be expedited by the safest method (usually Caesarean section after confirmation of normal clotting status). If clotting is abnormal, correction may be needed whilst delivery is being planned.

The mother must be intensively monitored in a high-dependency unit until the disease process has resolved (usually 24–48 hours after delivery).

If no signs of eclampsia are found, await spontaneous recovery under observation. Once the mother is recovered, a full re-evaluation of epileptic medication should be undertaken.

Factors that may have predisposed to the fit will include:

- missed medication (often because of concern about the effects on the fetus)
- sleep deprivation (not uncommon during the latter stages of pregnancy).

If there are worries that treatment doses are too low, serum levels can be checked. These are most helpful to ensure that therapy is actually being taken. There are no concerns regarding teratogenicity at this gestation, and the aim should be to manage the remainder of the pregnancy with no fits. Additional medication can be considered.

Question 10

There are a number of issues to address here:

- Is the fetus large?
- Is there any reason for the fetal macrosomia?
- Will induction of labour reduce the risks to the mother or fetus?
- What other strategies need to be employed to ensure safe delivery of mother and child?

Assessment of fetal size (see Chapter 13, Large for gestational age)

Both clinical palpation and ultrasound are prone to a large degree of error in the assessment of fetal size. If the predicted fetal weight is much above the 95th centile, the fetus palpates large on clinical examination and the mother reports the fetus as being larger than before, the probability of fetal macrosomia is higher. However, the mother must realize that there is a large error, and the fetus may turn out to be significantly smaller than expected.

Risk factors for fetal macrosomia (see Chapter 13)

- Advanced maternal age
- Prior or family history of diabetes
- Previous large infant (>4 kg)
- Unexplained stillbirth
- Previous shoulder dystocia
- Persistent glycosuria.

These risk factors should be sought. If the fetus is macrosomic, a random blood sugar can be helpful. If this is < 6 mmol/L, gestational diabetes is unlikely. If there is any doubt, a full glucose tolerance test can be performed. If gestational diabetes is confirmed and the fetus is macrosomic, induction of labour may be a valid option.

If the fetus is large but there is no sign of gestational diabetes, the management is contentious. Induction of labour is not without risk and there is no evidence that induction before the fetus has an opportunity to grow more is associated with a better fetal or maternal outcome. This must be explained to the mother.

Risks of induction of labour (Chapter 30)

Induction of labour at 38 weeks' gestation carries a significant risk of failure and Caesarean section. This risk is higher when the cervix is unfavourable. A vaginal examination will help to determine whether induction is likely to succeed. The mother must understand that even a favourable cervix does not imply an easy labour. The use of Syntocinon in multigravidae is also not without risk (Chapter 27, Failure to progress in the first stage).

A careful weighing up of all of the factors and discussion with the mother about her anxieties should be undertaken. Induction must only be considered if the benefits are thought to outweigh the risks.

Intrapartum management (Chapter 40)

If the fetus is macrosomic, whether labour is spontaneous or induced, strategies to watch for shoulder dystocia must be employed. The major requirements are that someone experienced in the management of shoulder dystocia must attend delivery, a paediatrician should be alerted in the second stage, and difficult instrumental delivery should be avoided.

Question 11

First identify the problems:

- The cause of the bleeding needs to be identified and treated.
- It has not been possible to exclude cervical neoplasia by screening with cervical cytology.

Identify the cause of the bleeding (see Chapter 52, Intermenstrual bleeding)

- Ask about pill taking, other medication, vaginal discharge, other intermenstrual bleeding and last menstrual period (LMP). Ask about previous treatment for cervical neoplasia and the results of previous smears.
- Perform a speculum examination of the cervix.
- Take vaginal and cervical swabs to exclude infection.

If the LMP was abnormal or is late, pregnancy must be excluded. Cervical malignancy must be excluded by visual inspection and colposcopy but the most likely cause in a woman of this age is a benign cervical lesion such as an ectropion or polyp. These can be treated by cervical cautery or removal. Lower genital tract infections should be excluded by taking swabs. The bleeding may also be coming from the uterus or as breakthrough bleeding on the pill. Remember this may have implications for the reliability of the pill for contraception. Ask about compliance and other medication, including antibiotics. Consider changing the type of pill.

Whatever the cause, the bleeding may be the reason why it has not been possible to obtain a satisfactory smear.

Exclude cervical neoplasia (see Chapter 45, The abnormal cervical smear test)

Refer the patient for colposcopic assessment. Cervical intraepithelial neoplasia (CIN) does not cause bleeding. Postcoital bleeding may be a presenting symptom of cervical carcinoma. Referral for colposcopy is indicated in this case, even if there were no symptoms, because there have been three unsatisfactory smears. Patients should be seen within 8 weeks of referral or within 2 weeks if the appearance of the cervix raises a suspicion of malignancy. She should be encouraged to stop smoking, as this is an additional risk factor for CIN. Further treatment will depend on the diagnosis made at colposcopy.

Question 12

The key issues to address here are:

- What is the cause of the infrequent periods and how is this likely to affect her fertility?
- What effect has the previous termination of pregnancy had on her current fertility?
- The need to exclude male factor causes.
- Making a plan of management for treatment.
- The need to involve both partners in the investigation and treatment of the infertility whilst respecting the need of one for confidentiality about her previous history.

Infrequent periods

- Ask about previous menstrual history, other medication and abnormal hair growth.
- Check FSH, LH, prolactin.
- Arrange pelvic ultrasound.

The most likely cause is polycystic ovarian syndrome. This would also be consistent with the history of weight gain. The diagnosis can be confirmed by ultrasound examination of the ovaries and an increased LH:FSH ratio and an increased free androgen level. If the androgen levels are markedly elevated, further investigations for androgen-producing tumours should be arranged. Other causes such as hyperprolactinaemia should be excluded and a CT or MRI scan of the pituitary arranged if the prolactin level is significantly raised.

Previous termination

- If possible, obtain a copy of the notes of the previous surgery.
- Ask about any associated infections.
- Arrange hysterosalpingogram or laparoscopy and dye test.

The perforation of the uterus which occurred at the time of the previous termination is unlikely to cause secondary infertility, and Asherman's syndrome (adhesions within the uterus) is also unlikely if menstruation was normal until recently. More importantly, the events following the termination may have resulted in tubal damage as a result of ascending infection and this should be excluded by hysterosalpingogram or laparoscopy. Laparoscopy would probably give more information about peritubular adhesions but may be more hazardous if there is a midline scar from the previous laparotomy.

Male factor causes (see Chapter 51, Infertility)

- Ask about any history of infertility with other partners.
- Arrange for semen analysis.

Despite the more 'obvious' potential female cause for infertility, this does not exclude the possibility of a male factor. In this case it would be useful to know whether her partner has not previously had children out of choice. Mumps orchitis is a potential cause of azoospermia. A minimum of two semen analyses should be carried out.

Plan management

- Check rubella immunity
- Ovulation induction
- Assisted conception.

This will depend on the diagnosis. Significant tubal damage or oligospermia will probably require treatment by *in vitro* fertilization techniques. If these can be excluded, the likely diagnosis will be of anovulation due to PCOS. The couple could be reassured that spontaneous conception might still occur and weight loss should be encouraged. However, bearing in mind her age, it may be appropriate to instigate treatment at this stage with agents to induce ovulation. Initially this could be with clomiphene citrate monitored by serum day 21 progesterone levels or ultrasound tracking of follicles. The couple should be warned about the risk of multiple pregnancy.

Before embarking on any treatment, immunity to rubella should be confirmed.

The need to involve both partners

There is an absolute duty to respect the woman's wishes for confidentiality with respect to her previous history. At the same time she may harbour feelings of guilt or anxiety about the previous pregnancy and may feel that this is somehow the cause of the current problem or 'punishment' for the termination. If more invasive treatment such as IVF is required, these feelings may put considerable strain on the relationship and encouraging the woman at an early stage to talk to her partner about this (especially if this can be combined with reassurance after investigation that this is not the cause of her infertility) may help to reduce this.

Question 13

First identify the main problems:

- The need to establish whether termination is the appropriate course of action.
- Determining whether she is able to give informed consent for termination.

- Potential medicolegal and child protection issues of underage sexual intercourse.
- The need to exclude any sexually transmitted infection.
- The need to ensure adequate contraception after termination.

Decide if termination is appropriate (see Chapter 61, Termination of pregnancy)

- Establish gestation by clinical examination or ultrasound.
- Discuss her reasons for requesting termination and an alternative course of action.
- Try to determine if it is her own decision or if it is due to external pressure.

First establish on what basis pregnancy was confirmed and, if necessary, repeat the pregnancy test. Remember that oligomenorrhoea is more common in young teenagers. Gestational age will have a bearing on both the practical and legal aspects of termination. For example, termination after 24 weeks is not legal under the amended 1967 Abortion Act for clauses C and D. Termination after 12 weeks is usually done medically. She may not be aware of the implications of this and some practitioners or units may not be prepared to support this even if they perform earlier surgical terminations.

There needs to be a discussion about the risks of termination (which may be greater in a girl of this age in her first pregnancy than in an older multiparous woman) as well as the problems associated with having a baby at 15. The alternatives, such as adoption, also need to be explored. External pressure may not only be from family or partners but from other health care or social work professionals.

Consent

- Encourage her to discuss the matter with her parents.
- Gillick principles.

She has a right to confidentiality but should be encouraged to talk to her parents wherever possible. If she can or will not do this, she may still be able to consent to treatment if she can demonstrate that she is able to understand and retain the information given to her about termination. This is assumed for any competent person over 16 and may be the case here if you are satisfied that she:

- understands that there is a choice and that choices have consequences;
- shows a willingness and ability to make a choice;
- understands the nature and purpose of the termination;
- understands the potential risks and side-effects of termination;
- understands the consequences and risks of the alternatives to termination;
- is making her own decision free from outside pressure.

Medicolegal aspects

Although prosecutions are rare in practice, it is important to remember that intercourse with a girl under 16 is an offence. Intercourse may have occurred without her consent, in which case there will be the issue of assault or sexual abuse. In someone of this age, this may in fact constitute a child protection issue which all health care professionals have a statutory obligation to report.

Vaginal discharge (see Chapter 64)

- Take triple swabs.
- Antibiotic prophylaxis.

If she has been having unprotected intercourse, she is also at increased risk of sexually transmitted infection. If this is not treated, there is an increased risk of pelvic infection occurring after termination and subsequent infertility. Swabs should be taken from the vagina and endocervix to screen for *Chlamydia*, gonorrhoea and bacterial vaginosis. If the results are not available by the time of termination, antibiotic prophylaxis should be given. If a sexually transmitted infection is identified, appropriate follow-up to confirm cure and contact tracing of partners should be arranged with the local genitourinary medicine (GUM) clinic.

Contraception (see Chapter 48)

Whatever the outcome of the current pregnancy, it is essential to counsel and provide adequate contraception. The contraceptive pill can be started on the day of termination but requires a fairly high degree of compliance. Intrauterine contraceptive devices (IUCD) tend to be avoided in this age group and the side-effects of injectables may be a problem, but these have to be balanced against the risk of further unplanned pregnancies. Whatever method is chosen, she should also be encouraged to use barrier contraception to protect against infection. The same criteria as used when determining consent for termination need to be applied before prescribing contraception. It is essential to ensure adequate follow-up with her GP or local family planning clinic.

Question 14

The key issues here are:

- the causes of the urinary incontinence and appropriate treatment
- the relevance of the vaginal prolapse to this
- the patient's own expectations for treatment.

Incontinence

- Ask about when incontinence occurs and other urinary symptoms and the effect on daily life.
- Send midstream urine for culture.
- Refer to continence team (physiotherapy).
- Anticholinergics.

The common causes are detrusor instability and genuine stress incontinence (GSI). Urge incontinence is suggestive of detrusor instability whilst stress incontinence can occur in either. Detrusor instability is usually associated with other symptoms, especially nocturia and frequency of micturition. Treatment of any coexisting urinary infection is the first step in the management of any patient complaining of urinary symptoms.

Bladder pressure studies should be considered before undertaking any surgical treatment for incontinence, especially if there is a 'mixed' picture clinically. The management of detrusor instability will almost always be medical, with a combination of bladder retraining and anticholinergic drugs. Patients with mild to moderate degrees of genuine stress incontinence may also gain adequate control with pelvic floor exercises or stimulation.

Surgery is indicated in more severe cases of GSI or in those who fail to respond adequately to physiotherapy. In this case, the operation of choice will usually be a suspension procedure. Vaginal repair operations for prolapse are less likely to control incontinence. Where there is a mixture of both, the detrusor instability should be treated first.

Relevance of the prolapse

Ask about any other symptoms that may be due to prolapse. A large cystocele may lead to incomplete emptying and associated leakage of urine after micturition and may be associated with the pelvic floor weakness causing genuine stress incontinence. It is not likely to be a significant factor in urge incontinence.

Other prolapse symptoms include a dragging sensation or feeling of something coming down in the vagina, typically worse towards the end of the day. If prolapse is asymptomatic, it does not require treatment. It is likely in this case that the urinary symptoms are due, at least in part, to detrusor instability so will not be improved by surgical treatment of the prolapse.

Patient expectations

The symptoms may have been present for some time before the patient sought advice from her GP and may be a cause of considerable distress and embarrassment. Fear of incontinence and the need to be near a toilet may have significantly restricted her ability to leave the house. At the same time, surgical treatments are not 100 per cent effective and are not without complications. Conservative treatment may be preferable as long as the urinary symptoms can be improved sufficiently to allow her to function normally. Equally, the patient may have been left with the impression by her GP that she needs a vaginal repair operation to cure her urinary symptoms, and the reasons why this is probably not the case will need to be discussed with her (and her GP).

Question 15

First, think about the likely causes:
- endometriosis
- chronic pelvic inflammatory disease
- benign or malignant pelvic neoplasm.

Take a history and in particular ask about:
- any previous history of pelvic pain and investigations for this
- treatment for pelvic inflammatory disease or infections
- any recent change of partner and method of contraception
- date and result of last cervical smear

- any family history of breast or ovarian neoplasia
- wishes for future fertility.

Any of the above diagnoses can be associated with a change in the pattern of menstruation and period pain. However, it is relatively uncommon for ovarian tumours to present with pain, and when they do, it is usually acute as a result of torsion or rupture. Pelvic inflammatory disease (PID) is less common in this age group but may still occur if there has been a recent change of partner(s). An inflammatory tubo-ovarian mass may also occur in association with an intrauterine device. Endometriosis can give rise to a pelvic mass (ovarian endometriomas) and is more common in older nulliparous women.

On examination, look for:
- fever or signs of acute infection
- any signs of primary breast cancer
- whether the mass is palpable per abdomen and if it appears to arise from the pelvis
- whether the mass can be separated from the uterus on pelvic examination
- whether the mass is fixed or mobile
- the presence of any associated ascites.

The presence of a significant pyrexia and raised white cell count is suggestive of an inflammatory cause for the mass, but a low-grade temperature may also occur after torsion of any ovarian cyst or leakage of the contents into the peritoneal cavity.

If the mass is mobile, it is more likely to be a benign ovarian tumour. A fixed ovarian mass is more likely to be a malignancy but is also consistent with findings in endometriosis and PID. The commonest cause of secondary tumours in the ovary is metastases from a breast primary.

Next arrange appropriate investigations:
- full blood count
- ultrasound
- tumour markers.

In most cases, ultrasound will distinguish ovarian from uterine masses and the appearance of endometriomas, simple benign and malignant ovarian cysts. Tumour markers such as CA125 may be useful as baseline recordings for later follow-up in malignant ovarian disease and can help to determine whether the pelvic mass is more likely to be a malignancy, but laparotomy will still be required to confirm the diagnosis. Remember that some tumour markers such as CA125 are also raised in endometriosis and PID.

Plan appropriate treatment; the options to discuss might include:
- antibiotics for PID
- laparoscopy to confirm the diagnosis and possibly remove the cyst laparoscopically
- laparotomy and unilateral ovarian cystectomy
- unilateral oophorectomy
- hysterectomy and bilateral oophorectomy.

Because of the need to exclude malignancy and the risk of acute surgical complications even in benign lesions, removal of the cyst will usually be indicated even if the patient is asymptomatic. A mass of this size is unlikely to be functional in nature or to resolve without treatment. Endometriomas of this size are unlikely to resolve with medical treatment alone. If there is evidence of an infective cause, treat with antibiotics and follow up with ultrasound to see if there is a clinical response before considering surgery. A cyst of this size would need to be drained to be removed laparoscopically. This would not be appropriate for a malignant lesion and dissection may be technically difficult in endometriosis or PID.

If an open approach is taken, the choice of whether to proceed to removal of both ovaries and the uterus will depend primarily on the likelihood of malignancy. This increases with age and cannot reliably be excluded by visual inspection of the cyst at the time of surgery. At the same time, if the likely diagnosis is benign, the patient's wishes and the risks of more extensive surgery need to be balanced against the risk of missing occult malignant disease and needing to do a second operation.

Index

Note: page numbers in *italics* refer to tables, page numbers in **bold** refer to figures.

abdominal circumference (AC)   89,
   90, 296
abdominal distension   14, 285–6
abdominal examinations
   gynaecological   13–14, 17, 272
   obstetric   8, 100, 113, 159–60, 278
abdominal pain
   acute   271–5
   in pregnancy   99–101, 272
Abortion Act 1967   250
abscess
   Bartholin's   263
   puerperal pyrexia   175
acetic acid jelly   297
acetylcholinesterase (AChE)   47
acidosis   121–2
acquired immune deficiency syndrome
   (AIDS)   57
   see also human immunodeficiency
     virus
acyclovir, oral   263, 299
adenomyosis   194, 195, 197, 206
adhesions   194, 197
adnexum   **15**, 274
   see also fallopian tube; ovary
age *see* gestational age; maternal age
Agnus castus fruit extracts   240
airway management   132
alcohol consumption   92, 93
allergies   13
amenorrhoea   188–93
   causes   189–90
   definition   188, 296
   diagnosis and clinical assessment
     190–92
   management   192–3
   primary   188, 189–90, 191, 192, 231
   secondary   188, 190, 191, 231
amniocentesis
   blood group incompatibility   22
   chromosomal fetal abnormality
     44–5, *44*, **44**
   in multiple pregnancy   65
   polyhydramnios management   62
   structural fetal abnormality   47
amnioinfusion   138
amniotic fluid   88, 137, 296
amniotic fluid embolism (AFE)   131,
   135
amniotic fluid index   61, 88, 296

amniotic fluid volume   84
   definition   296
   oligohydramnios   88, 137
   polyhydramnios   60, 61–2, 155
ampicillin   162
anaemia, in pregnancy   25–8, 65
anaesthesia   113
   see also analgesia
analgesia
   for acute abdominal pain   271–2, 274
   for assisted vaginal delivery   113
   caudal   71
   epidural   36, 71, 112, 144, 146, 150
   inhalation   149
   opiate   149–50, 284
   regional   150
aneurysm, splenic artery   135
anovulatory bleeding   205, **205**
antepartum haemorrhage (APH)
   102–5, 296
anti-D immunoprophylaxis   21,
   23, 251
antibiotics
   for pelvic inflammatory disease   197,
     273–4
   for preterm labour   158
   for puerperal pyrexia   176
   for rupture of membranes whilst
     not in labour   162
antibodies
   abnormal   21–4
   antiphospholipid   296, 300
anticholinergic drugs   254
anticoagulation therapy   54, 180
antidepressants, tricyclic   174, 254
antiemetic therapy   288
antifibrinolytics   207
antigens, red blood cell   21
antihypertensive medication   51,
   52, 54–5
antiphospholipid antibodies (APA)
   296, 300
antiphospholipid syndrome   74, 77,
   246, 247
aortocaval compression   132, **132**
Apgar score   140, *140*
appendicitis   272, 273, 274
   in pregnancy   99, 100, **100**, 101
Apt's test   104
arterial ligation   153

artificial rupture of membranes
   (ARM)   296
Asherman's syndrome   192, 280
asphyxia at delivery   72, 74
aspirin, low-dose   54, 247
asthma, in pregnancy   29, 30, 31
atosiban   158

babies
   see also neonates
   born before arrival   297
   breast-feeding difficulties   170
   hip dislocation   36
baby (maternity) blues   172, 173
bacterial vaginosis (BV)   246, 247,
   259–60, 296
bag and mask   140, 141
barrier methods   199, 203
Bartholin's abscess   263
Bartholin's gland   261, 262, **262**, 263
Beckwith-Wiedemann syndrome   60
bed rest
   for pelvic inflammatory disease   274
   for pre-eclampsia   54
Behçet's syndrome   262, 263
bereavement teams   128
beta human chorionic gonadotrophins
   (βhCG)   296
beta-sympathomimetics   35, 157, 296
bilateral salpingo-oophorectomy
   (BSO)   296
bimanual examination   15, **15**, 278
biophysical profile (BPP)   84, *85*, 296
biopsy
   cervical   184, 185–6, **186**
   cone   185–6, **186**
   vulval   263, 266
biparietal diameter (BPD)   296
birthweight-for-gestational age   73, 88
Bishop Score   75, 76, 124, *124*, 125
bladder   297
'bladder drill' therapy   254
bladder neck elevation   257
bladder pressure studies (cystometry)
   256–7, **256**
bleeding
   see also menstruation; postpartum
     haemorrhage
   anovulatory   205, **205**
   dysfunctional   205, 208

bleeding *(continued)*
in early pregnancy 276–82
causes 276–8
diagnosis and clinical assessment 278–9
management 279–81, **280**
estimated blood loss 298
intermenstrual 205, 206, 219–21
intraventricular haemorrhage 300
postmenopausal 224, 231, 234–7
postoperative 283, 286
blood counts, full 54, 160
blood films 26–7
blood glucose measurement 38, 39, 40
blood groups, incompatibility 21–4
blood pressure
see also hypertension
maternal hypotension 120
measurement 53
blood transfusion
exchange transfusions 23, 24
intrauterine 23
maternal 298
blood volume, in pregnancy 25
body mass index (BMI) 297
bone mass, post-menopausal changes 222
booking 297
born before arrival (BBA) 297
brachial plexus injury 163, 164
bradycardia, fetal 117–18, 120, 133
breast-feeding
contraindications 170
difficulties 169–71
as form of contraception 203
normal physiology of 169
technique 169, 170, **171**
breasts
see also nipples
engorgement 169, 170
examination 13, **13**
mastitis 170, 171, 175, 176
breathing management 132
breathlessness, in pregnancy 29–32
breech presentation 33–6
causes 33
diagnosis and clinical assessment 8, 33–4
management 34–6
in multiple pregnancies 67–8
preterm 158
types 34, **34**
bromocriptine 217
Burch colposuspension 257, **257**

Caesarean section
abnormal fetal heart rate 122
analgesia for 150
asphyxia at delivery 74
breech presentation 35–6
brow presentation 297
cord prolapse 106
diabetes in pregnancy 40
failure to progress in the first stage 110, 111

failure to progress in the second stage 113, 114
induction of labour 123, 125
intrauterine growth restriction 90
large for gestational age fetus 61
maternal infections 59
multiple pregnancy 66, 67, 68
placental problems 104–5
pre-eclampsia 55
previous 69–71
puerperal pyrexia 175, 176–7
rupture of membranes without labour 162
scar rupture 69, 70, 71, 152, 303
shoulder dystocia 164, 165
structural fetal abnormality 49
thromboembolic disease 180
types
classical (vertical upper segment) 69, **70**, 96
elective 69–71
lower segment 69, **70**, 300
unstable lie 96
urinary retention 286
vaginal birth after 69–71, 152, 303, 304
calcium channel blockers 157
Candida 14, 259–60, 261, 263, 265–6, 297
caput succedaneum 297
Carboprost 153
cardiac arrest 131, 135
cardiac disease
fetal 22
maternal 29, 30, 31, 131, 135
cardiotocograph (CTG) 115–22, **116**
abnormal 117–20, **118**, **119**, 121–2
normal **117**
suspicious 120–21
cardiovascular compromise, postoperative 283
catheters
intrauterine 300
urinary 257, 286
cefoxitin 273–4
cellulitis 285
cephalopelvic disproportion (CPD) 297
cerebrovascular accidents 131, 135
cervical cancer 183, 184, 231, 297
and human papilloma virus 183, 299
and intermenstrual bleeding 220
management 186–7
and postmenopausal bleeding 235
staging *187*
cervical caps 203
cervical cerclage 74, 158, 247
cervical dilation, rate of 108–9, **108**, 124–5, *124*, 142–3
cervical erosion (ectropion)
definition 14, 183
and intermenstrual bleeding 219, 220
and vaginal discharge 259
cervical excitation 272

cervical incompetence
fetal loss 73, 74, 246, 247
preterm labour 155, 158
cervical intraepithelial neoplasia (CIN) 184–6, 219, 297
cervical intraglandular neoplasia (CIGN) 184, 297
cervical polyps 219, 220
cervical smear 14, 235
abnormal 183–7
causes 183–4
diagnosis and clinical assessment 184–5
false negatives 183
grading 183
inadequate 183–4, 185
inflammatory 184
management 185–7
cervicitis 259
cervix
definition 297
effacement 298
examinations 14, 15, 272
see also cervical smear
intermenstrual bleeding from 219
torn 153
chancre 302–3
chemotherapy 232, 267
chest infections
postoperative 285
in pregnancy 29, 30, 31
chest X-ray 30
Chlamydia 14, 271, 277
cholecystitis 100, 101
cholestasis of pregnancy 80–81, 82
chorioamnionitis 128
choriocarcinoma 278
chorionic villous sampling (CVS) 44, *44*, **44**, 297
chorionicity 63, *64*, **64**, 65, **65**, 66
circulation management 132
clavicle, breakage in the neonate 165
climacteric 222, 223, 297
clindamycin 274
clomiphene citrate (Clomid) 192, 216, 297
clonidine 225
clotrimazole 260, 297
coagulation diathermy 185
coagulopathy 102, 105, 152
cocaine abuse 92–3, 155
collapse, maternal 130–36
colostrum 169
colporrhaphy 244
colposcopy 184–5, 186, 220
conception 214
condoms 203
confinement 297
congenital heart defects 29
contact tracing/treatment 274
contraception 199–204
see also specific methods; sterilization
and amenorrhoea 193
clinical assessment 199–200
definitions 199
enquiring about in history taking 12

failure rates 199, *199*
methods 200–204
controlled cord traction 297
cordocentesis 21, 22, 90
corpus luteum 189, 297–8
counselling 5
  regarding bereavement 128
  regarding breech delivery 34, 35–6
  regarding IUCD insertion 202
  regarding neural tube defects 48–9
  regarding preterm labour 158
  regarding prolonged pregnancy 76
  regarding shoulder dystocia 165
  regarding sterilization 248–9
  regarding termination of pregnancy 251
Crohn's disease 262, 263
crown–rump length (CRL) 298
cyclical bisphosphonate therapy 225–26
cyproterone acetate (CPA) 213
cyst *see* ovarian cyst
cytomegalovirus (CMV) 56, 57, 58–9

danazol 196–7, 209, 240
decidua 53
deep vein thrombosis (DVT) 175, 176, 178–80
dehydration 287, 288
delirium tremens 286
delivery
  see also Caesarean section; labour
  estimated blood loss 298
  estimated date of 6, 298
  premature 158
    fetal loss 72, 73, 74
    and haemolytic disease 23, 24
    and the large for gestational age fetus 61
    in multiple pregnancy 66–7
    and pre-eclampsia 55
    and rupture of membranes while not in labour 161
    treatment 296
  vaginal
    abnormal fetal heart rate 121–2
    assisted 36, 113–14
    breech presentation 35–6, *35*
    cord prolapse 106–7
    failure to progress in the second stage 112–14
    fetal well-being during 137–8
    fitting patient 134
    following Caesarean section 69–71, 152, 303, 304
    haemolytic disease 23, 24
    hypertensive mothers 51, 55
    induction of labour 124
    intrauterine fetal death 128
    intrauterine growth restriction 90
    maternal cardiac disease 31
    maternal diabetes 40
    meconium detection 137–8
    multiple pregnancy 66–8
    placental abruption 105
    pre-eclampsia 55

premature 23–4, 55, 61, 66–7, 72–4, 158, 161
  previous Caesarian section 70–71
  puerperal pyrexia 175
  rupture of membranes while not in labour 160–61
  shoulder dystocia 163, 164–5, **165**
  structural fetal abnormality 49
  thromboembolic disease 180
  unstable lie 96
  ventouse 113, 114
delivery team 67
denominator 298
Depo-provera 201–2
depression, postnatal 172, 173, 174
dermatoses, vulval 261, 262, 265, 266–7
detrusor instability 253, 254, 255
dextrose 40
diabetes
  gestational 37, 38
  in pregnancy 37–40
diaphragms 203
diathermy 185, 197
diazepam 133, 139
diet
  diabetes in pregnancy 39
  premenstrual syndrome 240
dilation & curettage (D&C) 208, 280, 298
dipstick tests 78
disseminated intravascular coagulation (DIS) 128, 298
diuretics 240
donor insemination (DI) 298
Doppler ultrasonography 84–5, **85–6**, 115
Down's syndrome (trisomy 21) 41–5, 72
  definition 303
  and diabetes in pregnancy 40
  history taking 43
  karyotype **42**, 43
  screening 41–5
doxycycline 273–4, 274
dural puncture 150
dysfunctional uterine bleeding 298
dysmenorrhoea, primary 194, 195
dyspareunia 227–29
  deep 227, 229
  primary 227
  secondary 227
  superficial 227, 228–29

early pregnancy assessment unit (EPAU) 298
eclampsia 130, 131, 133–4
ectocervix 183
ectopic pregnancy 272
  common sites **277**
  investigations for 279
  management 281
  presenting features 279
  risk factors 277, *277*
eczema, vulval 261, 265, 266
Edward's syndrome (trisomy 18) 41
effacement, cervical 298

electrophoresis, haemoglobin 26, 27
embryo transfer 217
emergency contraception 201, 203
endocrine disorders 190
endometrial ablation 190, 192, 197, 208–9
endometrial carcinoma 206, 231, 234–5, 236
  prognosis **237**
  staging *235*
endometrial hyperplasia 236
endometrial resection 208–9, *209*
endometriosis 194–7, 214, 233
endometrium
  amenorrhoea 190, 192
  intermenstrual bleeding of 219
  menstrual cycle 189
  mixed mesodermal tumour 301
endomyometritis 175, 176
endotracheal tubes 132, 135
engagement 144, 298
Entonox 149
epidural analgesia 150
  interference with the second stage of labour 112, 144, 146, 150
  and previous Caesarian section 71
  side effects 150
  and vaginal breech delivery 36
epilepsy, in pregnancy 130, 133–4
episiotomy
  forceps delivery 113, 114
  in normal labour 144, 146, 147
  vaginal breech delivery 36
  wound infection 175, 177
erythromycin 162
estimated blood loss (EBL) 298
estimated date of delivery (EDD) 6, 298
estimated fetal weight (EFW) 298
evacuation of retained products of conception (ERPOC) 298
evening primrose oil 240
examinations 4
  see also abdominal examinations; pelvic examinations; vaginal examinations
  breast 13, **13**
  gynaecological 13–16
  obstetric 7–10
exercise tolerance, reduced 30, *30*
external cephalic version (ECV) 34–5, 96

face presentation 298
factor V Leiden 178–9
faints 130
fallopian tube
  assessment 216, 299
  damaged 214, 215
  definition 298
  rupture 279, 281
  surgery 217, 296
fatty liver of pregnancy, acute 80, 81, 82
feeding
  see also breast-feeding
  artificial 171

Ferguson reflex 112, 144, 150
'ferning' 160
ferrous sulphate 27
fetal abnormality 139
  chromosomal 41–5
    as cause of fetal loss 72, 74
    causes 41
    diagnosis and clinical assessment
      41–5
    and intrauterine growth restriction
      90
    management 45
    in multiple pregnancy 65
    and recurrent miscarriage 246,
      247
    risk assessment 41
    soft markers of 43
  due to diabetes in pregnancy 37, 38
  structural 46–9
    as cause of fetal loss 72, 74
    causes 46
    diagnosis and clinical assessment
      46–8
    and intrauterine growth restriction
      90
    management 48–9
    in multiple pregnancy 65
  and termination of pregnancy 250
  and unstable lie 95
fetal alcohol syndrome 92
fetal blood sampling (FBS) 121–2
fetal heart rate 133, 137–8
  abnormal patterns in labour 115–22
    accelerations 115, 116, *116*,
      117, 122
    baselines 115, 116, *116*, 117
    decelerations 115, 116, *116*,
      118, 119, 120
      early **118**, 119
      late 119, **119**
      variable **118**, 119, 120
    diagnosis and clinical assessment
      119–20
    factors affecting 115–16, *116*
    management 120–22
    variability 115, 116, *116*, 117, 118
  continuous monitoring 84, **85**
  normal patterns in labour 117, **117**,
    145, 146
  in preterm labour 158
  and rupture of membranes while not
    in labour 160, 161
fetal lie
  assessment 8, **9**, 144
  definition 300
  in multiple pregnancy 67
  transverse 88, 95–6
  unstable 95–6
fetal loss
  due to prolonged pregnancy 75
  intrauterine death 126–9, 300
  previous 72–4
fetal movement
  charts 83, **84**
  definition 298
  reduced 83–7, **84**

fetal scalp blood sampling 67, 121–2
fetal scalp electrodes (FSEs) 67, 115,
  120, 298
fetal well-being, assessment 83, 84–5,
  90, 137–8, 160, 296
α-fetoprotein 46–7, 49, 296
fetus
  see also intrauterine growth
    restriction; products of
    conception
  abdominal circumference 89, 90, 296
  abdominal examination 8
  and antepartum haemorrhage
    102–4, 105
  assessment for delivery 144
  assisted vaginal delivery risks 114
  bleeding from 104
  blood group incompatibility 21–3
  bradycardia 117–18, 120, 133
  cord prolapse 106, 107
  engagement 144, 298
  estimated weight 298
  failure to progress in the first stage
    108, 109–10
  failure to progress in the second stage
    112, 113, 114
  head ballottability 33
  head circumference 89, 90, 296
  induction of labour 123
  internal rotation 143
  intraventricular haemorrhage 300
  karyotypes **42**, 43, 47–8, 127
  large for gestational age 60–62, 300
  lung maturation 90, 105, 156, 161
  macrosomic 37, 60, 61, 163, 164
  malposition 110, **110**, 300, 301
  and maternal diabetes 37, 39, 40
  and maternal infections 56–7, 58–9
  meconium 137–8
  miscarriage of 276–7
  in multiple pregnancy 63, 65–6
  and nausea and vomiting in early
    pregnancy 287
  in normal labour 143–4
  position 302
  postmortems 73, 127
  and pre-eclampsia 52, 54
  presentation
    assessment 145
    breech 33–6
    brow 297
    cephalopelvic disproportion 297
    definition 302
    denominator 298
    face 298
    malpresentation **109**, 110,
      110, 112, 300
    in rupture of membranes while not
      in labour 160
  presenting part 302
  and preterm labour 157, 158
  restitution 144
  and rupture of membranes while not
    in labour 159, 160, 161, 162
  sedation 139, 150
  selective fetal reduction 66

shoulder dystocia 163, 164
small for gestational age 73, 88–91
  and substance abuse 92–4
  vertex 304
fibroids 200, 230, 231
  and heavy periods 206, 207
  and irregular bleeding 220
  management 208, 232–3
  in pregnancy 99, 100, 101
  red degeneration of 99, 100, 101
  types of **233**
fistula formation 255, 256, 258
fits, maternal 130, 133–4
'flat babies' 139
fluconazole 260, 297
fluid balance 134
fluorescent treponemal antibody test
  (FTA) 303
Foley catheters 106
folic acid deficiency
  anaemia in pregnancy 25, 27
  neural tube defects 47
folic acid supplementation 27, 39, 48
follicle-stimulating hormone
  (FSH) 190
  definition 298
  and hirsutism/virilization 212
  in the normal menstrual cycle 188–9
  and polycystic ovary syndrome
    191–2
  and sperm count 216
  tests for 191
follicles 188–9
follicular phase 189, 299
forceps delivery 36, 113, **114**
functional residual capacity (FRC) 140

gamete intra-fallopian tube transfer
  (GIFT) 217
genital tract trauma 151, 153
  see also perineal trauma
gentamicin 273–4
gestational age
  see also large for gestational age fetus;
    small for gestational age fetus
  at time of fetal loss 73
  birthweight-for 73, 88
  definition 299
  in prolonged pregnancy 75–6
  uncertainty of 75
gestational trophoblastic disease (molar
  pregnancy/hydatidiform mole)
  277–8, 281, 303
  complete hydatidiform mole 278,
    281
  partial hydatidiform mole 278, 281
glandular cells, atypical 183, 184, 186
glucose metabolism 127
glucose tolerance test (GTT), oral 38, *39*
gonadotrophin therapy 193, 217
gonadotrophin-releasing hormone
  (GnRH) 188, 197, 217, 240, 299
granulosa cells 188–9
gravida 299
gravidity 12, 299
gut motility 285

haematoma 175, 176, 285
haemoglobinopathy 25–6
haemolytic disease 21, 22, 23
haemorrhage see bleeding; postpartum
    haemorrhage
hallucinogens 93
healthcare teams
  antepartum haemorrhage
    management 104
  bereavement management 128
  delivery management 67
  eclampsia management 133
  postpartum haemorrhage
    management 152
HELLP (haemolysis, elevated liver
    enzymes and low platelets)
    syndrome 299
helper T-lymphocytes 59
heparin 180, 247
hepatitis 57
hepatitis A 80, 81, 82
hepatitis B 80, 81, 82
hepatitis C 80, 81, 82
heroin abuse 93
herpes gestationalis 80, 81, 82, 299
herpes simplex virus (HSV) 57, 58,
    59, 261, 263, 266, 299
high vaginal swab (HVS) 299
hip dislocation, breech babies 36
hirsutism 211–13
history taking 4
  gynaecological 11–13, 16–17
  obstetric 6–7, 9
Homan's sign 179
hormone replacement therapy (HRT)
    208, 223, 224–26
  benefits 225, 225
  contraindications 224
  and irregular bleeding 219, 220
  oestrogen-alternatives 225
  and postmenopausal bleeding 235
  preparations 224
  side-effects 224–25, 225
  to prevent vulval pain 263
hot flushes 223
human chorionic gonadotrophin (hCG)
    217, 247, 279, 287, 296
Human Fertilisation and Embryology
    Authority (HFEA) 299
human immunodeficiency virus (HIV)
    57–8, 59, 93–4, 261, 263, 299
human menopausal gonadotrophin
    (HMG) 299
human papilloma virus (HPV) 183,
    299
hydralazine 133, 134
hydramnios 106
  oligohydramnios 88, 137
  polyhydramnios 60, 61–2, 155
'hydrops', fetal 22, 23, 59
hymen, imperforate 190, 191, 231
hyperbilirubinaemia 24
hyperemesis gravidarum 287
hyperprolactinaemia 190, 193
hypertension
  in pregnancy 50–55, 302

chronic 50–51, 51
high-risk patients 50, 51, 51
low-risk patients 50, 51, 51
management 51, 133, 134
non-proteinuric pregnancy-
    induced (PIH) 50, 51–2
pre-eclampsia 50, 52–5, 52
hypoglycaemia 38, 39, 40
hypotension 120
hypothalamus 188
  failure 189–90, 191, 192
hypoxia
  antenatal 139
  intrapartum 139
hysterectomy
  for adenomyosis 197
  for cervical intraepithelial neoplasia
    186
  complications 209, 209
  for endometrial carcinoma 236
  for endometriosis 197
  extended (Wertheim's) 186
  for fibroids 233
  for heavy periods 205, 208–9, 209
  for mixed mesodermal tumours 301
  for ovarian cancer 232
  for pelvic inflammatory disease 197
  for postpartum haemorrhage 153
  for primary dysmenorrhoea 196
  for uterine prolapse 244
  vaginal 209
hysterosalpingogram (HSG) 299
hysteroscopy 206–7, 229, 236, **236**

ibuprofen 240
ileus 285–6
in vitro fertilization (IVF) 217, 300
indomethacin 62, 157–8
induction of labour see labour, induction
infections
  see also sexually transmitted infection
  common in pregnancy 56–9
  and fetal loss 72, 74
  and intrauterine growth restriction 90
  neonatal 139, 141
  post-delivery 175
  postoperative 284–5
  and preterm labour 155, 156, 158
  and recurrent miscarriage 246, 247
  and rupture of membranes while not
    in labour 159, 160–61, 162
  caused by termination of pregnancy
    251
infertility 214–18
  and amenorrhoea 192–3
  causes 214–15
  diagnosis and clinical assessment
    215–16, 302
  female factor 214, 215, 216–17
  male factor 215–16, 217–18
  management 216–18, 298, 300
  normal conception 214
  primary 214
  secondary 214
injectables (hormonal contraception)
    201–2, 251

insulin therapy 39, 40
intercourse, painful 227–29
intermenstrual bleeding (IMB) 205,
    206, 219–221
internal podalic version 67–8
internal rotation 143
International Federation of Obstetrics
    and Gynaecology (FIGO) 300
intracytoplasmic sperm injection (ICSI)
    217, 300
intrauterine catheters 300
intrauterine contraceptive device
    (IUCD) 199, 200, 202–3,
    202, 219
  definition 300
  and ectopic pregnancy 277
  following termination of pregnancy
    251
  and heavy periods 206, 208
intrauterine fetal death (IUFD) 126–9,
    300
intrauterine growth restriction (IUGR)
    88
  as cause of fetal loss 72, 73
  causes 89
  definition 300
  diagnosis and clinical assessment 89
  and Down's syndrome 43
  late-onset 90
  management 89–90
  in multiple pregnancy 66
  and structural fetal abnormality 49
intrauterine insemination (IUI) 217,
    300
intrauterine system (Mirena) 300
  see also levonorgestrel-releasing
    intrauterine system
intrauterine transfer 158
intrauterine transfusion 23
intraventricular haemorrhage 300
intubation 132, 135, 140–41
iron deficiency 25, 26–7
irritable bowel syndrome (IBS) 194–5,
    197, 275, 300

jaundice, in pregnancy 80–82

karyotypes
  Down's syndrome **42**, 43
  intrauterine fetal death 127
  neural tube defects 47–8
ketoacidosis 38
Kielland's forceps 113, **114**
Kleihauer test 23, 101, 104
knee–chest position 106, **107**

labetalol 133, 134
labour
  see also delivery
  abdominal pain 99–100
  abnormal fetal heart rate during
    115–22
  augmentation 161
  definition 300
  failure to progress in the first stage
    108–11

labour *(continued)*
  failure to progress in the second stage
    112–14
  false 99–100
  induction 70–71, 123–5
    clinical assessment 124
    contraindications 124
    failure 125
    and fetal heart rate 121
    indications for 123
    and intrauterine fetal death 128
    management 124–5
    methods of 125
    in prolonged pregnancy 75, 76,
      123, 125
    risks 123–4
  and maternal cardiac disease 31
  and maternal diabetes 40
  mobility in 145–6
  in multiple pregnancy 67
  normal 142–7, **143**
    clinical assessment 144–5
    first stage
      active phase 142–3
      decelerative phase 142, 143
      latent phase 142
    management 145–7
    onset 142
    physiology 142–4
    progress 146
    second stage 143–4, 146
      active phase 144
      passive phase 144
    third stage 144, 146–7, 151
  pain relief 148–50
  and placental gas transfer 115–16,
    119, 139
  preterm 73, 74, 155–8, 302
  following previous Caesarian
    section 70–71
  primary dysfunctional 108, **108**, 110
  prolonged latent phase 108, **108**, 110
  rupture of membranes 162
  secondary arrest 108, **108**, 110–11
  and shoulder dystocia 164
  and unstable fetal lie 96
lactation 128
lactogen 87
laparoscopy
  abdominal pain investigation 272–3
  ectopic pregnancy management 281
  infertility investigation 216
  pelvic pain investigation 195, **195**
  sterilization 248, 249
laparotomy
  for ovarian cancer 232, *232*
  for postpartum haemorrhage 153
  for uterine rupture 134–5
large for gestational age (LFGA) fetus
  60–62, 300
large loop excision of the transformation
  zone (LLETZ) 185–6, **185**, 300
laser ablation 185, 190, 192, 197, 208–9
last menstrual period (LMP) 6, 12, 299
left ventricular failure (LVF) 284
leiomyosarcoma 300

levonorgestrel 201
levonorgestrel-releasing intrauterine
  system (IUS) 202, 208,
  208, 219, 300
libido, loss of 227–28, 229
lichen planus 261, 265
lichen sclerosus 261, 265, 266, 267
lichen simplex 266
lie *see* fetal lie
limb contractures 161
liquor 161
  see also amniotic fluid volume
  'ferning' 160
  meconium-stained 138, 145
lithium carbonate 174
liver disease, chronic 80
liver function tests 300
Lloyd-Davies position 273
lochia 300
lower genital tract, atrophy 234, 237
lower segment Caesarean section
  (LSCS) 69, **70**, 300
lung maturity, fetal 90, 105, 156, 161
lupus anticoagulant (LAC) 300
luteal phase 189, 300
luteinizing hormone (LH) 188–9,
  191–2, 212, 300
lymph nodes
  cervical cancer 186, 187
  endometrial carcinoma 236
  vulval cancer 265, 267
lysergic acid diethylamide (LSD) 93

magnesium sulphate 133, 134, 157
malposition 110, **110**, 300, 301
malpresentation **109**, 110, **110**,
  112, 300
Manchester repair 244
manual removal of placenta (MRP) 300
Marcain 150
Mariceau-Smellie-Veit manoeuvre 36
marijuana 93
mastitis 170, 171, 175, 176
maternal age, Down's syndrome 41, 43
maternal collapse 130–36
maternal confusion/withdrawal 172–4
maternal mortality rate (MMR) 301
maternal serum α-fetoprotein 46–7,
  49, 296
maternal well-being, investigations
  of 54
measles 57, 58
meconium 137–8, 140
  thick 137, 138
  thin 137
meconium aspiration syndrome
  (MAS) 137–8
medoxyprogesterone acetate 208
mefenamic acid 207
Mefigyne 280–81
mefipristone 251
membrane sweeping 124–5
menarche 301
menometrorrhagia 205
menopausal symptoms 222–26,
  263, 301

menorrhagia 205, 207–9, *207*, 301
menstrual calendars 238, 239–40, **239**
menstrual cycle 12, 188–9
  follicular phase 189, 299
  luteal phase 189, 300
menstrual history 12
menstruation
  see also amenorrhoea
  heavy 205–10, *207*, 301
  normal blood loss 205
mental state, altered 286
methadone 94
methotrexate 281
metronidazole 162, 260, 274
micturition 301
midwife 145
miscarriage
  anembryonic pregnancy 277
  complete 276
  definition 301
  diabetic mothers 37
  early embryonic demise 277
  incomplete 276, 280–81
  inevitable 276
  management 279–81
  recurrent 246–7
  threatened 276
mixed (Müllerian) mesodermal tumour
  301
moulding 145
multiparous women
  failure to progress in the first stage
    108, 111
  failure to progress in the second stage
    112
  induction of labour 125
  normal labour 142, 144, 146
  prolapse 242
multiple pregnancy 63–8
  chorionicity 63, *64*, **64**, 65, **65**, 66
  complications 63, *64*
  diagnosis and clinical assessment
    63–5
  management 65–8
  preterm labour 155
  selective fetal reduction 66
  twin types 63
myocardial infarction
  during pregnancy 131
  postoperative 284
myomectomy 208

naloxone 141, 284
nasogastric (NG) tubes 286
nausea/vomiting
  in early pregnancy 287–9
  postoperative 284
neck, fetal hyperextension 34
necrotizing fasciitis 285
Neisseria 14
neonatal death (NND) 301
neonatal resuscitation 139–41
  bag and mask 140, 141
  cardiopulmonary 141
  intubation and ventilation
    140–41

neonates
  see also babies
  haemolytic disease   21, 22, 23, 24
  infections   139, 141
  intraventricular haemorrhage   300
  maternal diabetes   38, 39
  meconium   138
  perinatal mortality rate   301
  preterm labour   155, 157, 158
nephropathy   38
neural tube defects   46–9, 301
Neville–Barnes forceps   113, **114**
New York Heart Association   30, *30*
nifedipine   157
nipples
  cracked/sore   169, 170–71
  flat/inverted   169, 170
nitric oxide donors   157
nitrous oxide   149
nocturia   253
non-steroidal anti-inflammatory drugs
  (NSAIDs)   196, 207
norethisterone   208
Norplant silastic rods   201–2
nulliparous women
  endometriosis   194
  failure to progress in the first stage
    108
  failure to progress in the second stage
    112
  induction of labour   125
  normal labour   142, 144
nutrition   145, 289

obesity, maternal   60
obstruction, signs of   111
occipitoposterior position   110, **110**,
  300, 301
oedema, caput succedaneum   297
oestradiol implants/patches   240
oestriol   87
oestrogen
  adrenal   212
  deficiency   192, 211, 222,
    224, 234, 237
  excess   234
  hormone replacement therapy   224,
    225
oestrogen alternatives (hormone
  replacement therapy)   225
oflaxacin   274
oligomenorrhoea   188–93, 301
oligospermic males   218
oocytes   214, 217, 301
oogenesis   301
oophorectomy   209, 232, 236, 240, 296
opiates
  abuse in pregnancy   93, 94
  pain relief in labour   149–50
  postoperative overdose   284
oral contraceptive pill   199–201, 251
  and amenorrhoea   193
  combined   199, 200–201, 207,
    213, 219, 230
  contraindications   201
  drug interactions   199–200, 220

and endometriosis   196
everyday (ED) preparations   200
for heavy periods   207
and hirsutism/virilization   213
and intermenstrual bleeding   219,
  220
and oligomenorrhoea   190
and premenstrual syndrome
  reduction   240
and primary dysmenorrhoea   196
progesterone-only   199, 200, 201
side-effects   201
osteoporosis   222, 225
ovarian cancer   230–32, *230, 232*
ovarian cyst   232, 233
  acute abdominal pain   271, 272, 274
  management   274
  types
    benign epithelial tumours   274
    corpus luteum cyst   274
    follicular cyst   274
    malignant epithelial tumours   274
    mature cystic teratomas (dermoid
      cysts)   274
ovarian failure   190, 192, 193, 222, 223
ovarian hyperstimulation syndrome
  217, 301
ovarian tumour   190–92, 211–13, 220,
  232, 234
ovary
  definition   301
  menstrual cycle   188–9
  surgical removal   296
  torsion   274
overdose, postoperative opiate   284
ovulation   188–9
  confirmation of   216
  failure   214
  induction   63, 216–17
ovum   188–9, 301
oxybutynin hydrochloride   254
oxytocin   125
  see also Syntocinon
  endogenous   144, 301
  and placental gas transfer   121, 139
  to limit postpartum blood loss   146
  and uterine rupture   70, 71
oxytocin antagonists   157, 158

paclitaxel   232
pain
  see also abdominal pain
  during intercourse   227–29
  pelvic   194–8
  'shoulder tip'   279
  vulval   261–4
pain relief
  see also anaesthesia; analgesia
  in labour   148–50
palpation   144
parity   12
paroxysmal supraventricular tachycardia
  29, 30, 31
partograms   **143**, 144, 145, 146
parvovirus   56, 57, 58, 59
Patau's syndrome (trisomy 13)   41

Pearl index   199
pelvic examinations
  see also vaginal examinations
  gynaecological   14–16, 17,
    206, 228, 272
  obstetric   8–9, 95, 100, 124
pelvic floor exercises   257
pelvic inflammatory disease (PID)
  acute   271, 272–4
  chronic   194, 195, 197
  definition   301
  diagnosis   273
  and ectopic pregnancy   277
  and intermenstrual bleeding   220
  and IUCDs   203
  management   273–4
pelvic mass   230–33, 272
pelvic pain, chronic   194–8
pelvimetry   34, 69–70
pelvis, size/shape   109, 112, 297
perinatal mortality rate (PMR)   301
perineum   301
  trauma   144, 147, **147**
  see also episiotomy
pethidine   139, 149
pH, fetal blood   121–2
phenothiazines   174
pituitary gland   188
  failure   189–90, 191
placenta
  delivery   144, 146–7, 297
  gestational trophoblastic
    disease   278
  low lying   300
  manual removal   300
  postmortem examination   73, 127
  retained   151, 153
  and uterine infection   175
placenta accreta   151, 153
placenta increta   151
placenta percreta   151
placenta praevia   102, 103, **103**,
  104–5, 151, 302
placental abruption
  and antepartum haemorrhage   102,
    103–4, 105
  concealed   103–4, **104**
  and preterm labour   155, 156
  small   99, 100, 101
placental gas transfer
  and fetal loss   72, 74
  and intrauterine growth restriction
    89
  in labour   115–16, 119, 121, 139
placental site bleeding   151
pneumoperitoneum   273
polycystic ovary syndrome (PCOS)
  189, 191–3, 211, 212, 246, 247, 302
polymenorrhoea   205
position   302
postcoital test   302
postmaturity *see* prolonged pregnancy
postmenopausal bleeding (PMB)   224,
  231, 234–7, 302
postmortem, fetal/placental   73, 127
postnatal depression   172, 173, 174

postoperative complications 283–6
early 283–4
late 284–6
postpartum haemorrhage (PPH)
151–4
and assisted vaginal delivery 114
causes 151–2
definition 302
diagnosis and clinical assessment
152
management 152–4
in multiple pregnancy 67, 68
normal levels 144
primary 151
secondary 151
pre-eclampsia 50, 52–5
as cause of fetal loss 72
causes 52, 53, **53**
complications 52
diagnosis and clinical assessment 53
and jaundice in pregnancy 80
management 54–5
and maternal collapse 131
and proteinuria 77, 78, 79
recurrence 55
symptoms 131
pregnancy
see also Caesarian section; delivery;
fetus; labour
abdominal pain 99–101, 272
and amenorrhoea 190
anaemia in 25–8, 65
antepartum haemorrhage 102–5,
296
bleeding in early 276–82
breathlessness in 29–32
breech presentation 33–6,
67–8, 158
cervical intraepithelial neoplasia
treatment in 186
chromosomal fetal abnormality
41–5, 65, 72, 74, 90, 246, 247
common infections in 56–9, 56
cord prolapse 106–7
and diabetes 37–40
ectopic 272, 277, 277, **277**,
279, 281
hypertension during 50–55, 302
intrauterine fetal death 126–9
irregular bleeding during 219–20
jaundice during 80–82
large for gestational age fetus 60–62
maternal collapse 130–36
meconium 137–8
multiple 63–8, 155
previous fetal loss 72–4
prolonged 75–6, 123, 125
proteinuria 77–9
pruritus 80–82
reduced fetal movement 83–7
rupture of membranes while not
in labour 159–62
small for gestational age fetus 73,
88–91
structural fetal abnormality 46–9,
65, 72, 74, 90

substance abuse during 92–4, 103, 155
termination 45, 58, 250–52
unstable lie 95–6
vomiting in early 287–9
pregnancy rates 199
pregnancy tests 272, 279
premenstrual syndrome (PMS) 238–41
definition 302
psychological problems in 238, 240
presentation see fetus, presentation
preterm 302
see also delivery, premature; labour,
preterm
preterm premature rupture of
membranes (PPROM) 159,
161, 302
procidentia 242
products of conception 276, 278,
280–81, 298
progesterone 189, 240
progesterone challenge test 191
progestogens
for heavy periods 208
for hirsutism 213
hormone replacement therapy 224,
225
for premenstrual syndrome reduction
240
for primary dysmenorrhoea 196
prolactin 169, 191, 302
see also hyperprolactinaemia
prolapse 242–5
causes 242
cystocele 242, 243, **243**, 244
diagnosis and clinical assessment
242–4
enterocele 242, **243**, 244
management 243–4
rectocele 242, 243, **243**, 244
and urinary incontinence 256
vault-type 244
prolonged pregnancy 75–6, 123, 125
prostaglandin analogues 280–81
prostaglandin synthetase inhibitors
157–8
prostaglandins 125, 153, 251
proteinuria 53, 77–9
pruritus
in pregnancy 80–82
vulval 265–8
psoriasis, vulval 261, 266
psychiatric disorders 172–4, 238
psycho-sexual clinics 229
psychological problems
new mothers 172–4
in premenstrual syndrome 238, 240
psychosis, puerperal 172, 173–4
puberty 302
puerperium 302
psychosis 172, 173–4
pyrexia 175–7
pulmonary embolism 29
diagnosis and assessment 30, 178, 179
management 180
pulmonary hypoplasia 161
'pushing' 112, 113, 146

pyrexia
fetal heart rate during labour
120–21
postoperative 284–5
puerperal 175–7

radiotherapy 186, 186–7, 267
reagent strips 78
red blood cells 21, 23, 25
red degeneration 99, 100, 101
renal failure, acute 77, 78, 79
renal function tests 27
respiratory depression 141
restitution 144
resuscitation
antepartum haemorrhage 104
maternal collapse 132, 135
neonatal 139–41
postpartum haemorrhage 152
retinopathy, proliferative 38, 39
Rhesus (Rh) group 22
Rh-negative women 21, 23, 104, 251
Rh-positive women 21
rheumatic heart disease 29
rhythm method 203–4
ritodrine 35, 157
round ligament pain 99, 100, 101
Royal College of Obstetricians and
Gynaecologists (RCOG) 302
rubella 56, 57, 58
rupture of membranes (ROM)
artificial 296
preterm premature 159, 161, 302
while not in labour 159–62, 302

sacrocolpoplexy 244
sacrospinous fixation 244
salpingectomy 281
salpingotomy 281
scabies 266
scar tissue
uterine 69, 70, 71, 152
vaginal 228
selective oestrogen receptor modulators
(SERMs) 225
semen analysis 216
see also sperm
serum folate estimations 27
sexually transmitted infection (STI)
examinations 14
swollen/painful vulva 261, 262–3
vaginal discharge 259–60
shoulder dystocia 37, 61, 163–5
drill 164–5
McRobert's position for delivery
164, **165**
'shoulder tip' pain 279
show 302
sickle cell haemoglobin disease 25, 26, 27
sling operations 257
small for gestational age (SGA) fetus
73, 88–91
smoking, in pregnancy 92, 93, 103, 155
speculums
Cusco's 14, **14**
Sims' 15, **15**, 243

sperm 214, 216, 217
spermatogenesis 215, 302
spina bifida 46
spinal anaesthesia 150
splenic artery aneurysm 135
squamocolumnar junction (SCJ) 183,
    184, 185, 302
Stamey operation 257
'station' 145, 302
sterilization 248–9, 251
steroids
    anabolic 211–12
    for fetal lung maturation 90, 105,
        156, 161
    for pre-eclampsia 55
    topical 266–7
stethoscopes, Pinnard's fetal 8, 120
stillbirth 72, 73, 302
Streptococcus, group B 72, 139
stroke
    non-haemorrhagic 131
    subarachnoid haemorrhage 131
substance abuse, in pregnancy 92–4,
    103, 155
suction evacuation 251
supraventricular tachycardia 29, 30, 31
sutures
    B-lynch 153, **154**
    polyglycolic acid 147
swabs, high vaginal 299
symphysiotomy 165
symphysis–fundal height
    definition 302
    large for gestational age fetus 60, 61
    in multiple pregnancy 65
    in prolonged pregnancy 75
    small for gestational age fetus 88
Syntocinon
    see also oxytocin
    failure to progress in the first stage
        110, 111
    failure to progress in the second stage
        113, 114
    fitting patient 134
    in multiple pregnancy 67, 68
    postpartum blood loss limitation 68,
        144, 153
    risks 123–4
    and uterine rupture 131
Syntometrine 144, 153
syphilis (Treponemum pallidum) 57,
    59, 303

tachycardia
    fetal 118, 210
    maternal 29, 30, 31, 120–21
TENS machines 149
tension-free tape 257
terbutaline 35
term 303
termination of pregnancy 45, 58, 250–52
testicular feminization syndrome 190,
    192
thalassaemia
    alpha-thalassaemia 25, 26, 27
    beta-thalassaemia 25–6, 27

thiamine 289
thromboembolic disease 178–80, 225
thrombophilia 178–9
tibolone 225
tinea 266
tocographs 115, 117
tocolytics 35, 40, 156–8
tolterodine 254
'TORCH' infections 56, 57, 58–9
toxoplasmosis 57, 58
tranexamic acid 207
transabdominal ultrasound
    transducer 67
transformation zone (TZ) 183, 303
transvaginal (transabdominal)
    ultrasound scan 303
trauma
    genital tract 151, 153
    perineal 144, 147, **147**
    vulval 263, 266
trial of scar 303
Trichomonas 14, 259, 260, 303
triple test 43
trisomy 303
    see also Down's syndrome
        (trisomy 21)
    Edward's syndrome (trisomy 18) 41
    Patau's syndrome (trisomy 13) 41
trophoblast 53, 303
trophoblastic disease see gestational
    trophoblastic disease
tubo-ovarian inflammatory mass 233
tumour
    mixed (Müllerian) mesodermal 301
    ovarian 190–92, 211–13, 220, 232,
        234
    uterine 233
Turner's syndrome 41, 189, 190, 191,
    192
'turtle sign' 164
twin pregnancies 63
    antenatal care 66
    chorionicity 63, 64, **64**, 65, **65**, 66
    complications 63, 64
    delivery 66, 67
    postnatal care 68
    zygosity 63
twin–twin transfusion 66

ultrasound
    abdominal pain 101, 272
    antepartum haemorrhage 103, 104
    definition 303
    Down's syndrome 43, **43**
    DVT diagnosis 179
    estimating gestational age 75–6
    haemolytic disease 22, 23
    heavy periods 207
    large for gestational age fetus 61
    meconium detection 137
    multiple pregnancy 63, 65, **65**, 67
    postmenopausal bleeding 236
    preterm labour 155
    recurrent miscarriage 247
    rupture of membranes while not
        in labour 160

small for gestational age investigations
    89, 90, **90**
structural fetal abnormality 46, 47,
    48–9, **48**
types
    Doppler ultrasonography 84–5,
        85–6, 115
    serial 89, **90**
    transvaginal (transabdominal)
        303
unstable lie 96
umbilical artery
    acid–base status 122
    Doppler ultrasonography 84–5,
        85–6
    pulsatility index (UAPI) 303
umbilical cord
    see also cordocentesis
    compression 119
    controlled cord traction 297
    prolapse 106–7
ureter 303
urethra 303
urinary frequency 253–4
urinary incontinence 255–8
    causes 255
    diagnosis and clinical assessment
        255–7
    genuine stress incontinence (GSI)
        255, 256, 257–8
    management 257–8
    mechanisms of normal urinary
        continence 255
    pelvic examinations 15
    urge incontinence 255, 256
    urinary fistula/overflow incontinence
        255, 256, 258
urinary retention 256, 286
urinary tract infection (UTI)
    definition 303
    during pregnancy 77, 78–9, 99,
        100, 101
    post-delivery 175, 176
    postoperative 285
urine analysis
    gestational diabetes 38, 39
    oestriol levels 87
    pre-eclampsia 53, 54
    proteinuria 77–8
urogenital triangle 303
uterine atony 151, 152–3
uterine contractions
    effects on placental gas transfer
        115–16, 119, 139
    first stage 109
    second stage 112
uterine hyperstimulation 121, 139
uterine inversion 152, **152**
uterine rupture
    causes 131
    management 134–5
    and postpartum
        haemorrhage 152
    and previous Caesarian section 69,
        70, 71, 152
    signs 134

uteroplacental hypofusion 53
uterus
    bimanual contraction 152–3, **153**
    bimanual examination 15,
        15, 16
    congenital absence 190
    definition 303
    dysfunctional uterine bleeding
        298
    infections 175, 176
    malformations 246, 247
    malignant tumours 233
    and postpartum haemorrhage 151,
        152–3
    retroverted 15
    size 8, **8**, 16

vagina
    see also delivery, vaginal
    definition 304
    post-menopausal changes 222
    prolapse 242, 243–4, **243**
    swabs 299
    tears to 146, 147, **147**
vaginal birth after Caesarean section
    (VBAC) rate 304
vaginal discharge 77, 159,
    259–60, 302

vaginal examinations 103, 109, 113,
    144–7, 155, 278–9
    see also pelvic examinations
    in theatre not under
        anaesthetic 298
vaginal pessaries 243–4
    ring-type 244, **244**
    shelf-type 244, **244**
vaginal sponges/rings 203
vaginismus 227, 228
vaginitis, atrophic 259, 260
varicella zoster virus 56
vasectomy 248
vasovagal episodes 132–3
venography 179
venous thrombosis 200–201
    see also deep vein thrombosis
ventilation 140–41
ventouse delivery 113, 114
vertex 304
vestibular glands 262, **262**
vibroacoustic stimulation 122
Virchow's triad of thrombosis 175
virilization 211–13
vitamin B$_6$ 240
vomiting see nausea/vomiting
Von Willebrand's disease
    (VWD) 152

vulva
    normal anatomy **262**, 304
    swollen/painful 261–4
vulval biopsy 263, 266
vulval cancer 262, 263, 265, 267
vulval intraepithelial neoplasia (VIN)
    265, 266, 267, 304
vulval pruritus 265–8
vulvectomy 267
vulvodynia 262, 263–4
vulvoscopy 263

warfarin 180
warm water, analgesic effects 149
wedges 132, **132**
withdrawal method 203
'wood screw' manoeuvre 165
wounds
    dehiscence 285
    postoperative infection 175,
        176–7, 284–5

X-ray pelvimetry 34, 69–70
X-rays
    chest 30
    pelvic 216

Zavanelli manoeuvre 165